AN ILLUSTRATED HISTORY OF BRAIN FUNCTION

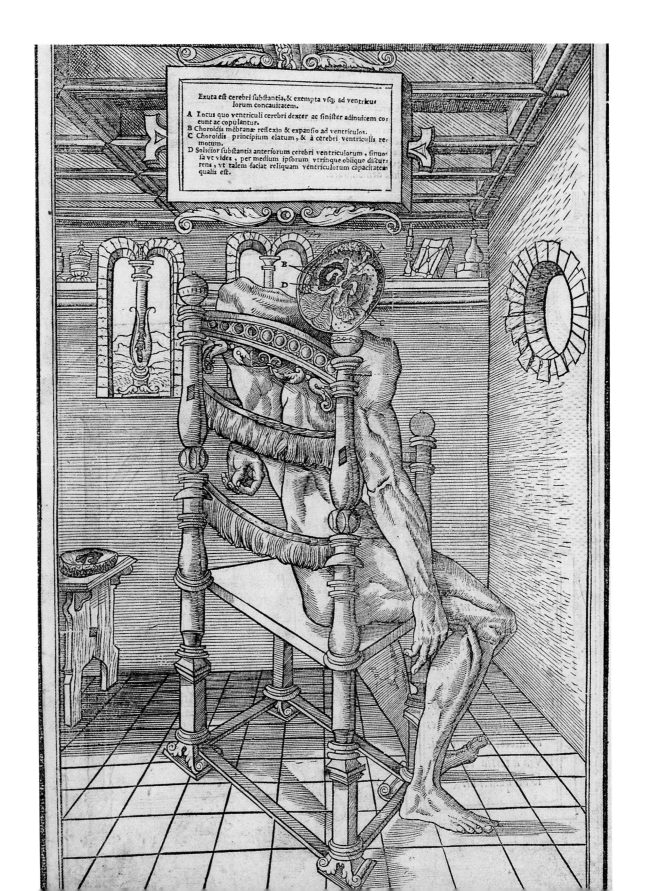

HISTORY OF BRAIN FUNCTION

Imaging the Brain from Antiquity to the Present

EDWIN CLARKE

M.D. F.R.C.P.

KENNETH DEWHURST

M.Litt D. Phil M.R.C.Psych

Second Edition, Revised and Enlarged

With a New Preface by Edwin Clarke

and a New Chapter Surveying Advances

in Imaging Technology

by Michael J. Aminoff, M.D. F.R.C.P.

NORMAN PUBLISHING SAN FRANCISCO 1996

Library of Congress Cataloging-in-Publication Data

Clarke, Edwin.

An illustrated history of brain function / by Edwin Clarke and Kenneth Dewhurst; with a new preface by Edwin Clarke and a
new chapter by Michael Aminoff.

p. cm. — (Norman neurosciences series ; 3)

Includes bibliographical references and index.

ISBN 0–930405–65–X

1. Brain—Localization of functions—History. 2. Brain—Anatomy—History. I. Dewhurst, Kenneth. II. Aminoff, Michael J.
(Michael Jeffrey) III. series.

[DNLM: 1. Brain—physiology—atlases. 2. Medical Illustration—history—atlases. W1 NO254TH no. 3 1995 / WL 17 C597i
1995]

QP385.C58 1995

612.8'2—dc20

DNLM/DLC

for Library of Congress   95–711

CIP

Norman Neurosciences Series, No. 3

This book is printed on acid-free paper and its binding materials have been chosen for strength and durability.

Manufactured in the United States of America.

Copies may be ordered from:

NORMAN PUBLISHING

720 Market Street

San Francisco, CA 94102–2502

Phone: 1–800–544–9359

Outside USA and Canada: (415) 781–6402

Fax: (415) 781–5507

E-mail: orders@jnorman.com

Frontispiece: Cross section of brain in an unusual Renaissance interior setting. Note the top of
the cadaverís head displayed on the table at the left. While it may have been typical to conduct
anatomical dissections indoors in anatomical theaters or dissection rooms, from the early 16th
century work of Berengario da Carpi onward, book illustrations usually depicted dissected
cadavers outdoors in a natural setting. One possible reason for this is that the artists preferred
to work in the open air because the smell of rotting flesh would have overcome even the
infrequently bathed participants of that era. This is one of eight dissections of brain appearing
in Charles Estienne's *De dissectione partium corporis humani libri tres* . . . . (Paris, 1545). The
imaginative arrangement of cadavers in some of the sixty-two full-page woodcuts in this work
have been the subject of considerable art and historical research. Its manuscript and illustrations were completed by 1539 but publication was delayed by a lawsuit. The book describes
numerous innovations in anatomical technique and contains many original observations. Had
its publication occurred on schedule in 1539, it would have stolen much of the thunder from
Vesalius' *De humani corporis fabrica* (Basel, 1543). See also figures 70 and 84.

In Memoriam: Kenneth E. Dewhurst

(1919–1984)

CONTENTS

In May 1961, during breakfast in a Chicago hotel, one of us (E.C) discussed plans with the late Professor C. D. O'Malley for the preparation of two books. The first was to be an iconography of the brain, the other an anthology of readings in the history of neuro-anatomy and neuro-physiology. Work on the former began at once and a considerable amount of material was collected. Then attention was turned to the second project, which culminated in *The human brain and spinal cord. An Historical Study Illustrated by Writings from Antiquity to the Twentieth Century* published in 1968 by the University of California Press.

For a variety of reasons it was not possible to proceed with the first book and after the untimely death of Professor O'Malley the idea was abandoned. Recently, however, we have resurrected the scheme, believing that there is a need for such a work. The end-result of our labours, however, differs considerably from the original plan, which was to present a wide variety of brain illustrations with no central them. We have thought it advisable to restrict ourselves to illustrating one topic only, the history of cerebral localization, extending from the primitive speculation of Classical Antiquity to the complexities of present-day cortical physiology.

We should like to thank the librarians through whose courtesy many of the illustrations are reproduced and to acknowledge with gratitude the advice given us by Dr. John McFie, Consultant Psychologist, Charing Cross Hospital, London, and the unremitting labours of Miss Mary Stevens in preparing the manuscript.

E. C.
K. D.
1972

It is said that history should be rewritten by each generation. Changing opinions and attitudes, the rejection or re-interpretation of accepted judgments and cherished beliefs, shifts in political, social, and religious forces, together with more concrete events such as the discovery of new source material, all contrive to make the periodical recasting of history inevitable. A recent example is the "revisionist" approach of some present-day historians, with the need to be "politically correct" in regard to gender, race, minorities, and fads, especially political and so forth. On the other hand, science must be reviewed at shorter intervals owing to the many advancements being made by an increasing population of scientists making use of the burgeoning field of technology, which provides them with an augmenting array of ingenious and powerful tools for their researches.

The present book is an attempt to juxtapose these disparate disciplines of history, a part of literature in the broadest sense of the word, and science, which are usually considered to be the classic incompatibles, identified by C.P. Snow in 1959 as the "two cultures".[1] Today, they remain to a large extent segregated, but even so any attempt to relate the full history of a limited bio-medical topic such as brain function must bring the story up to contemporary scientific achievements. To do so the intellectual barrier that separates the library from the laboratory must be crossed and the historical scene exchanged for the technocratic era of today. It is hoped that in whichever "culture" the reader's skills are based they will complete the journey as portrayed below and that they will find it rewarding.

An Illustrated History of Brain Function was first published in December 1972 with the intention of presenting a survey of the evolution of the ways in which the functions of the brain have been thought to operate, where they were located, and how they were represented pictorially, over a period of some eight hundred years from the thirteenth century to the year of publication. It was necessarily made up of two parts. The first and predominant of them traced these affairs up to the early twentieth century, and the second discussed the progress made thereafter in several pertinent areas of neuroscience which have increased our understanding of how the cerebral cortex acts, supplemented by appropriate illustrations when available. In its original form this book, therefore, presented iconographical material ranging from crude, medieval sketches of hypothetical structures (Chapter 3, for example) to those depicting notions of cortical localization current in 1972. Here then were the two dissimilar elements mentioned above: eleven chapters of history (Chapters 2–12) and one reporting researches too recent to permit meaningful assessments (Chapter 13). Just as their contents differed markedly so did the methods of handling them in the process of revision and modernization.

Regarding the historical chapters, little change has been necessary. The few minor errors have been eradicated, but on account of the paucity of research on the pre-twentieth century history of our subject carried out in the twenty-three years since publication, no emendations of note were needed. In fact, not one work of major significance has been added to the literature, but smaller contributions, as well as related ones, have been listed in Appendix 2, "Additional Bibliography" (pp. 183–184).[2] There may be several reasons for an apparent lack of interest in this area of research, but the suggestion that there is little need for further investigation of it is not one of them. Thus, in the case of ideas prevalent before 1800 (Chapters 2–9) explorations more thorough than those already attempted are requisite. In particular a wider search for further illustrative data in manuscripts and printed sources, both Western and Eastern, for additional interpretations of brain function as well as a comparative study of occidental and oriental views, and for the tracing of themes through the philosophy and literature of subsequent epochs, as well as in medicine and science, await the attention of appropriate scholars either solo or in collaboration.[3] Unfortunately, the number of individuals capable of undertaking such projects is today small, and it is this factor that has to a great extent determined the amount of deep scholarship devoted to the pre-nineteenth century aspects of our topic. Few recruits have come forward to labour on these and comparable problems in medical history, contrasted with the large number of historians engaged in the probing of social and psychological features of Western medicine of the nineteenth and twentieth centuries. However, although a person can select his own special area of endeavour to which he plans to apply his talents and energy, the choice is usually determined by the educational system to which he has been exposed. Nevertheless, there can be little doubt that it is much easier to undertake research using vernacular tongues, especially exclusively English, rather than classical and perhaps non-European languages. In addition, the scholarly investigations of earlier periods of medical history usually requires a competence in modern languages, in premodern history especially of science, philosophy, religion, and, in the present case, of art. Furthermore, modern history, even though it is expanding rapidly in volume, does not require its practitioners to grapple with archaic and obscure concepts, explications, and facts, or to acquire an intimate familiarity with ancient and abstruse cultural backgrounds. It is also apparent that the closer a historical enterprise is to the present day the greater is its relevancy, immediacy, lucidity, and thus attractiveness.

In the case of the second portion of this book, which was entitled "Modern aspects of cortical localization" (Chapter 13), plans to bring it up-to-date revealed a situation the reverse of that posed by the first. Thus, because of the many potent increments to our concepts of the function and form of the cerebral cortex since 1972, brought about by an expanding band of workers, it was clear that refurbishing this chapter would be inadequate and the rewriting was demanded. Regrettably, Dr. Kenneth Dewhurst whose main role in preparing the original edition was to write chapter 13, died in December 1986 and the author of the new Chapter 14, which reviews the most recent research into the physiology of the cerebral cortex, is Professor Michael J. Aminoff, M.D., F.R.C.P., a clinical neurologist. His demanding task has been to peruse and appraise the vast amount of recent literature generated by the study of the body's most enigmatic and complicated organ, made even more perplexing by species differences and by its protective osseous ramparts, which form a barrier to the intimate scrutiny of its activities. Dr. Aminoff has also had to select suitable illustrations, in particular those stemming from the revolutionary methods of revealing cortical processes, based on ingenious imaging and other techniques. Because this field of research is developing so rapidly, all that can be provided at this time is a review of the literature, accompanied by only tentative comments, guarded opinions, and prudent inferences in regard to the likely significance and future of the data revealed. All that can be said with certainty is that the anatomical and physiological intricacies of the cerebral cortex mirror the growing complexity of neuroscience itself. Dr. Dewhurst in 1972 described this frustrating yet challenging situation as follows:

"The extensive literature on the localization of cortical function is still lacking in coherence and abounds with inconsistencies. It covers a wide range of disciplines and without mastery of all of them a balanced and critical appraisal is well nigh impossible."[4]

Nearly a quarter of a century later his judicious observation is still expedient and is likely to remain so well into the future. Moreover, it can be discerned that as neuroscientific research, like that in most biological disciplines, becomes increasingly technical the chasm separating the "two cultures" is widening.

Neuroscience today is a vast undertaking of which cortical structure and activity are but small components. It has become one of the most extensive and vibrant components of modern bio-medicine, but, like any growing and composite endeavour, the correlation and reciprocation of its several strands create problems of integration and communication. However, it is of interest to note that in historiography beneficial symbioses are occasionally achieved. Thus, in the "Preface" to his French translation of this book the distinguished French neurologist, Henri Hécaen (1912–1982), made reference to an anthology of classic neuroanatomical and neurophysiological texts.[5] He proposed that the present work can be used as a helpful companion to it:

"Indeed, concerning the more limited theme of cerebral localization its valuable illustrations allow a better understanding of the ancient texts, which present the modern reader with difficulties because of the terms used and the methods of reasoning."[6]

Finally, the librarians and others who allowed the reproduction of many of the illustrations in the book deserve our thanks, as does William Schupback for his helpful advice.

Edwin Clarke
September 20, 1995

NOTES

1. C.P. Snow, *The two cultures and the Scientific Revolution. The Rede Lectures 1959*, Cambridge, at the University Press.

2. E. R. Harvey's monograph *The inward wits* (1975), listed in Appendix 2, "Additional Bibliography", deals with the ancient concept that mental faculties or "wits" were located in the cerebral ventricles (see Chapter 3 below). In his review of it (*Isis*, 1976, 67:630) David E. Leary made the following comment: "Unfortunately, the history of these 'wits' remains to be written. . . ." Today it is still incomplete.

3. An example of the penetrating scholarship required when attacking problems relating, for example, to the cell doctrine of psychological functions (Chapter 3) is apparent in H.A. Wolfson's "The internal senses" (1935) included in Appendix 2, "Additional Bibliography". It has been referred to by Leary (note 2, above), but seems to be unknown to historians of neuroscience. Its sequestration in a theological periodical and its objective of addressing the subject only from a comparative philological and philosophical viewpoint, with no anatomical or psychological details, nicely demonstrate the dichotomy between the "two cultures". Although the results of this and other research techniques are indispensable, a synthesis of data from various fields will eventually be needed.

4. K. Dewhurst in E. Clarke and K. Dewhurst, *An illustrated history of brain function* (1972).

5. E. Clarke and K. Dewhurst, *Histoire illustrée de la fonction cérébrale*, Paris, Les éditions Roger Dacosta, 1975, p. 7.

6. E. Clarke and C. D. O'Malley, *The human brain and spinal cord. A historical study illustrated by writings from Antiquity to the Twentieth Century*, Berkeley & Los Angeles, University of California Press, 1968.

7. *Histoire illustrée* (1975)—note 5 above, p. 7.

"The evolution of our knowledge of cerebral localisation is one of the most astonishing stories in the history of medicine."

Henry Head*

The history of medical illustrations is inextricably interwoven with the general history of art. Its earliest origins are reflected in prehistoric man's attempts to draw his own shape and in various art forms of the early Mediterranean civilizations, together with those of America and the Far East. Likewise during Classical Antiquity and in the Middle Ages the human body and parts of it were represented by both artists and physicians, using various media. However, the purposeful and accurate depiction of anatomical structures is of relatively recent date and begins with the Renaissance of anatomy and art in the 16th century.

We are concerned here with the history of anatomical illustrations, which is only a part of the history of medical illustrations in general, a topic that has received some, but by no means adequate, attention. In fact, the sole comprehensive work presently available is by the late Professor Robert Herrlinger of Kiel, and this deals only with the period from Antiquity to 1600.[1] Herrlinger is not only concerned with the illustration itself but with the idea it may portray, as is evident from his statement, "Medical illustration is, therefore, part of the history of art, which is in turn part of the history of thought".[2] We

*Aphasia and kindred disorders of speech, Vol. 1, Cambridge University Press, 1926, p. 1.

endorse this general interpretation of the study of medical illustrations, and in this work we intend to reproduce a pictorial history of the brain based upon the evolution of corresponding ideas of function.

A number of authors have written on the history of anatomical illustrations, the most important being Choulant, whose book was revised by Frank.[3] Wagner[4] and De Lint[5] also provide general treatments of the subject, but Garrison,[6] MacKinney,[7] and Wolf-Heidegger and Cetto[8] have written on special aspects. Occasionally the evolution of the iconography of a single organ has been studied, such as the elegant work by Weindler on the history of gynaecological anatomy, dealing mainly with the uterus.[9] There is also Schott who, in his iconography of the heart, pointed out the value of the pictorial method of surveying the growth of knowledge concerning a single organ or system of the body.[10] The history of diseases of organs has also been investigated in this way, as for example, the thyroid gland by Merke.[11]

The nervous system was first presented pictorially in an interesting book published in 1750[12] by Pierre Tarin (c. 1725–1761), who was in charge of all contributions to the great *Encyclopédie* on anatomy and physiology. It is a survey of illustrations mainly of the brain from Magnus Hundt of 1501 (Figure 32) to those of his own. There is a wealth of description but no connecting theme, other than a chronological progression, all the illustrations having been redrawn, usually for the worse. More recently, Artelt[13] has briefly discussed drawings of the brain, and Grünthal has been concerned with depicting the history of the cerebral localization of psychological activity, supported by twenty-eight illustrations.[14] There is also a recent pictorial history of psychology and psychiatry.[15] However, no attempt has so far been made to use anatomical illustrations primarily to trace in depth the evolution of concepts concerning an organ's function, in contra-distinction to the converse of simply illustrating a text.

The object of our book is, therefore, chronologically to survey carefully chosen pictorial representations of the brain in order to illuminate one aspect of medical thought: the localization of function within it. The story is of particular fascination and relevance because it not only reveals a sequence of intriguing notions but also contributes to our understanding and appreciation of modern views. Our survey has therefore been from Classical Antiquity to the present day, with the selection from a large amount of graphic material of only those most germane to our central theme. Thus, a consideration of the crude ideas of Antiquity will be followed by a discussion of the equally primitive medieval concept of the localization of mental activity within the ventricles of the brain. Thereafter, we shall deal with the 17th century idea that the solid parts of the brain are of greater functional significance. At this stage, owing to the ever-growing dimensions of our topic, selection becomes essential and the rôle of the cerebral convolutions with their cortical mantle will alone be traced. The final portion will treat exclusively localization of function within the cerebral cortex, one of the most fascinating yet perplexing problems of modern neurophysiology and psychology.

Although most of the book is devoted to the evolution of Western ideas of brain function, the Asian contribution has not been omitted. In the medieval period Islamic illustrations will be included on account of the great historical consequences of Arabic medicine. Later, in the 17th century, the effect of the scientific revolution which was providing the West with new facts, will be contrasted with contemporary Asian knowledge as reflected in illustrations from the Near and Far East.

Although the main aim of the book is the portrayal of an idea, the techniques whereby anatomists and artists have attempted to achieve their purposes are also relevant and form a vital part of the history of art.[16] This aspect of the study, although receiving less attention, has not been neglected.

NOTES

1. R. Herrlinger, *History of medical illustrations from Antiquity to 1600*, London, Pitman, 1970. A translation of *Geschichte der medizinischen Abbildung*, 2nd edition, Munich, H. Moos, 1967. Continued by Marielene Putscher, *Geschichte der medizinische Abbildung. 2. Von 1600 bis zur Gegenwart*, Munich, H. Moos, 1972.

2. *Ibid.*, p. 7

3. L. Choulant, *History and bibliography of anatomic illustration in its relation to anatomic science and the graphic arts*, translated and edited by M. Frank, Chicago, Ill., University of Chicago Press, 1920. Hereafter, referred to as Choulant-Frank.

4. R. N. Wagner, *Das Anatomiebildnis. Seine Entwicklung im Zusammenhang mit der anatomischen Abbildung*, Basel, B. Schwalbe, 1939.

5. J. G. De Lint, *Atlas of the history of medicine. I. Anatomy*, London, H. K. Lewis, 1926.

6. F. H. Garrison, *The principle of anatomic illustration before Vesalius. An inquiry into the rationale of artistic anatomy*, New York, P. B. Hoeber, 1926.

7. L. MacKinney, *Medical illustrations in medieval manuscripts*, London, Wellcome Historical Medical Library, 1965.

8. G. Wolff-Heidegger & A. M. Cetto, *Die anatomische Sektion in bildlichen Darstellung*, Basel, S. Karger, 1967.

9. F. Weindler, *Geschichte der gynäkologisch-anatomischen Abbildung*, Dresden, von Zahn & Jaesch, 1908.

10. A. Schott, "Historical notes on the iconography of the heart", *Cardiologia*, 1956, 28:229–268.

11. F. Merke, *Geschichte und Ikonographie des endemische Kopfes und Kretinismus*, Stuttgart, F. Enke, 1971.

12. P. Tarin, *Adversaria anatomica, de omnibus corporis humani partium, cum descriptionibus, cum picturis. Adversaria anatomica prima, de omnibus cerebri, nervorum . . .*, Paris, J. F. Moreau, 1750.

13. W. Artelt, "Gehirnsabbildungen vom 13. bis 18. Jahrhundert", *Leopoldina* (Halle/Saale), 1960–1961 [1963], 6–7 (3rd Series): 137–139.

14. E. Grünthal, "Geschichte der makroscopischen Morphologie des menschlichen Grosshirnreliefs nebst Beitragen zur Entwicklung des Ideen einer Lokalisierung psychischer Funktionen", in, *Beiträge zur Geschichte der Psychiatrie und Hirnanatomie*, Basel, S. Karger, 1957, pp. 94–128 (*Bibliotheca Psychiatra et Neurologia*, supplement to *Psychiatria et Neurologia*, Fasc. 100).

15. A. A. Roback & T. Kiernan, *Pictorial history of psychology and psychiatry*, New York, Philosophical Library, 1969.

16. Books such as these and many more can be consulted: C. D. Clarke, *Illustration. Its techniques and application to the sciences*, Baltimore, Md., J. D. Lucas, 1939; G. Lapage, *Art and the scientist*, Bristol, J. Wright, 1961.

It is now generally thought that anatomical illustrations were first produced in Hellenic Alexandria about 300 B.C.[1] The tradition, owing much to Herophilus *(fl. c.* 290 B.C.) and to Erasistratus *(fl. c.* 280 B.C.), has been traced by way of Byzantium to the Medieval West and East, where their descendants are now represented by a group of figures first studied by the great German historian of medicine, Karl Sudhoff (1853–1938).[2] These drawings, depicting osseous, muscular, nervous, arterial and venous systems, are now found in both Western and Eastern medical manuscripts and will hereafter be referred to as "the Alexandrian Series". They are crude in design, as can be seen in those of the brain (Figures 1, 2, 99).

There is, however, no evidence that illustrations were used to illuminate a medical text prior to the Ancient Greeks.[3] At about the beginning of the Alexandrian period, Aristotle (384–322 B.C.) made occasional references to geometric diagrams to facilitate the understanding of bio-mechanical phenomena such as animal movement.[4] He also referred to sketches,[5] and anatomical drawings on walls of a lecture room[6] but, unlike the Alexandrian figures, as far as is known, none has come down to us. In any event, such illustrations would only have an indirect bearing on our theme as Aristotle confined his dissections to animals.

Galen (A.D. 130–200), the greatest anatomist of Antiquity,[7] did not, however, encourage his students to rely on illustrations, believing that direct visualization and handling of structures was the only way to appreciate their form and relationships,[8] a laudable attitude by modern standards. In his great treatise, *On the usefulness of the parts,* Galen described the construction of a geometric diagram to illustrate the optics of the eye,[9] and, as

will be seen below, similar drawings were produced much later (Figures 59–66). Likewise, in his *On anatomical procedures,* he referred twice to graphic methods of complementing his text on muscles,[10] but like Aristotle, he studied animal rather than human anatomy.

Another Graeco-Roman art form, that of sculpture, must be mentioned briefly. It has been claimed by Major[11] that the convolutions of the brain are depicted on a terra-cotta votive offering. These sculptures were of the part of the patient's body afflicted by disease and taken by them to the temple of healing, where they sought relief. Sculptural representations of the brain have never been reported[12] and descriptions of so-called convolutions have been found, on closer inspection, to be the artist's representation of hair covering the sculptured head.[13]

In Classical Antiquity there were three main attempts to identify and localize brain function. The earliest was to regard the brain as the repository of the soul.[14] This was about the 6th century B.C. and the fourth ventricle was favoured as a precise location (see p 8).[15] Thereafter, a controversy constantly waged throughout Classical Antiquity, the Middle Ages and beyond as to whether the soul was sited in the brain or in the heart.[16] This uncertainty is neatly reflected in this couplet from the *Merchant of Venice* (1596):

"Tell me where is fancie bred,
Or in the heart, or in the head". (III, ii, 64)

Shakespeare's question remained unanswered and this important issue, which obviously does not lend itself to graphic representation, persisted for several centuries, reappearing in modified form in the works of Descartes (Figures 92–95) and again at the end of the 18th century in the curious notion of Soemmerring (Figure 109).

A contribution to the more exact placing of function in specific parts of the brain was made by Galen who, following the Alexandrians Herophilus and Erasistratus, identified motor and sensory nerves and traced the former to the cerebellum and the latter to the cerebrum.[17] Thus two functional areas were created.

Although this concept likewise cannot be supported by illustrations, the last example of functional brain localization in Classical Antiquity has been amply depicted. This is the *rete mirabile,* or "marvellous net", described first by Herophilus and incorporated by Galen into his general theory of human bodily function.[18] According to him "vital spirits" were produced in the left ventricle of the heart and distributed to all parts of the body. On reaching the cranial cavity by way of the internal carotid arteries, the blood entered a rich network of fine vessels at the base of the brain. This was the *rete mirabile* wherein the vital spirits underwent conversion into "animal spirits" by a subtle process of refinement. These varieties of "spirits" are somewhat difficult to comprehend. As its name suggests, "animal spirits", or "psychic pneuma", was regarded as the life force, the word "animal" being used in the sense of *animus,* the spiritual principle of life. Their actual physical form was never made clear but possibly they were thought to have ethereal qualities. Animal spirits were stored in the ventricles of the brain and from thence entered the nerves (thought to be hollow) where they mediated both movement and sensation. Galen, who often contradicted himself, also postulated the ventricles as the site of production for the animal spirits. This, in its simplest form, is his theoretical concept of nervous system function, and it is important to realize its remarkable longevity in holding sway with minor modifications, until the beginning of the 19th century.

The *rete mirabile* provides a fascinating story, which will be started here and continued in Chapter 5 (pp. 59–64). Galen did not dissect the human body and when studying the brain usually used the pig or ox. These animals, together with other ungulates, have a well-developed *rete* occupying the position of the Circle of Willis in man; its function is not thoroughly understood even today.[19] Unfortunately, in the Middle Ages, it was wrongly assumed that Galen had described the anatomy of man and so, until the 16th, and in a few instances, the 17th century, the *rete* was accepted and depicted as a feature of the human brain in many illustrations. Here are two examples:

FIGURE 1[20]

The text of this manuscript, composed in the early 13th century, is illustrated by a number of crude drawings, including the Alexandrian Series (see p. 5). This one of the arterial system is of interest here because the two arteries running to the cranium, presumably the internal carotids, terminate in a criss-cross area representing the *rete mirabile.* The picture typifies medieval anatomy, for teachers unquestioningly accepted the animal studies of Galen and applied them directly to man, without carrying out any confirmatory practical investigation. As is usually the case with medieval drawings, animal structures and functions were crudely and schematically drawn and superimposed on an outline of the human body. Similar representations of the *rete* are to be found in other manuscripts of the period.[21]

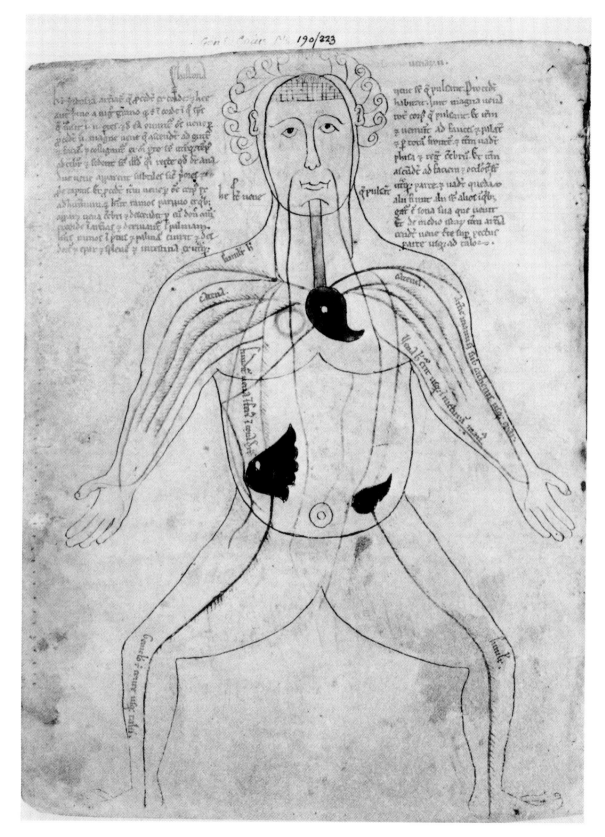

FIGURE 1

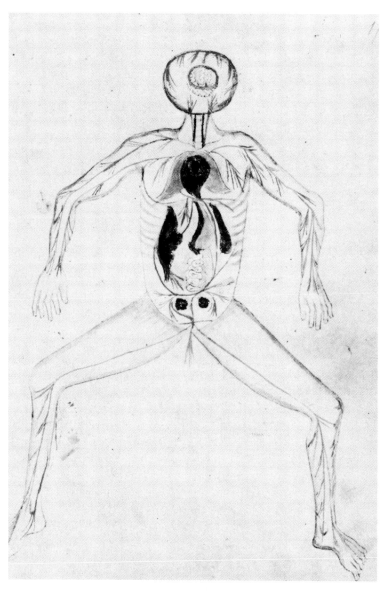

FIGURE 2[22]

This is a unique drawing of around 1250 which, according to Sudhoff, may have originated in Salerno.[23] It is part of the Alexandrian Series and depicts the venous system. While two vessels enter the cranial cavity from below, others dip in from the periphery. In the centre is an oval shape consisting of three wavy structures, the significance of which is impossible to elucidate from the drawing alone. The text, written in Catalan, describes three chambers in the brain, thus referring to the Cell Doctrine of ventricular localization of mental functions (see Chapter 3), although it is not readily apparent where these are sited other than possibly between the worm-like structures. The cross-hatching below the oval shape presumably represents the *rete mirabile*.

There can be no doubt, however, concerning the *rete mirabile,* represented by a criss-cross area below the central oval and reminiscent of that shown in Figures 32 and 36. Owing to this certainty, together with our inability to identify the oval shaped structure, this figure has been included here, rather than among other illustrations depicting the Cell Doctrine of Brain Function discussed in the next chapter.

It is of considerable interest to note that an abbreviated version of Galen's *De usu partium,* entitled *De juvamentis membrorum,* containing a description of the *rete,* became available in Latin about 1250, which coincides exactly with the dating of this and the previous manuscript.

Although Galen was inconsistent over the site of formation of the animal spirits, he was in no doubt concerning the possible function of the cerebral convolutions—they had none, and he refuted Erasistratus' contention that in the animal scale their complexity was directly proportional to intelligence.[24] He thus relegated them to a position of neglect which lasted until the be-ginning of the 19th century. As will be shown, not even the attempts of Willis and of the investigators of cortical microstructure to rehabilitate them functionally produced much change of opinion. It was the advent of phrenology about 1800 that gave the gyri a function and until the 1830's they were thought to adopt no standard pattern of arrangement.

NOTES

1. There is an excellent brief account of the early history of anatomical illustrations in Herrlinger (*op. cit.,* Chapt. 1, note 1), pp. 10–13. The claim that they may have originated in China has been made (see p. 76 below).

2. His *Kurzes Handbuch der Geschichte der Medizin* (Berlin, S. Karger, 1922, p. 129) contains a brief list of his more important contributions to the literature on this *Fünfbilderserie,* as he called it. See also C. Singer, "A study in early Renaissance anatomy, with a new text: the *Anothomia* of Hieronymo Manfredi (1490)", in, *idem* (editor), *Studies in the history and method of science,* as in ch. 3, n. 64 [vol. 1], Oxford, Clarendon Press, 1917, pp. 79–164, see p. 87, note 1.

3. Models of the liver used by the Mesopotamian priest to teach the art of divination, together with votive offerings (p. 5) and other early

sculptures, depict anatomical structures but do not qualify for consideration here (see C. Singer, *The evolution of anatomy,* London, K. Paul, Trench & Trubner, 1925, pp. 3–9).

4. "De motu", 9; 702b, 29–37 (see footnote for further examples): *ibid.,* 11; 703b, 29–35, in, J. A. Smith & W. D. Ross (editors), *The works of Aristotle,* Vol. 5, Oxford, Clarendon Press, 1912.

5. "Historia animalium", III, 5; 515a, 32 in, *ibid.,* Vol. 4, 1910.

6. "De generatione animalium", II, 6; 743a 1–3 in, Smith & Ross, *op. cit.* above, note 4.

7. George Sarton, *Galen of Pergamon,* Lawrence, Kansas, University of Kansas, 1954, pp. 43–44, note 52.

8. C. Singer, *Galen on anatomical procedures,* London, Oxford University Press, 1956, p. xxii.

9. "On the usefulness of the parts", Book X, Chapt. 12, in Margaret T. May (translator), *Galen on the usefulness of the parts of the body . . . "De usu partium",* Vol. 2, Ithaca, N.Y., Cornell University Press, 1968, pp. 492–495.

10. "On anatomical procedures", I, II, and IV, 6. (Singer, *op. cit.* above, note 8, pp. 28 and 105).

11. Ralph H. Major, *A history of medicine,* Vol. 1, Springfield, Ill., C. C Thomas, 1954, Figure on p. 133; legend states, "Votive from Asklepieion in Corinth. This votive shows the brain with its convolutions". It is described by F. J. de Waele, "The sanctuary of Asklepios and Hygieia at Corinth", *Amer. J. Archaeol.,* 1933, *37* :417–451.

12. Works such as those by W. H. D. Rouse (*Greek votive offerings. An essay in the history of Greek religion,* Cambridge, University Press, 1902), L. Stieda ("Anatomisches über alt-italische Weihgeschenke (Donaria)", *Anat. Hefte: Beitr. Ref. z. Anat.u.Entwicklungs.* (Wiesbaden), 1901, *16* (I.Abt.): 3–83, see pp. 22–23), and T. Meyer-Steineg (*Darstellungen normaler und krankhaft veränderter Körperteile an antiken Weihgaben, Jenaer medizin-historische Beiträge,* Heft 2, 1912) make no reference to votive offerings depicting the brain.

13. R. Bernard & P. Vassal, "Étude médicale des ex-voto des sources de la Seine", *Rev. Archéologique* (Dijon), 1958, *9*:328-359; see Fig. 96 on p. 331.

14. For the history of attempts to localize the soul, see: G. W. Corner, "Anatomists in search of the soul", *Ann. Med. Hist.,* 1919, *2*:1–7 who covers Antiquity to the 17th century; H. M. Brown, "The anatomical habitat of the soul", *ibid.,* 1923. *5* :1-22, mainly "Hammurabi to Harvey"; there is also the large work by the phrenologist, B. Hollander, *In search of the soul and the mechanism of thought, emotion, and conduct,* 2 vols., London, K. Paul, Trench, Trubner, n.d., and although encyclopaedic is virtually a history of psychology with no references.

15. By Herophilus of Alexandria. See, E. Clarke & C. D. O'Malley, *The human brain and spinal cord. A historical study illustrated by writings from Antiquity to the Twentieth Century,* Berkeley & Los Angeles, University of California Press, 1968, pp. 713–714; 2d ed., San Francisco, Norman Publishing, 1996.

16. *Ibid.,* pp. 1–26.

17. *Ibid.,* pp. 460–461.

18. Galen derived the *rete* from Herophilus, and described it in, *De usu partium,* Book IX, Chapt. 4; see May (1968), *op. cit.* above, note 9,

pp. 430–434 (Kühn, 1822, 3:696–703). He likened it to several superimposed fisherman's nets. He also discussed it in *Galeni de Hippocratis et Platonis placitis,* Book VII, Chapt. 3 (Kühn, 1823, 5:607–609). See Clarke & O'Malley (*op. cit.* above, note 15), pp. 757–760.

There is an excellent history of the *rete* by L. Belloni, "Rete mirabile (Introduzione storica)" in, S. B. Curri & L. Martini (editors), *Pathophysiologica diencephalica. Symposium internazionale, Milano, Maggio 1956,* Wien, Springer-Verlag, 1958, pp. 3–17. See also, D. H. M. Woollam, "Concepts of the brain and its functions in Classical Antiquity", in, F. N. L. Poynter (editor) *The history and philosophy of the brain and its functions,* Oxford, Blackwell, 1958, pp. 5–18.

19. The *rete* in the ox is depicted by S. Sisson, *The anatomy of domestic animals,* 3rd edition, Philadelphia, W. B. Saunders, 1938, Fig. 594 on p. 722.

20. Cambridge, Gonville & Caius College Ms. 190/223, F.2^{V} (courtesy of the Librarian). It is described in detail by M. R. James in, *A descriptive catalogue of the manuscripts in the Library of Gonville & Caius College,* Vol. 1, Cambridge, University Press, 1907, pp. 218–219. Our illustration is reproduced in De Lint (*op. cit.,* Chapt. 1, note 5), Fig. 23 on p. 29.

21. (1) Bodleian Ms. "Cod. ex Museo 19", from mid-14th century; see E. Seidel & K. Sudhoff, "Drei weitere anatomisch Fünfbilderserien aus Abendland und Morgenland", *Arch. Gesch. Med.,* 1909, 3:165–187, see Taf. III, 1.

(2) Bodleian Ms. Ashmole 399, F.19^{R}, from second half of 14th century (see K. Sudhoff, "Weitere Beiträge zur Geschichte der Anatomie im Mittelalter. 4. Die Oxforder anatomische Fünfbilderserie des Cod. Ashmole 399 . . .", *Arch. Gesch. Med.,* 1914, 7:363–366, see Tafel X). Reproduced by B. H. Hill, Jr., in, "The grain, the spirit in medieval anatomy", *Speculum,* 1965, *40*:63–73, Fig. 2.

(3) Raudnitz Ms., VI.Fc.29, of the last quarter of the 14th century (K. Sudhoff, "Abermals eine noeue Handschrift der anatomischen Fünfbilderserie . . .", *Arch. Gesch. Med..,* 1910, *3*:353–368, see Tafel IX).

22. Basel, Universitäts-Bibliothek, Provençal Ms. D.II, i, 1, F.170^{R} (courtesy of the Librarian). See pp. 181–182 of, Walther Sudhoff, "Die Lehre von den Hirnventrikeln in textlicher und graphischer Tradition des Altertums und Mittelalters", *Arch. Gesch. Med.,* 1913, 7 :149–205. Referred to hereafter as "W.S." (Also published as, *Inaugural-Dissertation,* Leipzig, J. A. Barth, 1913, p. 60, with additional illustrations).

23. K. Sudhoff, "2. Ein provenzalischer anatomischer Traktat aus dem 13. Jahrhundert", in *Ein Beitrag zur Geschichte der Anatomie im Mittelalter speziell der anatomischen Graphik . . .,* which is Heft 4 of *Studien zur Geschichte der Medizin,* Leipzig, J. A. Barth, 1908, pp. 11–23. Our illustration is reproduced in Tafel II.

24. Clarke & O'Malley, *op. cit* above, note 7, p. 631.

The seat of the soul, the localization of motor and sensory activities, and the *rete mirabile* were three Ancient Greek concepts of brain function which were handed down to the Middle Ages. Another idea was also widely accepted by medieval writers: the localization of mental processes in the ventricles or cells of the brain. Although this concept had not fully matured during Classical Antiquity, its basic elements can be traced in Galen's works. The Early Church Fathers, in particular Nemesius, Bishop of Emesa (*fl. c.* A.D. 390) and St. Augustine (A.D. 354–430), first proposed what we have termed the Cell Doctrine of Brain Function.

The functional role of the ventricles began with Herophilus of Alexandria (*fl. c.* 300 B.C.) who placed the soul in the fourth (see p. 3). Galen, in the second century A.D., gave a detailed description of them and vaguely hinted at their association with intellectual functions which he preferred to locate in the brain substance. Imagination, reason, and memory he thought were the three constituents of intellect and thought and, although they could be affected separately, he avoided indicating their precise localization. These basic components were brought together by the Early Church Fathers in the 4th and 5th centuries to form the Cell Doctrine. Essentially, it asserted that the faculties of the mind were contained within the ventricular system of the brain. The lateral ventricles were considered as one cavity, the first cell; our third ventricle was the second cell, and our fourth, the third. The first cell received sensation from the special senses and from the rest of the body and thus accommodated the "sensus communis" or "common sense". Images were created from this sensation and so "imaginativa" (imagination) and "fantasia" (image for-mation = imagination) were either in the posterior part of the first cell or in the second. The latter, however, was also the seat of reasoning: "aestimativa" (judgement), "cogitativa" (thought) or "ratio" (reason). "Memorativa" (memory) was contained within the third cell. This was the Cell Doctrine in its simplest form but, as might be imagined, such a system was liable to variations and more complicated rearrangements. Thus the first cell could have two parts ("sensus communis" and "imaginativa"), or the second might be duplicated ("aestimativa" and "cognitiva"); occasionally the third cell was in control of motion ("motiva") as well as of memory. The teachings of the masters such as Galen, Avicenna, the Church Fathers, and others determined these variations of the central theme which need not be treated in unnecessary detail here; for example Avicenna's interpretation favoured a five-cell scheme (cf. Figure 40). The most important development in the theory, however, was the addition of a dynamic element to the original static model and this appears to have taken place in the 10th century A.D. A sequence of events, occasionally compared with the process of digestion, was thought to take place, starting in the first cell and ending in the third. Thus the images created by the sensations ("sensus communis") in the first cell were manipulated in cell two (reasoning) and whatever was left over was stored in cell three (memory).

This intriguing speculation, founded on the established anatomy of the ventricular system of the brain, was virtually universal in the medieval West and East, so that there are many examples both in manuscripts and in early printed books of the way in which authors have illustrated their accounts of it. A number of historians have discussed this material,[1] the most comprehensive contribution be-

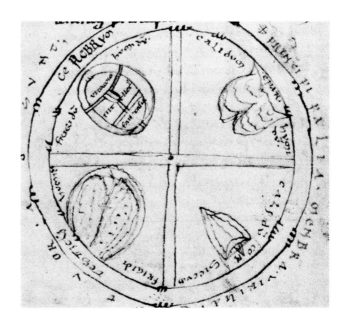

FIGURE 3

ing that of Walter Sudhoff; in 1913, hereafter referred to as "W. S.".[2] It has not, however, all been collected together before, nor has a grouping based on the increasing complexity of the illustrations been presented previously. The material may be arranged into the following four categories:

1. The mental faculties are written on the head, with or without partitioning into three parts representing the three ventricles. Rarely the head may be partitioned without labelling.
2. Simple shapes, usually circles, to represent the ventricles, are drawn on the head and usually their contents are identified.
3. The shapes (ventricles) are now linked together, indicating a connection necessary for dynamic thought processes.
4. Eye–brain diagrams. Here the primary purpose was to illustrate the eye but in so doing the Cell Doctrine was often depicted.

Each group has been arranged in chronological order.

1. HEADS LABELLED OR PARTITIONED

The easiest way to represent the Cell Doctrine was merely to name or letter the head appropriately, thus indicating very simply and imprecisely the localization of mental functions. A slightly more advanced method was to divide the cranium into the three parts, anterior, middle, and posterior, corresponding to the three cells. The areas so outlined could then be labelled with their alleged activities or they could be left unlabelled.

FIGURE 3[3]

This is from an 11th-century manuscript and is, therefore, the earliest known Western illustration of brain function. The design is reminiscent of the Celtic stone cross found in Anglo-Saxon diagrams, such as the Circle of Pythagoras, the Circle of Columcille,[4] and others of contemporary date. Around the circle is written, "There are present four principal human members", which are, in clockwise sequence from 12 o'clock, liver, heart, testes, and brain ("cerebrum"). The last is, in fact, a drawing of the skull facing inwards and seen from above, with the coronal, sagittal, and lamdoid sutures represented by double lines.[5] The mental faculties inscribed on it centrifugally are, "fantasia" (imagination), "intellectus" (reasoning), and "memoria" (memory). In accordance with the Ancient Greek theory of qualities, the brain is labelled cold and moist, whereas the heart is the opposite, hot and dry; these designations were given great prominence by Aristotle and his followers. The picture, therefore, transmits traditional Greek ideas as well as the concept of the ventricular localization of mental functions.

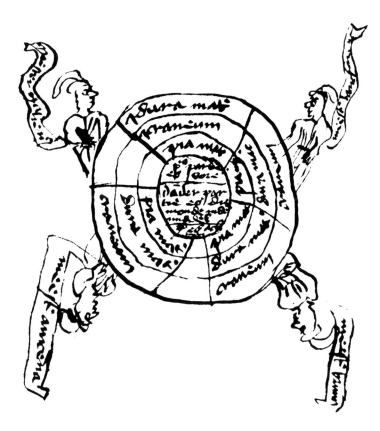

FIGURE 4

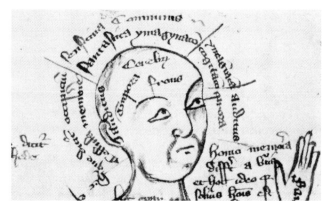

FIGURE 5

FIGURE 4[6]

This extraordinary drawing is in one of the manuscript versions of a book on surgery compiled in 1328 by the famous Flemish surgeon, Jehan Yperman (1295–1351).[7] The central nucleus is divided from above downwards into three divisions, named "the front part", "the middle part which is mutual", and "the third part". It is surrounded by three layers, from within outward, "pia mater", "dura mater", and "cranium"; in the upper segment the last two are transposed. The four figures of men are named, from two o'clock clockwise, "Lanfranc" (of Milan, d. c. 1306), "Meester Bruun" (probably Bruno of Longoburgo of the 13th century). "Avicenna" (980 A.D.–1037), and "Galen" (130 A.D.–200).

In the text the functions of the three parts of the brain are enumerated: the front presides over visual, gustatory and olfactory discrimination (the "sensus communis"), the middle over intelligence and hearing (the site of idea formation), and the posterior over memory. The location of hearing is unusual but can also be seen in Figure 43.

FIGURE 5[8]

This is the head from a full length figure of a "Disease Man", that is, a figure around, and on which, are written the names of diseases. It is in a manuscript dating from probably about 1380. On it are the words in Latin from the right side to the left: "Auditory, temples, brain, forehead." The ray-like lines proceeding from the head make four divisions in which are written, beginning with the one beside the left eye: "auditus, prora [?]", "ymaginativa cogitatio", "sensitiva communis, fantastica, ymaginacio" and, "memory cell which is called occiput". Between the chin and the upraised left hand is written, "Man differs in memory from brutes, and the reason why is because there is record only of man", a very reasonable statement. There is obvious confusion here over the grouping of the mental faculties.

FIGURE 6[9]

This curious diagram is dated about 1400 A.D. Below it is written: "Here is imagined to be the whole brain in animals." The inter-crossing lines on the left of the circle are labelled "optic nerves" and probably also represent the optic chiasma. The circle is divided into five columns, representing the brain ventricles. The first two have a compartment above them labelled "anterior part", the middle two have one named "middle part", and the last, "posterior part". A horizontal line divides the five columns into upper and lower compartments and the inscriptions in them can be summarized thus, from left to right:

1. First ventricle [of the first part of the brain]: "sensus communis". 2. Second ventricle of the first part of the brain: "Imaginativa or fantasia faculty which is the reservoir of appearances perceived and things not perceived . . . ." 3. First ventricle of the second part of the brain: "fantasia or imaginativa". 4. Second ventricle of the second part of the brain: "Estimativa or cogitativa, which from things perceived elicits the appearances of things not perceived and composes and separates them precisely, which fantasia cannot do." 5. (Upper compartment blank): "Memory, which preserves the appearances of things perceived and not perceived, which imagination and fantasy cannot do." 2. and 3. seem to be identical and together with 1. represent the psychological functions of the first cell. This together with Figure 42 seem to be only drawings which apply the Doctrine to animals.

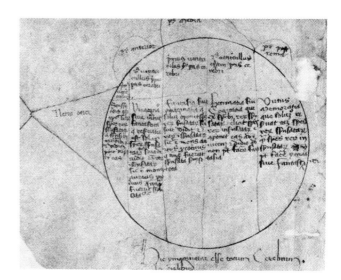

FIGURE 6

FIGURE 7[10]

This is the head from a Disease Man, drawn about 1400 (cf. Figure 5). The disease names around the head are like beams of light arranged in the fashion of a halo. The head is divided into four compartments labelled: "sensus communis", "cellula imaginativa", "cella aestimativa rationis" [rational judgement], "cella memorativa". It has been suggested that the diminutive "cellula" was used in the case of the second because this ventricle (our third) was thought to be the smallest.[11]

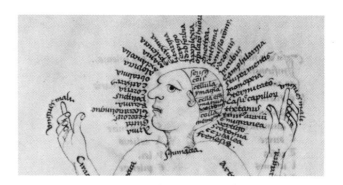

FIGURE 7

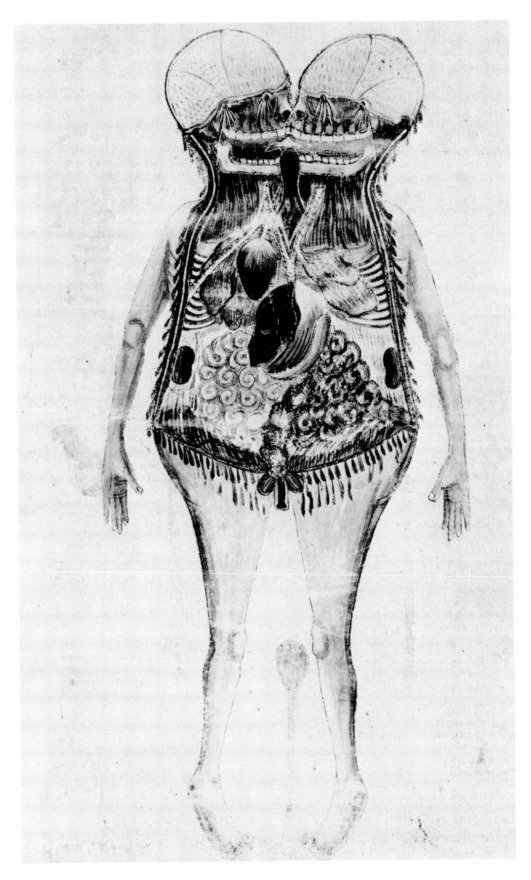

FIGURE 8

This drawing appears in a long vellum roll written probably about 1412 and is unique in all medieval anatomical art.[13] The text epitomizes the teachings of John of Arderne (1307 to end of century), who was a surgeon in Newark from 1349 to 1370. Instead of following the usual schematic form the artist has attempted to draw structures as they are seen during dissection, at a time when perceptual art was almost unknown. The sagittal splitting of the head reveals the cranial cavity, which is divided into three parts, anterior, middle, and posterior, thus implying the localization of mental functions.

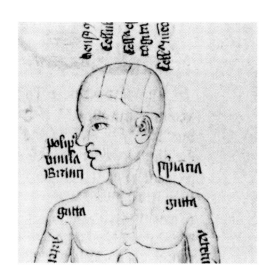

FIGURE 9

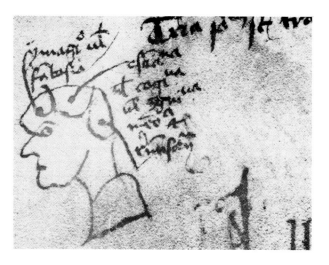

FIGURE 10

FIGURE 9[14]

This is dated c. 1420 and is similar to Figure 7. It is the head of a Disease Man which has four divisions, from anterior to posterior: "sensus communis", "cellula ymaginativa", "cella aestimativa vel cogitativa rationalis" and "cella memorativa".

FIGURE 10[15]

Again from the early 15th century (1435–40) and said to be the work of Professor Martin Guldeln of Vienna.[16] The head is divided into three parts, labelled from anterior to posterior: "ymaginatio vel fantasia", "aestimativa vel cogitativa [reflexion] vel cognitiva", and "memorativa vel reminiscentia [remembrance]".

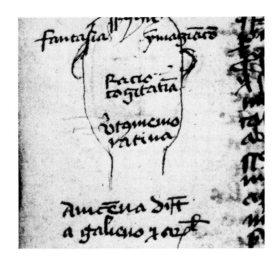

FIGURE 11

FIGURE 11[17]
This manuscript can be precisely dated to 1444. The head is viewed from behind and on it is written, from above downwards: "sensus communis", "fantasia" and "ymaginatio" on the same line, "ratio [reasoning]", "cogitativa", and "virtus memorativa". Below is written, "Avicenna disagrees with Galen and Aristotle". It was through Avicenna's teaching as much as anyone else's that the Cell Doctrine became canonical[18] and he favoured a five-cell scheme as perhaps is being suggested here (cf. Figures 24, 25, 39, 40, 41, 42).

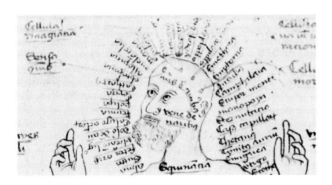

FIGURE 12

FIGURE 12[19]
Originating from the first half of the 15th century, this is from another Disease Man with a halo of disease names. The head is labelled from before backwards thus: "sensus communis", "cellula ymaginativa", "cellula aestimativa vel cogitativa rationalis", and "cellula memorativa" (cf. Figure 13).

FIGURE 13 (OPPOSITE)
The Cell Doctrine is also illustrated in printed books. Here is an elegant Renaissance drawing in the *Fasciculus medicinae* of Johannes Ketham, published in 1491, acclaimed as the finest illustrated medical book of the 15th century.[20] It is once more of a Disease Man and four balloons give the brain functions, as in previous examples: "sensus communis", "cellula ymaginativa", "cellula estimativa seu cogitati[va] rationalis", and "cellula memorativa". The first two are contained in the first cell. This and other fine wood-cuts in the book are in the style of Gentile Bellini (c. 1429–1507) of the famous Venetian family of painters. The influence of Andrea Mantegna (1431–1506) has also been noted.

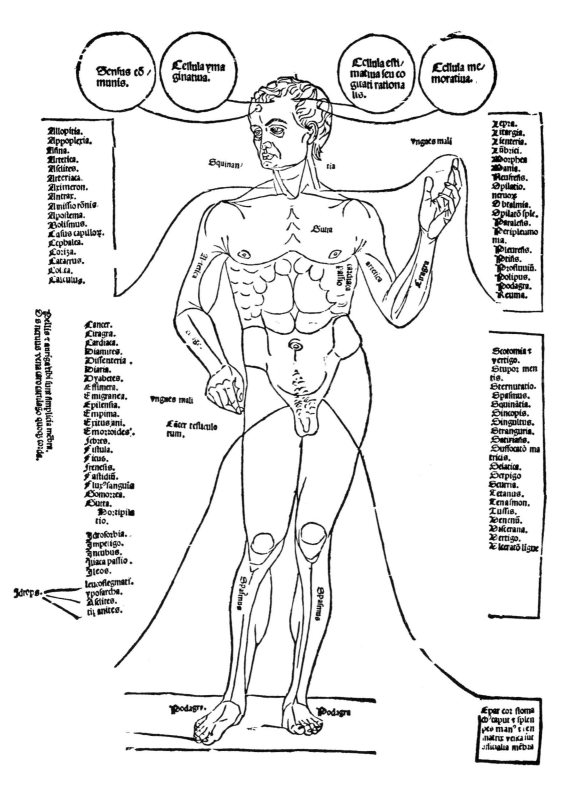

FIGURE 13

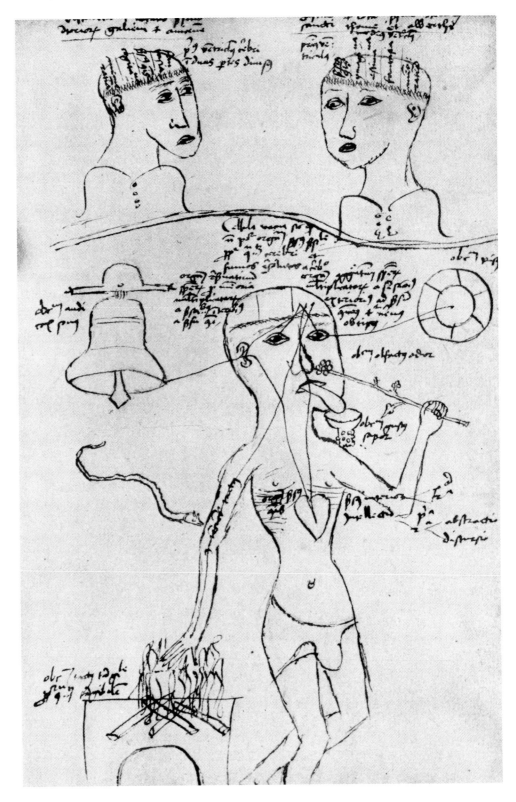

FIGURE 14

FIGURE 14 (OPPOSITE)

This crude drawing is on a blank leaf (KK6) preceding the printed work "De sensu" in the *Epitomata* of Gerard de Harderwyck (d. 1503) of 1496.[21] The upper two heads show the usual divisions and labelling. The one on the left is said to represent the teachings of Galen and Avicenna and has four compartments: "sensus communis", "phantasia", "cogitativa", and "memorativa". The first ventricle has two parts and contains the first two of these faculties. The one on the right has five: "sensus communis", "imaginativa", "estimativa", "phantasia", and "memorativa", and is said to accord with the tenets of St. Thomas Aquinas and Albertus Magnus.

The lower figure is of greater interest for it depicts not only the cranial divisions but also various sensations, special and peripheral, impinging upon the first cell to form the "sensus communis". But, in addition, there are connections between the ear, the first cell, and the heart, which illustrates the Aristotelian concept that the heart, not the brain, is the chief organ of the body and seat of the soul.[22] To it go all sensations, as is partly shown in the drawing.

FIGURE 15

This is another example of a manuscript drawing of brain functions in a printed book. It is of 1497 by a Dominican friar of Frankfurt and accompanies Aristotle's *De anima*.[23] It illustrates both sensory organs and mental faculties. The latter, which are located precisely to four points on the head, are labelled "organum sensus communis", "organum virtutis ymaginativa", "organum virtutis cogitativa", and "organum virtutis memorativa", in ribbons around the head. The use of the word "organ" is reminiscent of phrenology (see Chapter 10).

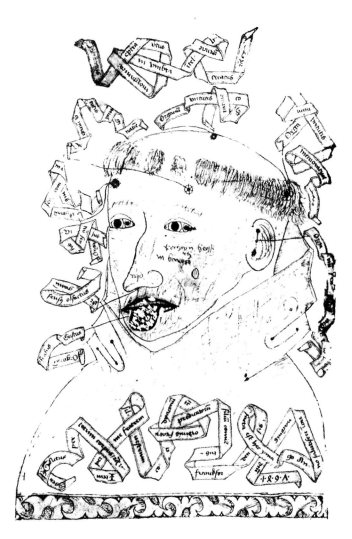

FIGURE 15

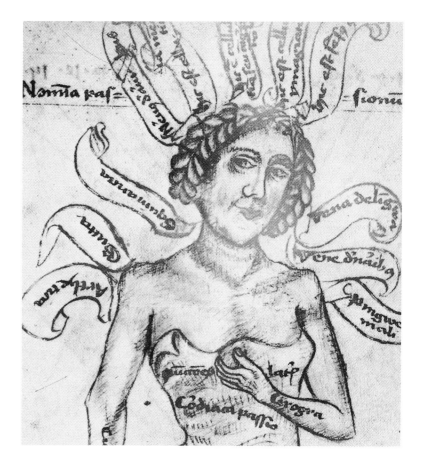

FIGURE 16

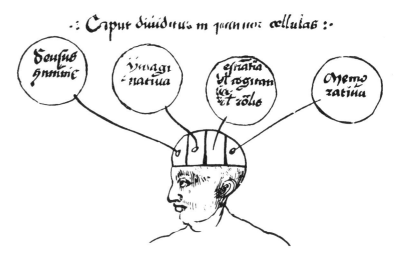

FIGURE 17

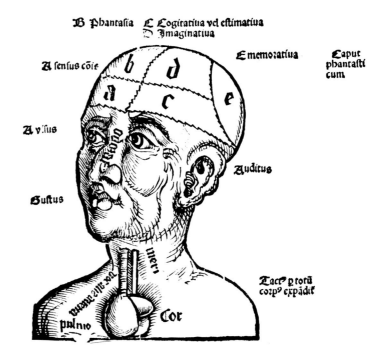

FIGURE 18

FIGURE 16 [24] (OPPOSITE TOP)
A drawing of a Disease Woman which cannot be dated more precisely than to the 15th century. The four ribbons labelling the skull carry, from the left of the head to the right: "hic est sensus communis", "hic est cellula ymaginativa", "hic est cellula aestimativa seu cogitativa rationalis" and "hic est cellula memorativa" (cf. Figure 7). The upper margin of the manuscript is defective but these readings are reliable.

FIGURE 17 [25] (OPPOSITE BOTTOM)
Again, dating is difficult but 1500 has been suggested for this Disease Man. The head has four compartments, labelled by means of balloons which read from left to right: "sensus communis", "ymaginativa", "estimativa vel cogitativa vel rationalis", "memorativa". Above the drawing is written "The head is divided into four little cells."

FIGURE 18 (TOP RIGHT)
From Aristotle's *Parvula philosophiae naturalis cum comment,* published in Haguenau in 1513[26] and edited by Matthias Qualle, about whom nothing seems to be known. The special senses are named and the key to the precisely delineated areas of the head is: a. "sensus communis", b. "phantasia", c. "cogitativa vel estimativa", d. "imaginativa", e. "memorativa".

FIGURE 19 (RIGHT)
This is an even simpler representation than Figure 18. There are five mental qualities and a key to them. It appears in a book on physiognomy published in 1630 by Cornello Ghiradelli (*fl.* 1630).[27]

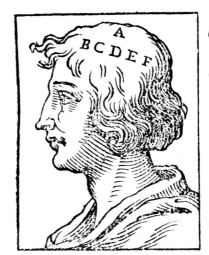

FIGURE 19

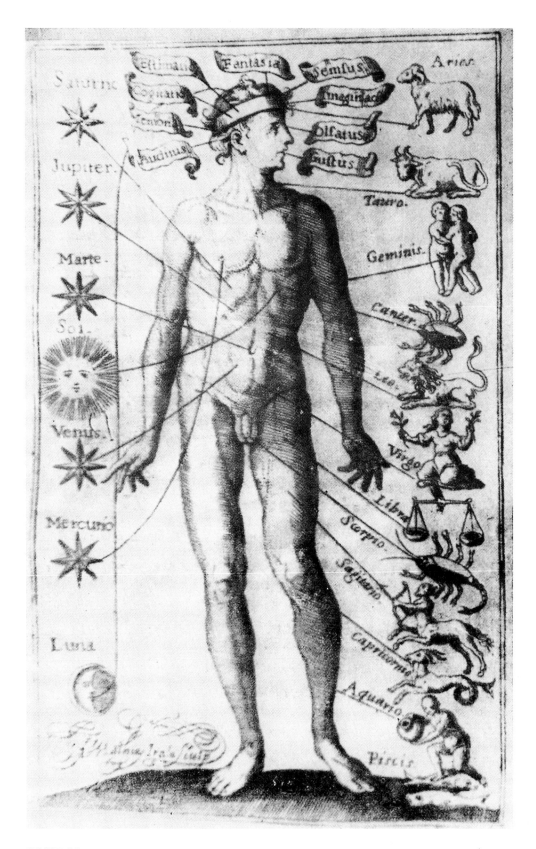

FIGURE 20

It is of considerable interest that labelling the head to indicate the medieval localization of brain function was still being used in the West during the 18th century. This is in a book on surgery and anatomy by Francisco Suárez de Rivera (1548–1617), published in Madrid, 1728.[28] The head is from a figure of a Zodiac Man, relating the zodiacal signs to various parts of the body. On a band circling the head, the psychological functions are indicated, from front to back, "imaginae", "sensus [communis]", "fantasia", "estimatio", "cognatio", "memori" (cf. Figure 56).

2. CELLS OUTLINED

A slight refinement in the technique of depicting the medieval concept of ventricular localization of mental qualities schematically was to draw shapes, usually circles, on the head to represent the ventricles.

FIGURE 21 [29]

In a manuscript copy of a book, Al-Mansūrī by the Persian physician Rhazes (A.D. 860–922), dating from the second half of the 14th century, there occurs the simplest possible diagram of the ventricular system. The text dates from the 9th century so that this is the earliest diagram of brain cells illustrating the theory of ventricular localization. As can be seen, there are four small circles, and reading from right to left, the first two are the lateral ventricles. These are in the part of the text dealing with the brain (Chapter 8) but appear only in this manuscript and not in printed versions or Latin translations of the text. Rhazes briefly cited Galen's anatomical findings concerning the ventricles[30] and in Chapter 1 stated, "The brain, besides being the source of sensation and movement, is also, according to Galen, the seat of imagination, of thought and of memory. Imagination resides in the two anterior [lateral] ventricles, thought in the middle [third] and memory in the posterior [fourth]".[31]

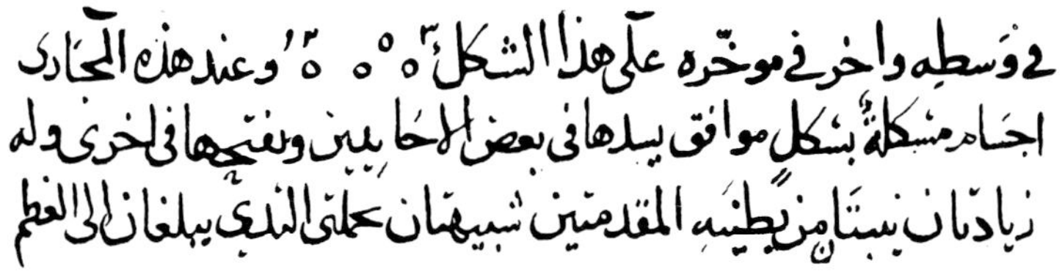

ودُسطه واخرنف موخره على هذا الشكل ٥ ٥ ٥ ٥ وعندهن المجادك
اجامر منبكة بنكل موانق يبدهانى بعض الجا بين وفتحها فى لخرى وله
زبادنان بسنًا من يطنه المقدمين سبهان حلنى الثلق يبلغان الى العظم

FIGURE 21

FIGURE 22 [32]

This manuscript contains a brief discourse on anatomy by Guido da Vigevano (c. 1280 – c. 1349) written in 1345 and illustrated by a series of interesting drawings. The fifteenth, seen here, shows the head after layers covering the brain have been removed, which, as Leonardo puts it, is like peeling off the layers of an onion (see Figure 43). Three circular cavities grouped together represent the ventricles, but they are not drawn as in nature. They are described in the text as being where "the mind and spirit are located, giving sensibility and motion to the whole body". The first contains "virtus apresensiva sive fantastica", the second "virtus raciocinatium [sic]", and the third, "virtus memorativa". The first is connected to the eyes and ears. On the left of these three, there are two more circular shapes, said to be concerned with the sense of smell for they represent the olfactory nerves. This is not found in any other medieval drawing but the text does not help us to understand the artist's intentions.

There is vague patterning on the surface of the exposed brain which may possibly be an attempt to draw the cerebral convolutions. If so, it is the earliest portrayal of them (see p. 65).

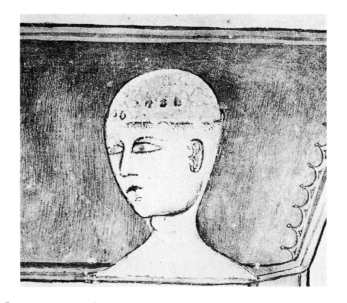

FIGURE 22

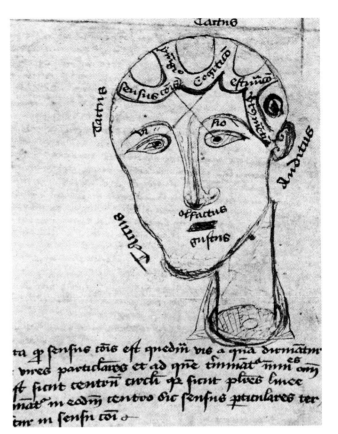

FIGURE 23

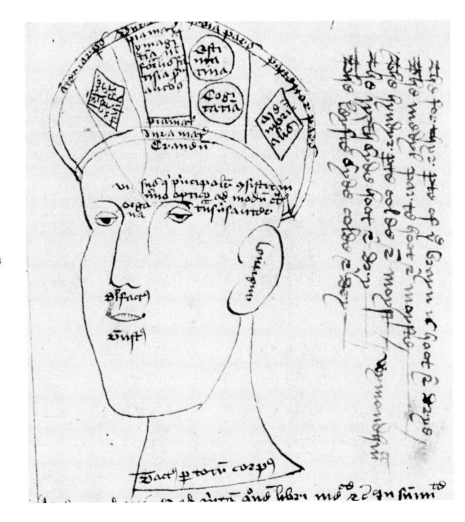

FIGURE 24

FIGURE 23 [33] (OPPOSITE TOP)
This manuscript is from the 15th century. Four areas are delineated on the head, from left to right: "sensus communis" relates to the first, "ymaginativa" to the first or second, "cogitativa" to the second, "estimativa" to the third, and "memorativa" to the fourth. Lines from each eye intersect in the mid-line to indicate the optic nerves and optic chiasma, but their central connections are not clear.

Below the head is written, "note that the *sensus communis* is a certain power from which are derived all the other particular powers and in which they terminate. It is like the centre of a circle because just as there are many lines that end in it so all the particular senses end in the *sensus communis*".

FIGURE 24 [34] (OPPOSITE BOTTOM)
This dates from about 1410 and is similar to Figure 25. It is as though the figure is wearing a head-dress, along the top of which, within a double line, is written from left to right "anterior part, dura mater, middle part, posterior part"; under the word "dura mater" is "pia mater". At its lower limits, above the left eye, are the words "pia mater, dura mater, cranium", one upon the other from above downwards. The "head-dress" or area enclosed by double lines has five compartments of various shapes. To the left is a rhomboid marked "sensus communis vel fantasia" with lines from the eyes which cross in the mid-line running to its sides. To the right is a rectangle containing "ymaginativa vel formalis fantasia secundum aliquos". Next come two circles, one above the other, the upper labelled "estimativa", and the lower, "cogitativa". The fifth compartment, another rhomboid, is "memorialis".

The special senses are also marked and where the optic connections cross (optic chiasma) is written, "organ of vision which mainly consists in the optic nerve, also in large degree trans-versely[?]"; and on the neck, "touch through the whole body". To the right of the head is written, "the forthyr parte of ye brayn is hoot and drye, the medyl parte hoot and moyste, and hyndryr parte colde and moyste, the rygth syde hoot ande dry, the leyft syde cold ande drey". This use of the Greek theory of qualities was of common occur-rence at that time in the works of medieval writers and can be compared with its use in relation to the ventricles and their storage potentials. It also occurred in Figure 3. The vermis ("virguncula serpentina") is mentioned in the text but is not in the diagram (see Figures 25, 39, 48, 57).

The five cell scheme was characteristic of Avicenna's interpretation of the Doctrine (cf. Figures 25, 39, 40, 41, 42).

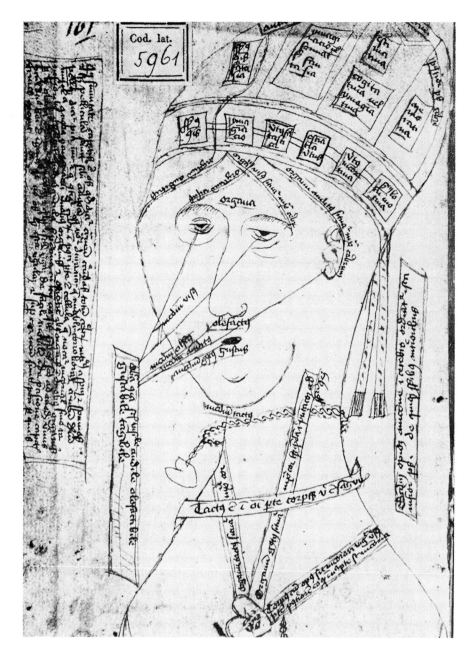

FIGURE 25

FIGURE 25 [35] (OPPOSITE)

This drawing, dating from 1441, is very like Figure 24. The head-dress, of a woman, is similar and the narrow strip over the top reads: "anterior part of the brain", "middle part of the brain", and "posterior part of the brain". The head-dress is divided into four sections. The first (on the left) has a panel containing "sensus communis fantasia", the second "ymaginatio vel formalis [form or pattern of images, cf. Figure 39] vel fantasia". The third section has two panels, an upper labelled "estimativa" and a lower "cogitativa vel ymaginativa". The fourth is "memorativa". The band across the forehead has six small squares linked together by two lines; they are inscribed, from left to right, "sensus communis, ymaginatio, virtus phantastica estimativa virtus, virtus incorporativa, secundum locum motiva". Why the ventricular functions are duplicated is not clear. Lines join together on their way to the brain from the left ear and right eye, the right ear and the left eye; the writing on them merely states their origins. The special senses are also named, both on the head and in the rectangle to the left of the head upon which lines from them converge. Round the neck is written "touch is located in all parts of the body" (cf. Figure 24). There are also connections, said to be from touch and taste, with the heart, reminiscent of those in Figure 14 and conforming to Aristotelian statements such as ". . . the heart constitutes the sensory centre . . . two of the senses, namely touch and taste, are manifestly in immediate connexion with the heart . . .".[36]

To the right of the figure is written in a rectangle, "According to the opinion of Avicenna the inferior part of the five inferior senses is arranged in the brain"; the significance of this is not clear. To the left of the head, also in a rectangle, is a lengthy description of the cranium, dura mater, pia mater, the brain cells, the vermis between cells two and three (see Figures 24, 39, 48, 57) and the hair of the head. There is a very similar passage in the text accompanying Figure 24.

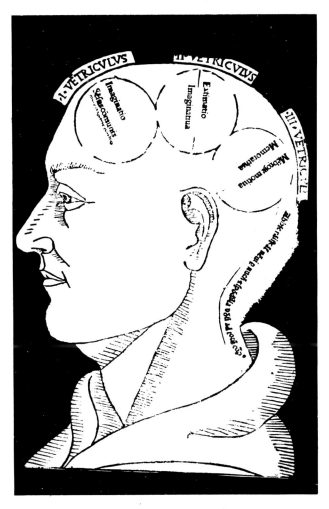

FIGURE 26

FIGURE 26

The manuscript tradition was carried over into the early printed books (cf. Figure 13) and Albertus Magnus (1206 – 1280) used simple circle drawings in several editions of his *Philosophia pauperum* when dealing with the soul. This one is from the edition of 1490.[37] The usual functions are allotted to the ventricles, an important difference from all previous examples, however, being the inclusion of "membrorum motiva" ("the power that moves the limbs") in the third cell (our fourth ventricle). This is explained by the fact that Galen localized motor function to the cerebellum (see p. 3) and thus some placed it also in the cerebellar, or fourth, ventricle (third brain cell).

On the neck is written, "The nerves radiate through the neck and all the vertebrae to the whole body" (cf. Figure 33).

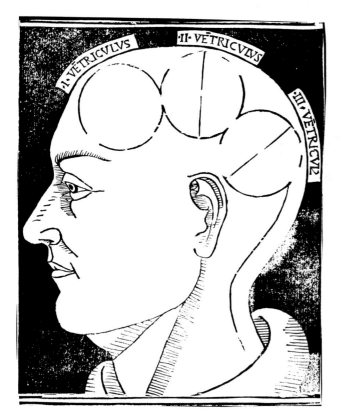

FIGURE 27

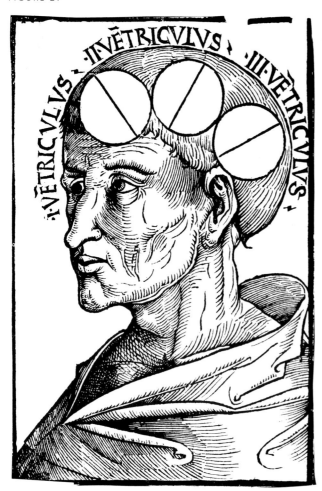

FIGURE 28

FIGURES 27 AND 28 (LEFT, TOP AND BOTTOM)
These are closely similar drawings found in the
1493[38] and the 1506[39] editions, respectively. Each
cell is divided into two, except the first in Figure
27.

FIGURE 29 (OPPOSITE TOP)
In addition to the drawing in Figure 15, the
National Library of Medicine possesses another,
also in an incunable.[40] It likewise illustrates
Aristotle's *De anima,* this edition having been
published in 1494. The four circles on the head are
labelled from anterior to posterior: "sensus
communis", "virtus cogitativa", "virtus
imaginativa", "memoria".

It is interesting to contrast this sketch, the
product of a skilled Renaissance artist, with the
almost contemporary one seen in Figure 15 which
follows the medieval tradition of art. This illustrates
well the revolution that was taking place in
anatomical drawing towards the end of the 15th
and the beginning of the 16th centuries (see
Chapter 4).

FIGURE 30 [41] (OPPOSITE BOTTOM)
This crude sketch is in a manuscript said to date
from 1497. However, there is adequate evidence
to show that its drawer was copying from Peyligk's
Philosophiae naturalis compendium published in
Leipzig, 1499 (see Figure 44) and thus it must have
been produced later than 1497. The alternative, of
suggesting that this was Peyligk's source, seems
very unlikely. The drawing is similar to Figure 47 for
it is headed by "The three powers are separate",
and the writing around the head is also comparable. The four cells depict "organs" (cf. the organs
of phrenology, Chapter 10): from left to right they
are labelled, "sensus communis", powers of
"cogitativa or estimativa", power of "imaginativa",
and power of "memorativa".

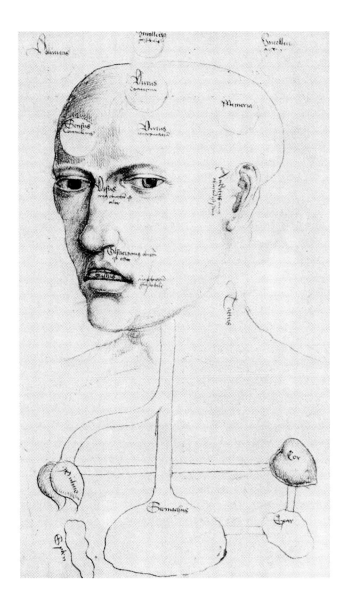

FIGURE 29

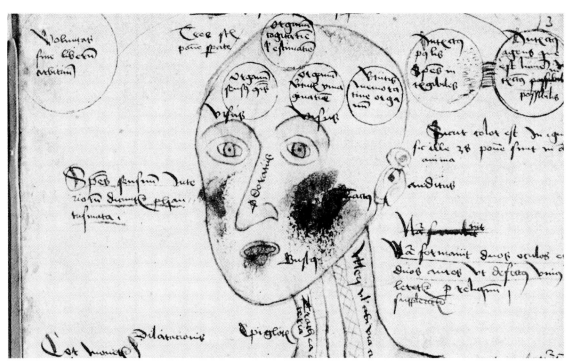

FIGURE 30

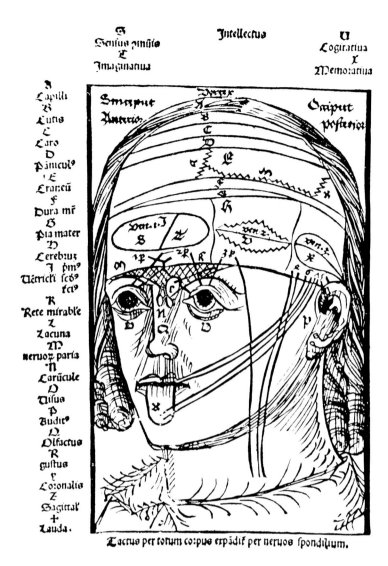

FIGURE 32

Tactus per totum corpus expādif per neruos spondiliuim.

FIGURE 31 (BELOW)
This wood engraving appears in the *Trilogium animae* of Ludovicus Pruthenus, or, de Prussia, published in 1498.[42] "Sensus communis" and "imaginatio" (B, C) are assigned to the first cell, "fantasia" and "estimativa" to the second (D, E), and "memoria" to the third (F).

Some evidence suggests that the drawing is by Albrecht Dürer (1471–1528) and that it portrays his friend Wilibald Pirckheimer (1470–1530), humanist and fellow citizen of Nuremberg.[43]

FIGURE 32 (LEFT)
Magnus Hundt (1449–1519), a professor in Magdeburg, graduated in both medicine and theology,[44] and published his *Anthropologium,* in 1501,[45] containing some of the rarest anatomical illustrations of this period.[46] They are crude woodcuts and include the one shown here, which shows brain coverings (A to G), the special senses (O to R) with their connections, and the ventricular system; in the first cell are "sensus communis" and "imaginativa", in the second, "cogitativa" and in the third, "memorativa". An unusual feature is the *rete mirabile,* shown as cross-hatching between the eyes (see Figures 1, 2, and Chapter 5). This drawing was copied by several authors, as for example Dryander (Figure 36).

Caput phificum

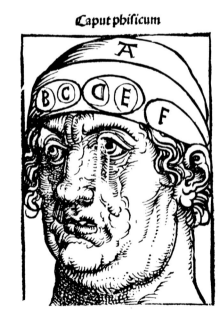

A
Cerebrum
per totum
B
Sensus cõis
C
imaginatio
D
Fantasia
E
Estimativa
F
Memoria

FIGURE 31

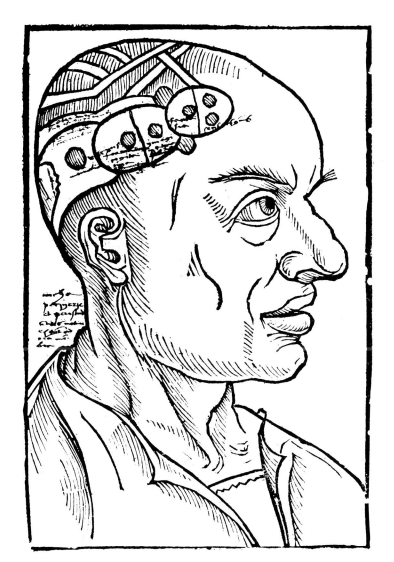

FIGURE 33

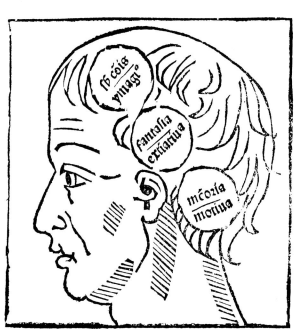

FIGURE 34

FIGURE 33 (LEFT)

Johannes Versor (d. c. 1485), professor of philosophy at Cologne, is here illustrating a 1501 edition of Aristotle's *De anima*[47]. There are three cells, the first two being each divided into two; in the copy of the book used they have been labelled by a previous owner: "sensus communis" is in the anterior half of the first cell, "phantasia" in the posterior; "imaginativa" is in the anterior part of the second cell, "estimativa", in the posterior. The third cell is single and on it is written "memorativa". At the back of the neck, written in Latin, is, "nerves go to all the members of the body to serve motion and sensation" (cf. Figure 26).

This is one of the few examples where the head is looking to the right and not to the left. Despite the comments of W. Sudhoff[48] there can be no significance in this, other than the fact that a right-handed person finds it easier to draw a face with the profile on the left, and *vice versa*. Versor's artist may therefore have been left-handed but reversal by means of the block is equally, if not more, likely. In the 1514 edition,[49] Versor scrapped this drawing and copied from Reisch (Figure 48).

FIGURE 34 (LEFT)

Alessandro Achillini (1463–1512), a famous Renaissance anatomist of Bologna,[50] reproduced this drawing in his 1503 revision of a book by Triumphus Augustinus de Anchona.[51] The usual functions are named in the circles, with the addition of "motiva" in the third cell (cf. Figure 26).

It is typical of the transitional period between the Middle Ages and the Renaissance that anatomists should be involved with the characteristic traditions of both periods. Thus Achillini who, on the one hand contributed to the upsurge of Renaissance anatomy, nevertheless included an illustration of a medieval concept.

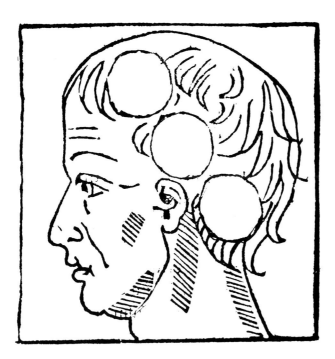

FIGURE 35

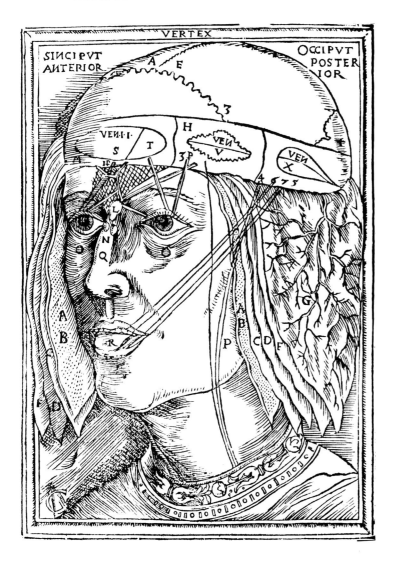

FIGURE 36

FIGURE 35 (LEFT)

It was much the same with another famous Renaissance figure, Berangario da Carpi (c. 1457–1530), who, although an outstanding pre-Vesalian anatomist,[52] reproduced Achillini's drawing, but without the intra-cellular names, on the title-page of his famous book on head injuries of 1518.[53] An edition of 1629 still carried this emblem of medieval medicine.[54]

FIGURE 36 (LOWER LEFT)

Johann Eichmann (1500–1560), professor of mathematics and medicine at Marburg, better known as Dryander, copied from Magnus Hundt's drawing of the ventricular system (see Figure 32) for his book of 1537.[55] It was redrawn less crudely, with the patterned collar giving it a Renaissance quality. The faculties in the cells are as in Figure 32.

Dryander, like Achillini (Figure 34) and Berengario (Figure 35), belongs to the transitional period between the medieval conceptual representation of anatomy and the perceptual art of the Renaissance. Thus he has life-like drawings of the brain, a product of the new art of anatomical illustration, along with this medieval figure (see Chapter 4).

FIGURE 37 (OPPOSITE TOP)

This is from a broadside published by Augustinus Darius Vincentinus in 1543,[56] about whom nothing is known. On the left of the head the five senses are detailed, on the right the elements, qualities, and heavenly bodies (cf. Figure 57). On the head itself the three cells are drawn, with details of their contents connected by guide lines. The psychological faculties are much the same as in Figure 57 and include "virtus motiva" in the third cell. It has been suggested that the head represents the anatomist Andreas Vesalius (1514–1564) and there may be some similarity; its date, 1543, is the same as that of his *De fabrica* (Figure 69).

FIGURE 38 (OPPOSITE RIGHT)

The mystic Paracelsian alchemist, Robert Fludd (1574–1637),[57] published this drawing in 1619.[58] The brain cells are outlined and the eye of the imagination in the first is creating the five pictorial images on the right; as we say "in the mind's eye". Fludd insisted on the prime importance of imagination. Five was his favourite number for a group of memory places, in this instance, an obelisk (the central image), the Tower of Babel and Tobias and the Angel on the left, with a ship and the Last Judgement on the right. He does not elucidate this selection, merely using it to propound his memory system.[59]

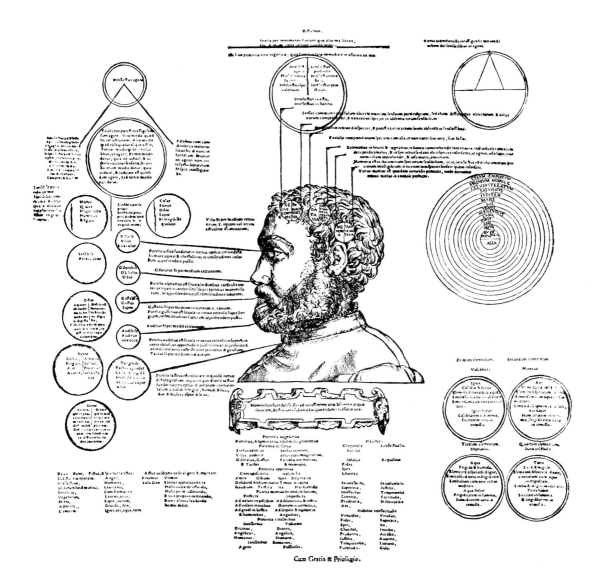

FIGURE 37

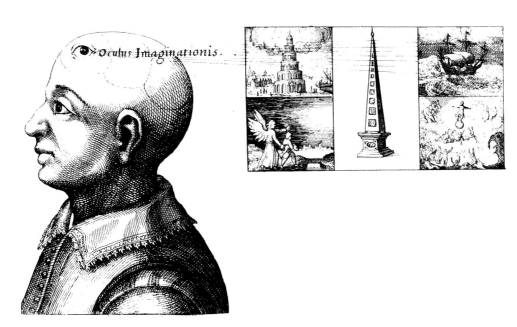

FIGURE 38

The next step in improving the pictorial representation of ventricular functions, was to incorporate links between the ventricles, thus introducing a dynamic element into the Cell Doctrine (see p. 8). Those by Reisch (Figure 48) and Romberch (Figure 53) have been the most popular and the most frequently reproduced drawings of the Doctrine.

This introduces the vermis ("worm") which though nowadays and originally refers to the mid-line cerebellar structure, was applied by most medieval authors to the choroid plexus of the lateral ventricles. At either site it regulated the flow of mental activity between two ventricles and so was an important feature of the Dynamic Cell Doctrine of Brain Function (see Figures 24, 25, 39, 48, 57).

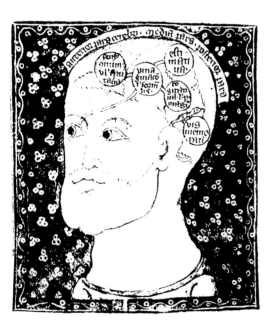

FIGURE 39

FIGURE 39[60]

This drawing dates from about 1310.[61] Above the head is inscribed, "anterior part of the brain, middle part, posterior part". There are five cells and the first two (first cell) immediately above the face are connected to the eyes, by means of crossing channels representing the optic nerves and the optic chiasma (cf. Figures 23, 24, 25). They are labelled "sensus communis vel sensatio", and "ymaginatio vel formalis"; "formalis" implies form or pattern of images (cf. Figure 25). Behind are two cells, one above the other (second cell) inscribed "estimativa" in the upper, and "cogitativa vel ymaginativa" in the lower. The fifth circle (third cell) is named "vis memorativa" and, between it and the lower of the two which form the second cell, the vermis of the cerebellum is depicted, drawn here as a worm, including an eye! (See Figures 24, 25, 48, 57.) In the text which this drawing illustrates the dynamic element added by Costa ben Luca (864–923) to the Cell Doctrine is mentioned (see p. 10). Thus the vermis of the cerebellum in this instance acted by opening or closing the channel between the middle and the posterior cell according to the needs of the thought processes.[62]

Comparison with Figures 24, 25, 40, 41, 42 can be made on account of the five-cell scheme.

FIGURE 40[63]

This crude diagram is at the end of a treatise by Avicenna, *De generatione embryonis,* copied probably in 1347. There is no legend, other than the statement, "This is the anatomy of the head for physicians", and so a full elucidation is not possible. However, the five senses are indicated and are connected to the first of five interconnected cells. The first two are the anterior ventricle, the second two the middle, and the last the posterior. Around the cranium is inscribed "sensus communis, fantasia, ymaginativa, cogitativa seu estimativa, memorativa". The five cell variety conforms closely to Avicenna's interpretation of the Cell Doctrine (cf. Figures 24, 25, 39, 41, 42).

FIGURE 41[64]

This is found in a manuscript copy of *De scientia perspectiva* by Roger Bacon (*c.* 1219–*c.* 1292) prepared in 1428.[65] It is very similar to Figure 40 showing five interconnected circles with much the same labelling and it accords with Avicenna (cf. Figures 24, 25, 39, 40, 42). In the accompanying text there is an interesting discussion of brain function which seems unique. It concerns the four humours of Ancient Greek medicine, blood, phlegm, yellow bile, and black bile which are said to be excreted from cranial apertures: blood from the mouth, phlegm from the nose, yellow bile from ears (cf. ear wax), and black bile from the eyes as tears. On the drawing these functions are recorded, close to each special sense organ. They do not seem to have been discussed by others, before or since.

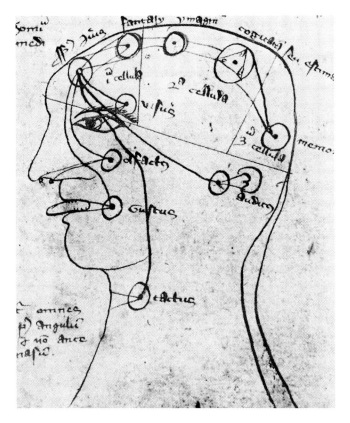

FIGURE 40

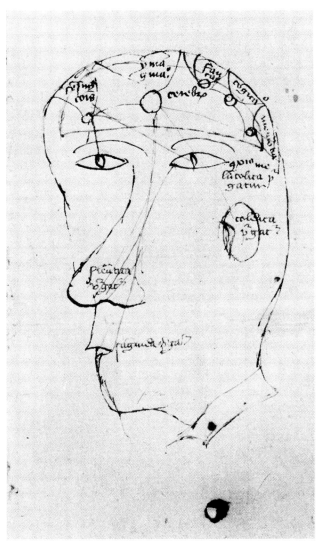

FIGURE 41

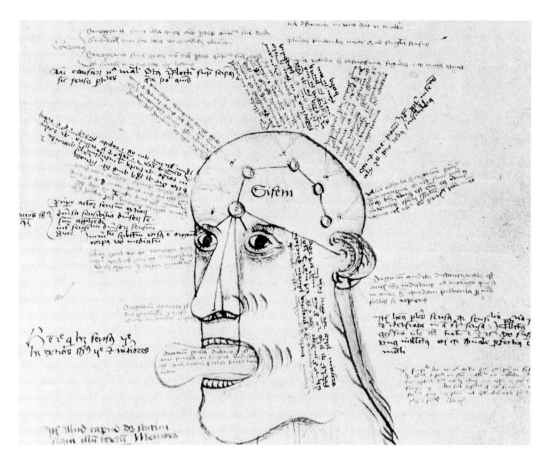

FIGURE 42

FIGURE 42[66]

Another version of the Avicenna scheme (cf.
Figures 24, 25, 39, 40, 41) accompanies an
incomplete and abridged version of Albertus
Magnus' *Parvulus philosophiae naturalis,* dated
1473 (cf. Figures 26–28). Comments concerning
the five cells radiate from the head and describe
the function and quality of each. Thus the first of
the anterior two is "sensus communis" and, being
moist, its contents do not stay long there but pass
on to the next cell, imagination, which is dry and
therefore more able to preserve mental matter.
The third cell, the organ of fantasy is also dry, but
the fourth is again moist and controls "estimativa"
in man and "cogitativa" in animals. Memory is the
fifth cell which is dry and thus well-suited for
storage.

The dynamic nature of ventricular functions is
again introduced, this time by the qualities of the
cells in relationship to the time taken by each
thought process.

FIGURE 43[67] (OPPOSITE)

These drawings in red crayon outlined with ink
were executed by Leonardo da Vinci (1452–1519)
in c. 1490.[68] The larger is of a sagittal section of
the head and the lower on the right is the open
cranium seen from above. Leonardo was attempting to illustrate Avicenna's description of the brain
and he depicted and labelled in the usual way the
various structures that envelope the brain. In these
two sketches the three ventricles connecting one
with the other labelled 0, M, N are shown, the first
being linked to the eyes by means of channels
representing the optic nerves, and to the ears by
similar connections. On another leaf,[69] however,
there is a view of the ventricles from above
indicating that the middle cell is the seat of the
"sensus communis".

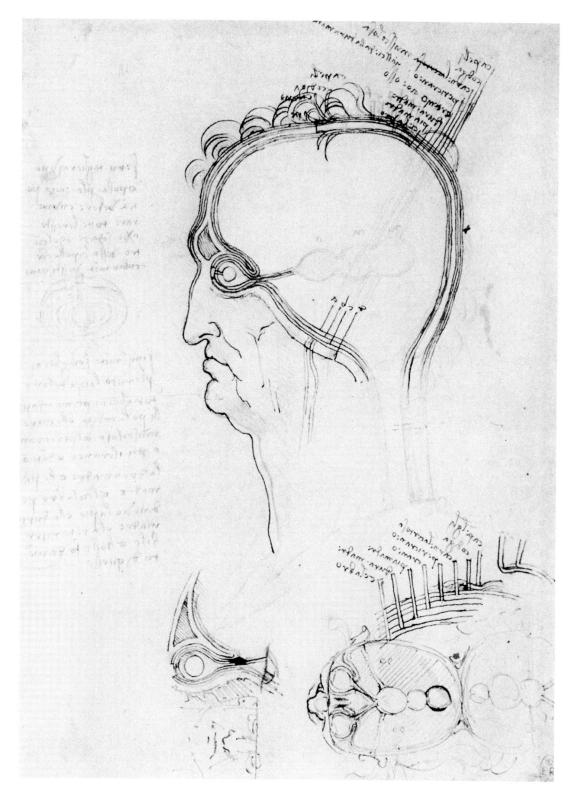

FIGURE 43

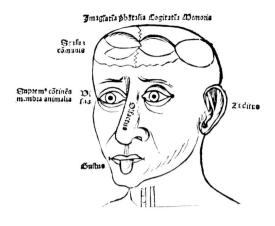

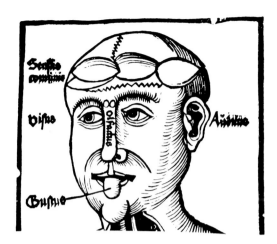

FIGURE 44

FIGURE 45

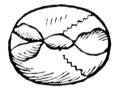

(a)

(b)

FIGURE 46

FIGURE 44 (TOP LEFT)
This is from a book by Hans Peyligk (1474–1522) of Leipzig, *Philosophiae naturalis compendium,* a commentary on Aristotle's medical treatise published in Leipzig, 1499.[70] The last seven leaves comprise an illustrated summary of anatomy, the text being entirely medieval. The eleven illustrations, however, "are the first series of anatomical figures specially prepared for a printed book".[71] Four ventricles are depicted with functions inscribed from right to left: "Sensus communis, imaginativa, phantasia, cogitativa, memoria". For the first time the two lateral ventricles are seen side by side.

FIGURE 45 (TOP RIGHT)
There were several editions of the *Compendium* of Peyligk and in them modifications of the illustrations were introduced. This is from the 1516 edition[72] where the ventricles and their labelling are much the same as in Figure 44.

FIGURE 46 (LEFT)
Also in Peyligk's book of 1499[73] there are these sketches of the brain ventricles: (a) from above showing them superimposed on the skull; note the two lateral ventricles; (b) a lateral view of the isolated ventricles with connections joining them to the *lacuna cerebri* or pituitary, through which waste products drained from the ventricles into the posterior naso-pharynx as phlegm, a concept derived from the classical Greek anatomists.[74]

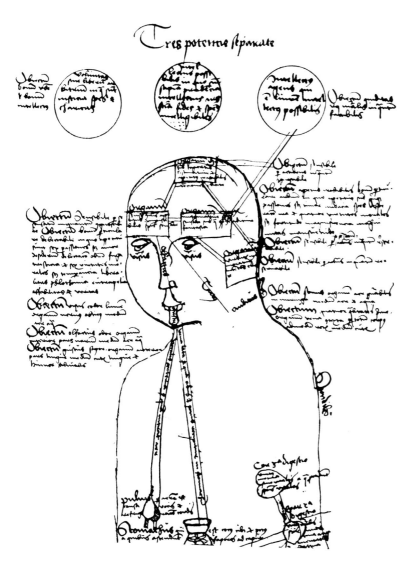

FIGURE 47

FIGURE 47

From a manuscript of about 1500, *Tractatus de potentiis animae et corporis organis et modo intelligendi* (p. 135), bound with tracts on Aristotle and Thomas Aquinas. It was advertised in a book catalogue of J. Halle of Munich in 1928 but its present location has not been traced.[75] The writer may have been Petrus Tozler.

It is headed by "The three powers are separate" and the three circles below this from left to right contain comments regarding will or free-will, potential intelligence, and active intelligence. The squares on the head represent four cells and are connected to each other. Although it is very difficult to decipher the writing in them, they seem to represent the usual mental faculties (cf. Figure 30). The lower of the two squares forming the second cell is linked to the circle labelled "active intelligence . . .". The writing around the head describes the senses.

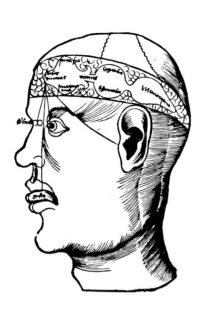

FIGURE 48

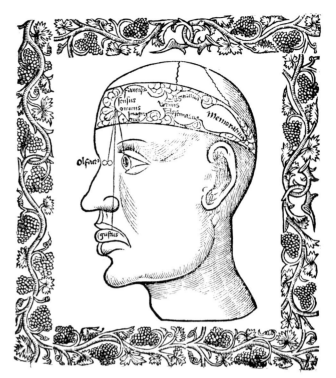

FIGURE 49

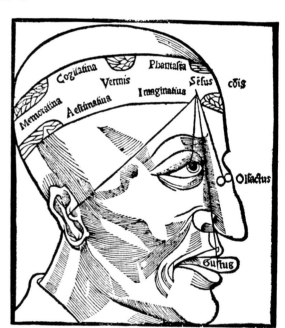

FIGURE 50

FIGURE 48 (OPPOSITE TOP LEFT)
This is one of the most popular portrayals of the
Cell Doctrine. In 1503 Gregor Reisch (c. 1467–
1525) a Carthusian prior of Freiburg and Confessor
to Emperor Maximilian I, published his compendium of grammar, science, and philosophy,
Margarita philosophica, the first notable modern
encyclopedia.[76] This drawing appeared in it[77] and
has been reproduced on many occasions since.

There are three freely communicating cells: the
first is inscribed "sensus communis, fantasia,
imaginativa", the second "cogitativa, estimativa";
and the third "memorativa". The special sense
organs are connected with the first cell and
between it and the second is the word "vermis".
To the modern anatomist this refers to the mid-line
portion of the cerebellum, thought by Galen to act
as a valve between the third and fourth ventricle
(see Figures 24, 25, 39, 57). In the present context,
however, it is applied to the worm-like choroid
plexus as it passes through the foramen of Monro
and controls the flow between cells one and two.
Manfredi in his *Anothomia* of 1490 described it in
this location and stated that thinking is arrested
when it blocks the passage and begins again when
it unblocks it.[78]

The patterning around the cells may conceivably
be intended to portray cerebral convolutions.

FIGURE 49 (OPPOSITE TOP RIGHT)
Reisch's drawing was soon plagiarized and a
sequence of publications from the 16th to the 19th
centuries contained various forms of it. One of the
first was in the 1523 edition of a book by Ramon
Lull (c. 1235–1316),[79] *Practica compendiosa artis,*[80]
in which the illustrations were drawn by Guillaume
Leroy II, the son of Lyons' first printer.

FIGURE 50 (OPPOSITE BOTTOM)
A version much cruder than the Reisch original was
published also in 1523 by Gulielmus Leporeus
(Guillaume Le Lievre, *fl. c.* 1520).[81] In this instance
the head looks to the left which is rare in drawings
of ventricular functions (cf. Figure 33).

FIGURE 51[82] (RIGHT)
This appears in a manuscript dated 1524 which
contains many illustrations but few of artistic merit.
Most have been copied from other sources, and in
our figure a crude Reisch-type ventricular system
has been superimposed on a drawing of a man's
head.

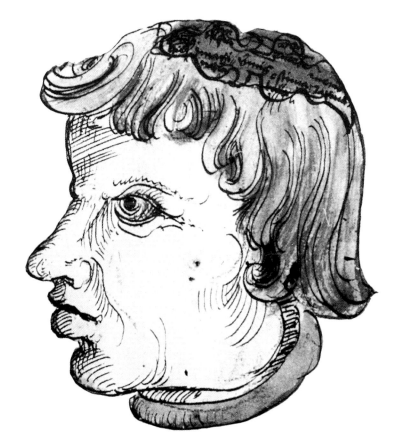

FIGURE 51

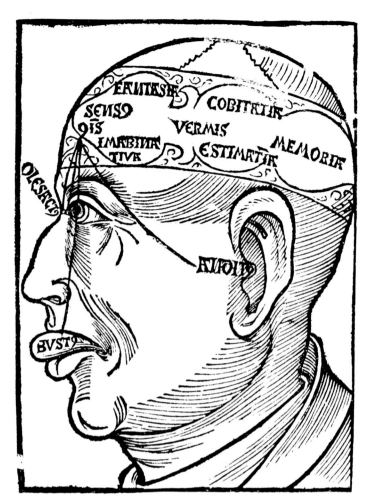

FIGURE 52

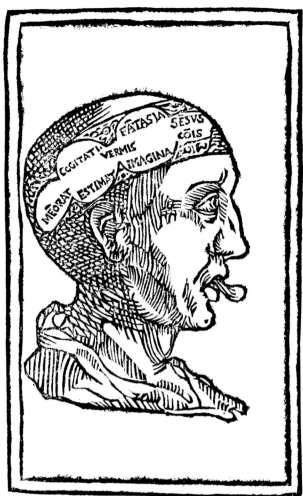

FIGURE 54

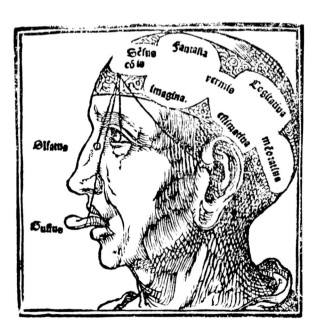

FIGURE 53

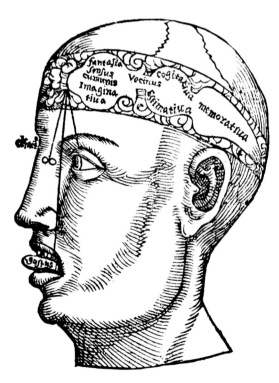

FIGURE 55

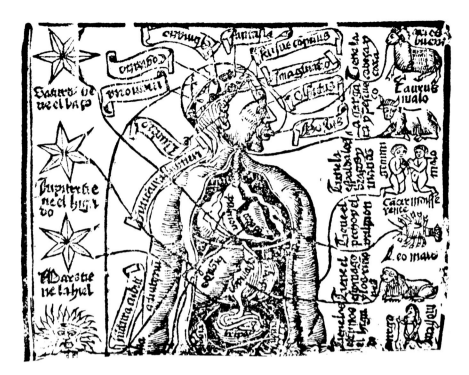

FIGURE 56

FIGURE 52 (OPPOSITE TOP LEFT)
An English variant appeared in 1525 in a book on
surgery by Hieronymus Brunschwig of Strassburg
(1450–1512),[83] first published in German in 1497.

FIGURE 53 (OPPOSITE BOTTOM LEFT)
A popular variant of the Reisch figure first
appeared in a book by Joannes Romberch de
Kyrspe (fl. 1520) of 1520[84] and Lodovico Dolce
(1508–?1568) used the same configuration in a
book very similar to Romberch's but in the form of
a dialogue, published in 1586.[85]

FIGURE 54 (OPPOSITE TOP RIGHT)
In 1579 the Thesaurus of Cosma Rosselli (d. c.
1577) was published in Venice.[86] It included a
Reisch/Romberch head, redrawn, reversed, and
with the connections between special sense organs
and the first cell omitted.

FIGURE 55 (OPPOSITE BOTTOM RIGHT)
The Lull (1523) version shown in Figure 49 was
slightly modified and used in his Opera omnia of
1612.[87]

FIGURE 56 (ABOVE)
This is a very crude presentation of the Reisch
model but the basic scheme can be recognized;
faculties and senses are named on medieval banner
labels. It is in a book published by Geronimo Cortès
of Valencia (d. 1615) in 1614.[88] Like Figure 20, the
head is part of a Zodiac Man and very similar to it.

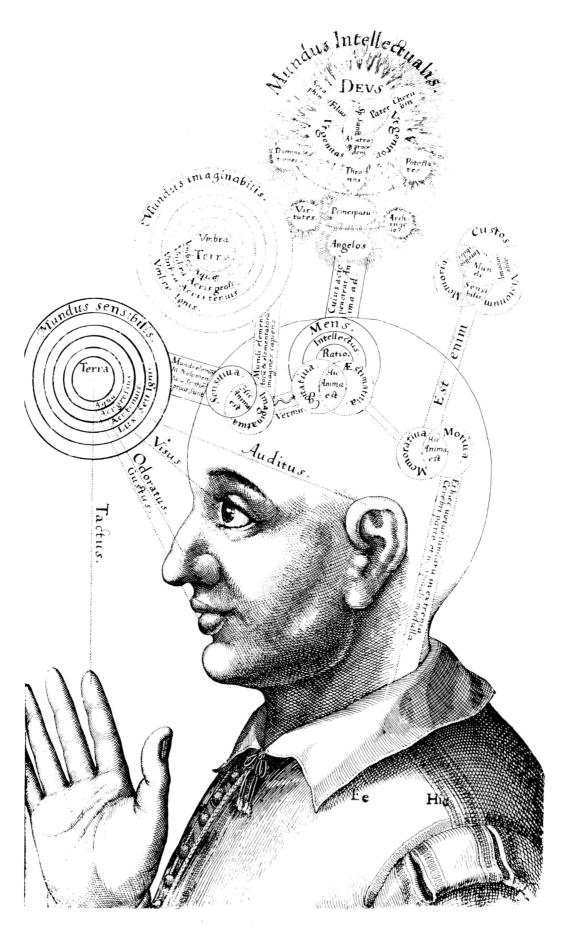

FIGURE 57

FIGURE 57 (OPPOSITE)

This intricate diagram of Fludd (1619)[89] is similar to that in Figure 37. It is not possible to explain here the whole system but the cranial elements are readily recognizable. Each of the three cells is double: "sensitiva" and "imaginativa"; "cogitativa" and "aestimativa"; "memorativa" and "motiva". Where they overlap is written, "The soul is here". They are not only linked to each other but also to extra-cerebral constellations. The first cell links with the material and imaginary worlds of sensation and imagination, respectively. It is labelled "sensitiva" and "imaginativa" because it observes true images and likenesses such as shadows of corporeal and sensible things. The middle cell is concerned with mind, intellect, and reasoning which in turn communicates with the intellectual world, with celestial things and with God. The third cell conceals, guards, and records the objects of vision, of the sensible world and of the world of imagination and intellect; it is labelled "memorativa" and "motiva". It also sends motion to any part of the microcosm by way of the spinal cord.[90] The "vermis" is between cell one and two (cf. Figures 24, 25, 39, 48).

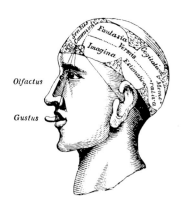

FIGURE 58

FIGURE 58

Phrenology is a system in which mental faculties are localized on the cerebral surface (see Chapter 10). When first introduced in the early 19th century, its proponents looked back into history to find support for their concept and were in sympathy with the theory of ventricular localization of psychological function. They, therefore, often published the Reisch figure (Figure 48), modified by Romberch (Figure 53). This example is taken from a translation by John Elliotson (1789–1868) of J. F. Blumenbach's *Institutiones physiologicae* published in 1840.[91]

4. EYE-BRAIN DIAGRAMS

The iconography of the eye is another fascinating part of the history of anatomical illustrations. Frequently the brain was included in the curious diagrams drawn and these are grouped here for convenience. They are all abstract compositions but only the parts depicting the brain will be elucidated.

FIGURE 59[92]

This drawing is probably from the late 12th or early 13th century. From a small circle, which represents either the brain or the first cell, extend three channels. The two lateral ones are the hollow optic nerves to the eyes, which are made up of five concentric layers, like an onion. The central canal is the nose channel ending in the "cartilage". Other organs of the body are depicted in diagrammatic form in this and in other manuscripts (Figures 60, 61). They represent anatomical features schematically and their main purpose is to illustrate contemporary physiological theory.

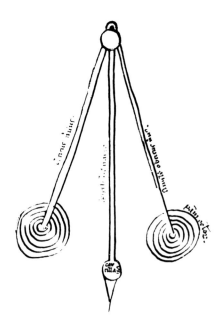

FIGURE 59

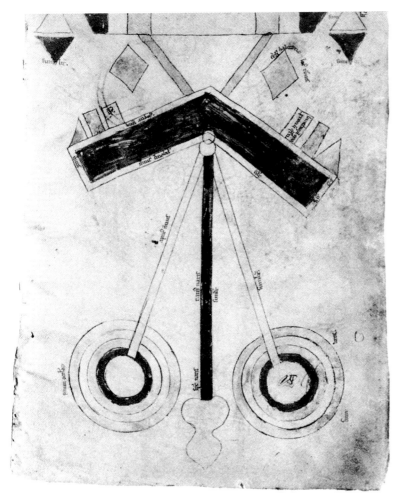

FIGURE 60

FIGURE 60[93]
A more elaborate form of the previous crude figure and probably contemporary with it. As the labelling is limited and the text unhelpful, it has never been adequately elucidated.

The eyes, optic nerves, and nose channel are the same as in Figure 59. In addition, however, there is a group of geometric shapes above them which represent at the top the coverings of the brain (pericranium, cranium, dura mater, pia mater) and the cells contained within it. The four rhomboids which depict the latter are reminiscent of those in Figure 24 and there are also similarities to the complex patterns of Figure 25. The diamond shape on the right is labelled "dwelling place of the brain or the place of reason", perhaps the middle cell. On the left piece of the angulated rectangle is written "auditus" above, "nervus" on the end, and "nervus immobilis" below. The significance of this is obscure. In the small rectangle on the right is "junction of the covering of the fourth thing", an equally mysterious comment. The diverging mid-line strips may represent the crossed optic nerves central to the optic chiasma.

FIGURE 61[94] (OPPOSITE)
Exactly the same geometric figure is found in this well-known manuscript. It is drawn with a little more accuracy, but carries no explanation. Like the previous manuscript it contains other organs depicted elsewhere. The stomach[95] and the sexual organs[96] are presented in the same curious schematic fashion and it seems likely that Islamic influences are responsible. Similar diagrams of established eastern origin are known (Figures 62, 99, 100).

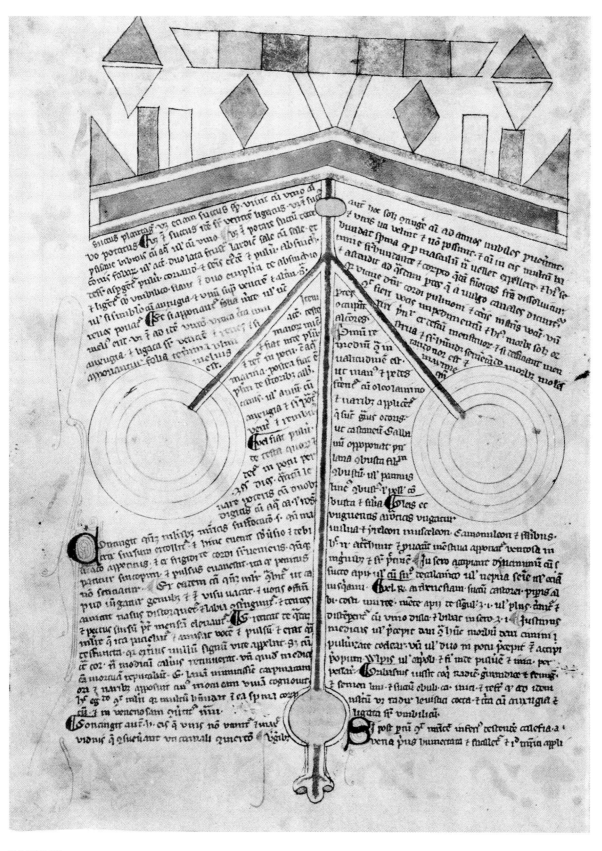

FIGURE 61

MEDIEVAL CELL DOCTRINE 45

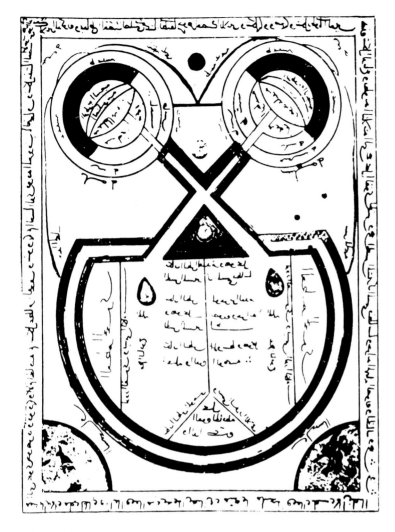

FIGURE 62

FIGURE 62[97]

This well-known schematic figure of the eyes and brain is of Islamic origin. It seems to have originated in a treatise on ophthalmology written in the second half of the 13th century by a Syrian, Halīfa, but may date back further, to at least A.D. 1000. It is, therefore, probably the oldest figure of its kind that has come down to us.[98] The present manuscript, however, is dated A.D. 1560. The drawing has been reproduced on many occasions but is described fully only by K. Sudhoff,[99] and J. Hirschberg.[100] The geometric form of this and other Arabic figures was presumably determined by the hostility of orthodox Moslems towards representations of the human form and by the religious restrictions which prevented Arabs dissecting and producing life-like pictures of parts of the body.[101]

The brain cavity is represented by the lower shape, which has an outline consisting of pericranium, bone, dura mater, and pia mater and to which are attached anteriorly the hollow optic nerves crossing in the optic chiasma to the eyes. Inside it are four ventricles or cells which are the site of the five mental faculties: the two black oval shapes are the first cell (left and right) which contains "sensus communis called phantasia" and visual perception; the second cell is the black triangle between the optic pathways and here imagination and judgement take place; the third is the triangular shape outlined posteriorly for memory, together with retention.

FIGURE 63[102] (OPPOSITE TOP)

Equally curious, but perhaps slightly less schematic, is this drawing from the second half of the 14th century, labelled: "The figure of the eye in the human head", taken probably from a treatise on ophthalmological medicine written by Magister Zacharias of Salerno and Constantinople in the 12th century.[103]

Our interest is limited to the posterior part where the onion-skin layers of cranium, dura mater, and pia mater are once more depicted. The brain, marked "cerebrum", is but a crescent-shaped slit. Although no reference is made here to the ventricles and to their functions, this drawing can be legitimately included in the schematic eye-brain diagram tradition.

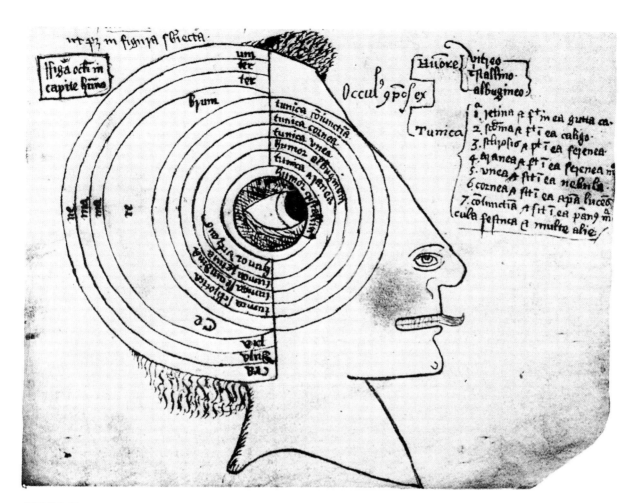

FIGURE 63

FIGURE 64[104]

Independently of the Islamic tradition, the longitudinal section of the eyeball was perpetuated in the medieval West. Thus the diagrams of Roger Bacon, Pecham and Witelo were widespread in the late Middle Ages and amongst them were some which included the brain.[105] John de Pecham (early or mid-1230's to 1294) was consecrated Archbishop of Canterbury in 1279.[106] He wrote prolifically on theology and science, his famous *Perspectiva communis* being amongst the latter.[107] There are many manuscripts of it and eleven printed editions,[108] but only three drawings from them qualify for inclusion here. First there is the figure shown, dating from the end of the 14th century.[109] The eyes are connected posteriorly to a circle, the cranium, in which there are four communicating chambers labelled from before backwards, "cerebrum, fantasia, memoria, cogitacio" thus showing some deviation from the usual pattern.[110]

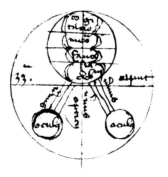

FIGURE 64

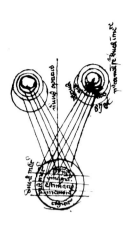

FIGURE 65

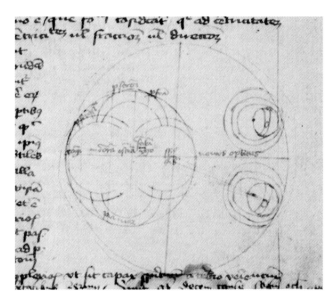

FIGURE 66

FIGURE 65[111]

This geometric pattern was drawn in 1367. The brain is surrounded by dura mater and pia mater and divided into slices labelled from before backwards, "sensus communis", "imaginativa", "estimacio", "memoracio", and "cogitacio".

FIGURE 66[112]

The third Pecham drawing dates from 1430. The brain consists of four cavities surrounded by pia mater. The anterior cell is labelled "sensus communis", and on a sagittal line from behind forwards is written "cogitativa, memorativa [in the posterior cell], estimativa, sensitiva ymago, sensus communis [in the anterior cell]". Again there are deviations from the usual arrangement. Written along the upper edge of the head (the left side of it) is "perfectissima perfectior perfecta", the significance of which is not clear.

NOTES

1. J. Leyacker, "Zur Entstehung der Lehre von den Hirnventrikeln als Sitz psychischer Vermögen", *Arch. Gesch. Med.* 1927, *19*:253–286. This is a deeper analysis of the theory and it supplements W. S. (Chapt. 2, note 22); W. Pagel, "Medieval and Renaissance contributions to knowledge of the brain and its function", in, Poynter, *op. cit.* Chapt. 2, note 18, pp. 95–114; H. W. Magoun, "Early development of ideas relating the mind with the brain", in, G. E. W. Wolstenholme & C. M. O'Connor (editors), *The neurological basis of behaviour,* London, J. & A. Churchill, 1958 (Ciba Foundation Symposium), pp. 4–27; E. Clarke, "The early history of the cerebral ventricles", *Transactions & Studies of the College of Physicians of Philadelphia,* 1962, *30*:85–89; Clarke & O'Malley (*op. cit.,* Chapt. 2, note 15) pp. 461–469.

2. W. Sudhoff, *op. cit.,* Chapt. 2, note 22.

3. Cambridge, Gonville & Caius College Ms. 428 F.50[R] (courtesy of the Librarian.) It has been published already by C. Singer, *Evolution of anatomy,* London, Paul, Trench & Trubner, 1925, Fig. 31 on p. 66 and by Grünthal (*op. cit.,* Chapt. 1, note 14), see Abb. 1.

4. J. H. G. Grattan & C. Singer, *Anglo-Saxon magic and medicine illustrated specially from the semi-pagan text 'Lacnunga',* London, Oxford University Press, 1952, pp. 48, 65–66. See also Fig. 44 on p. 94.

5. The writer of the Hippocratic book *On wounds of the head* described the types of skull suture patterns. His third variety which is shown in our Figure 3, is in the shape of a capital H, the cross-stem

representing the sagittal suture, the uprights the coronal and lambdoid sutures. See, "On wounds in the head", I, in, *Hippocrates with an English translation* by Dr. E. T. Withington, Vol. 2, London, W. Heinemann, 1927, pp. 6 & 7.

6. Ghent, Universiteits Bibliotheek, Ms. 1263, F.3^V (courtesy of the Librarian).

7. See W. S., pp. 182–183. The text and the drawing are reproduced by E. C. van Leersum, *De "cyrurgie" van Meester Jan Yperman,* Leiden, A. W. Sijthoff's Uitg., 1912, pp. 34 & 7 respectively, the text only by A. De Mets, in, *La chirurgie de Maître Jehan Yperman (1260?–1310?) Livres I et II,* Paris, Editions Hippocrate, 1936, pp. 26–27. See also, F. A. Snellaert, "Rapport sur le travail intitulée: La chirurgie de Maître Jean Yperman, le père de la chirurgie flamande (1295–1351)", *Annales de la Société Royal de Médecine de Gand,* 1854, *32*:149–158.

8. British Museum, Arundel & Burney Ms. 251, F.37^R (courtesy of the Librarian). See W. S., pp. 191–192, and K. Sudhoff, "Neue Beiträge zur Vorgeschichte des Ketham. B. Ein Krankheitsmann aus ein Arundel-Handschrift des Britischen Museums", *Arch. Gesch. Med.,* 1911, *5*:287–288.

9. Bodleian Library, Ms. Canon Misc. 366, F.1^V (courtesy of the Librarian). See W. S., pp. 194–196.

10. Bibliothèque Nationale, Ms. Latin 11229, F.37^V (courtesy of the Librarian). See W. S., p. 192. Also described by K. Sudhoff in greater detail in, "Eine Pariser 'Ketham'—Handschrift aus der Zeit König Karls VI. (1380–1422)", *Arch. Gesch. Med., 1909,* 2:84–100, see pp. 93–97 and Tafel IV, 4; reproduced by Magoun *(op. cit.,* above, note 1).

11. K. Sudhoff, *ibid.,* note 10 above.

12. Stockholm, Kungliga Biblioteket Ms. XII8 (courtesy of the Librarian).

13. See, W. S., p. 198. Sir D'Arcy Power translated the whole Ms. in, *De arte phisicali et de cirurgia of Master John Arderne, Surgeon of Newark, dated 1412,* London, J. Bale, Sons & Danielsson, 1922; this drawing is not described. See also, K. Sudhoff, "Weitere Beiträge zur Geschichte der Anatomie im Mittelalter. IV. 7. Die graphische Weiterbildung der anatomischen Fünfbilderserie aus Alexandrinerzeit und eine anatomische Serie aus Stockholm", *Arch. Gesch. Med.,* 1914, *8*:135–139. See pp. 137–139 and Tafel IV.

14. Wellcome Historical Medical Library, Ms. 49, "The Apocalypse", F.39^V (from the original Ms. in the Wellcome Library, by courtesy of the Trustees). See S. A. Moorat, *Catalogue of Western manuscripts on medicine & science in the Wellcome Historical Medical Library,* London, Wellcome Historical Medical Library , vol. 1, 1962, pp. 32–37. It is discussed in detail by F. Saxl in, "A spiritual encyclopaedia of the later Middle Ages", *J. Warburg & Courtauld Inst.,* 1942, *5*:82–137 and by O. Kurz, "The medical illustrations of the Wellcome MS."

ibid., pp. 137–142, see p. 140.

15. Munich, Hof- und Staatsbibliothek Codex latinus 73, inside front cover (courtesy of the Librarian).

16. W. S., pp. 198–199. See also, K. Sudhoff, in, *Tradition und Naturbeobachtung in den Illustrationen medizinischer Handschriften und Frühdrucke vornehmlich des 15. Jahrhunderts,* Heft 1 of *Studien zur Geschichte der Medizin,* Leipzig, J. A. Barth, 1907, p. 59.

17. Wolfenbüttel, Herzogliche Bibliothek, Codex Augustanius 42, 1st folio, F.264^V (courtesy of the Librarian). W. S., p. 201. This sketch accompanies the *Anatomia* of Mondino de Luzzi (1270–1326), placed in the margin beside the statement, "In man, when the membranes have been removed, the brain will appear."

18. Artelt *(op. cit.,* Chapt. 1, note 13).

19. Heidelberg, Bibliothek Universitäts, Codex Pal.Germ.644, F.2 (courtesy of the Librarian). W. S., p. 193; K. Sudhoff, "Neue Beiträge zur Vorgeschichte des 'Ketham'. A. Eine Heidelberger Kethamhandschrift aus der ersten Hälfte des 15. Jahrhunderts", *Arch. Gesch. Med.,* 1911, *5*:280–287, Tafel IV.

20. J. Ketham, *Fasciculus medicinae,* Venice. J. & G. de Forlivio, 26 July 1491, There is a facsimile of this edition, by K. Sudhoff & C. Singer, *The Fasciculus medicinae of Johannes de Ketham,* Milan, Lier, 1924. See Choulant-Frank, *op. cit.,* Chapt. 1, note 3, pp. 115–122. This figure was redrawn for J. de Ketham, *Thesoro universale della medicina di Pietro Montagnana,* Venice, A. Vidali, 1668, p. 6, but it is artistically inferior.

21. G. de Harderwyck, *Epitomata seu reparationes totius philosophiae naturalis Aristotelis,* Cologne, H. Quentell, 29 Feb. 1496 (See F. N. L. Poynter, *A catalogue of incunabula in the Wellcome Historical Medical Library,* London, Oxford University Press, 1954. No. 283.) Also reproduced in K. D. Keele, *Anatomies of pain,* Oxford, Blackwell, 1957, Plate II; and in Pagel *(op. cit.,* above, note 1) Fig. 1. (From the original book in the Wellcome Library, by courtesy of the Trustees.)

22. E. Clarke, "Aristotelian concepts of the form and functions of the brain", *Bull. Hist. Med.,* 1963, *37*:1-14.

23. H. E. Sigerist, "Two fifteenth century anatomical drawings", *Bull. Hist. Med.,* 1943, *13*:313–319. The drawing is on the blank verso of the last leaf (F.105^V) of the second of two books which are bound together; they were each published in Cologne in *c.* 1485. This volume is now in the National Library of Medicine, Bethesda, Md. as Incunabula 274, *Copulator super tres libros Aristotelis de anima . . .,* [Cologne (D. Molner)], *c.* 1485 (courtesy of the National Library of Medicine).

24. Munich, Hof- und Staatsbibliothek, Codex latinus 4394, F.115^V (courtesy of the Librarian). See W. S., p. 193; K. Sudhoff, "Neue Beiträge

zur Vorgeschichte des 'Ketham'. D. Ein Lasstellenmann und eine Krankheitsfrau in einer Münchener Handschrift des 15. Jahrhunderts", *Arch. Gesch. Med.*, 1912, 5:298–300, Tafel VI, Fig. 2.

25. Copenhagen, Ms. Ney. Kgl. Saml., 84b, E.5^R (courtesy of the Librarian). See W. S., p. 193.

26. [Aristotle,] *Habes hic amande lector textū Parvuli, qd' aiūt, ph'i natural' cū comentariis . . . matthie Qualle Carniolani*, Haguenau, J. Rynmann & H. Granciuis, 1513, Tractatus III, Lectio XII, Sig.K.vi.^{R}.

27. *Cephalogia fisonomica divisa in dieci deche . . .*, Bologna, C. Ferroni for the heirs of E. Dozza, 1630, p. 87.

28. F. Suárez de Rivera, *Theatro chyrurgico anatomico . . .*, Tomo primo, Madrid, 1728. The only copy of this book available in Britain was published in 1730 but is incomplete, the plate of the Zodiac Man having been removed. See, Luis S. Granjel, *Anatomiá española de la ilustración,* Salamanca, Universidad de Salamanca, 1963, Fig. 54 and also pp. 52–53.

29. Bibliothèque Nationale, Ms. arabe Slane 2866, F.15^V (courtesy of the Librarian).

30. See, P. De Koning, *Trois traités d'anatomie arabes*, Leyden, E. J. Brill, 1903, pp. 46–49.

31. *Ibid.*, pp. 8–9.

32. Chateau de Chantilly Bibliotheque (musée Condé), Ms. 569. See, W. S., pp. 162–163; E. Wickersheimer, "'L'anatomie' de Guido de Vigevano, médecin de la reine Jeanne de Bourgogne (1345)", *Arch. Gesch. Med.*, 1913, 7:1–25, see pp. 10 (lines 186–212) and 22 and Tafel III; also in, *idem, Anatomies de Mondino dei Luzzi et de Guido de Vigevano*, Paris, E. Droz, 1926, p. 75.

33. Durham, University Library, Ms. Cosin V.IV.7, F.47^R (courtesy of the University Library, Durham).

34. Cambridge, Trinity College, Ms.0.2.40, F.57^V (courtesy of the Librarian). See W. S., pp. 196–198. Reproduced by Magoun *(op. cit.* above, note 1).

35. Munich, Hof- und Staatsbibliothek, Codex latinus 5961, inside page of front cover (courtesy of the Librarian). See, W. S., pp. 199–200; also reproduced in K. Sudhoff, *Tradition und Naturbeobachtung in den Illustrationen medizinischer Handschriften und Frühdrucke vornehmlich des 15. Jahrhunderts,* Leipzig, J. A. Barth, 1907 (Heft 1 of *Studien zur Geschichte der Medizin),* pp. 60–61.

36. *The works of Aristotle,* Vol. V, *De partibus animalium* by William Ogle, Oxford, Clarendon Press, 1912, II, 10; 656a 29–31.

37. *Philosophia pauperum sive philosophia naturalis,* Brescia, B. Farfengus, 10 September 1490, Sig.aa.viii^V.

38. *Ibid.,* 13 June 1493.

39. *Philosophia naturalis,* Basle, M. Furter, 1506. Another edition, (Venice, G. Arrivabenus, 31 August, 1496, Sig.g.vi^R) has the same arrangement of the ventricles but a different head, one that is similar to Fig. 27.

40. Sigerist, *op. cit.* above, note 23. The drawing is on the blank verso of the last page (F.47^V) of, *Positiones circa libros physicorum et de anima Aristotelis . . .,* [Cologne, H. Quentell] 16 May 1494. This book is now in the National Library of Medicine, Bethesda, Md. (Incunable 379) and the drawing appears in D. M. Schullian & F. E. Sommer, *A catalogue of incunabula and manuscripts in the Army Medical Library,* New York, H. Schumann, 1950, Plate 6, facing p. 168 (by courtesy of the National Library of Medicine).

41. Manchester, University Library, Ms. Medical AN.1 (courtesy of the Librarian).

42. Ludovicus Pruthenus, *Trilogium animae,* Nürnburg, Koberger, 6 March 1498, Capitulum XXIII, Sig.E.i.

43. E. Reicke, "Die Deutung eines Bildnisses von Brosamer in der kaiserlichen Gemäldegalerie in Wien, nebst Beiträgen zur Dürer- und Pirckheimer-Forschung", *Jb. kunst-hist. Samml. allerhöchsten Kaiserhauses* (Wien/Leipzig), 1911, 30:228–255; N. Weisbach, *Der junge Dürer. Drei Studien,* Leipzig, Hiersmann, 1906 and review of it in *Kunst-geschichtliche Anzeigen (Beiblatt der Mitth. des Inst. f. österr. Geschichtsforschung)* Innsbruck, 1906, 3:79–88. The cut is described by W. Kurth (editor), *The complete works of Albrecht Dürer.* London, 1936, p. 18, No. 93 and is reproduced in J. Jacobi (editor), *Paracelsus. Selected writings,* London, Routledge & K. Paul, 1951, p. 197.

44. K. Sudhoff, *Die medizinische Fakultät zu Leipzig im ersten Jahrhundert der Universität,* Leipzig, J. A. Barth, 1909 (Heft 8 of *Studien zur Geschichte der Medizin),* pp. 115–121.

45. *Anthropologium de hominis dignitate, natura et proprietatibus; de elementis, partibus et membris humani corporis,* Leipzig, W. Stoeckel, 1501.

46. Choulant-Frank *(op. cit.,* Chapt. 1, note 3), pp. 125–126.

47. *Quaestiones librorum de anima Aristotelis,* Metz, C. Hochfeder, 1501, Sig.x8^V.

48. W. S., *passim.*

49. *Questiones librorum de anima,* Cracow, J. Haller, 1514, F. CXXIX^R.

50. "Achillini: Aristotelian and anatomist", in, L. Thorndike, *A history of magic and experimental medicine,* Vol. 5, New York, Columbia University Press, 1941, pp. 37–49.

51. *Opusculum perutile de cognitione animae et eius potentiis Augustini de Anchona cum quadam questione Prosperi de Regio,* Bologna, J. J. de Benedictus, 1503, sig.f.[viii]^R.

52. See, L. J. Lind, *Jacopo Berengario da Carpi. A short introduction to anatomy (Isagogae brevis),* Chicago, University of Chicago Press, 1959.

53. *Tractatus de fractura calve sive cranei a Carpo editus,* Bologna, H. de Benedictus, 1518.

54. The same. *Ed. nova,* Leyden, J. Maire, 1629.

55. *Anatomiae hoc est, corporis humani, dissectionis pars prior,* Marburg, E. Cervicornus, 1537, Sig.d.ii^R and g.iv^R. See Choulant-Frank (*op. cit,* Chapt. 1, note 3), pp. 148–149.

56. *Opus de mente peripatetichorum collectum noviter impressum dedicatum Petro Lando . . .,* Venice, 4 May, 1543. This was listed in a bookseller's catalogue (*L'Art Ancien,* S. A., of Zürich, Cat. No. 21) of about 1938 but its present whereabouts cannot be traced.

57. See, A. G. Debus, *The English Paracelsians,* London, Oldbourne, 1965, pp. 104–127, 132–136, and elsewhere. Also, W. Pagel, "Religious motives in the medical biology of the XVIIth century", *Bull. Inst. Hist. Med.,* 1935, 3:265–312, see pp. 265–297.

58. It is on the first page of "Ars memoriae" in his *Utriusque cosmi maioris scilicet et minoris metaphysica, physica atque technica historia,* Tomus secundus, Oppenheim [Hesse-Darmstedt], Aere J.-T. de Bry; Typis H. Galleri, 1619, pp. 326–327. Reproduced by F. A. Yates, *The art of memory,* London, Routledge & K. Paul, 1966, Plate 15, and discussed by her on pp. 326–327.

59. *Ibid,* pp. 320–367.

60. Cambridge, University Library, Ms.Gr.g.1.1, F.490^V (courtesy of the Librarian). See W. S., pp. 184–189.

61. It is reproduced by R. Dunglison, (*Human physiology,* 3rd edition, Vol. 1, Philadelphia, Carey, Lea & Blanchard, 1838, Fig. 50 on p. 292) who states it is "in the *Book Rarities* of the University of Cambridge". Also in De Lint (*op. cit.,* Chapt. 1, note 5), Fig. 20 on p. 27.

62. Galen described the vermis of the cerebellum in *De usu partium,* Book VIII, 14; see, M. T. May, *Galen on the usefulness of the parts of the body . . .,* Vol. 1, Ithaca, N.Y., Cornell University Press, 1968, pp. 419–423. He implied that the name was not his (*De anatomicis administrationibus,* Book IX, 5; see, C. Singer, *Galen on anatomical procedures,* London, Oxford University Press, 1956, p. 236).

63. Munich, Hof- und Staatsbibliothek, Codex latinus 527, F.64^V (courtesy of the Librarian). See W. S., pp. 189–191.

64. British Museum, Ms. Sloane 2156, F.ll^R (courtesy of the Librarian). It was reproduced by C. Singer, "A study in early Renaissance anatomy, with a new text: The *Anothomia* of Hieronymo Manfredi (1490)", in, C. Singer (editor), *Studies in the history and method of science* [vol. 1], Oxford, Clarendon Press, 1917, pp. 79–164, see Fig. 14 on p. 116; also by Magoun (*op. cit.* above, note 1).

65. For Bacon, see, *Dictionary of scientific biography,* Vol. 1, New York, Scribners, 1970, pp. 377–385.

66. Wellcome Historical Medical Library, Ms.55, F.93. (From the original Ms. in the Wellcome Library, by courtesy of the Trustees.) See, Moorat (*op. cit.* above, Note 14), pp. 39–41. It is dated 1472–1474 and was probably written by the historiographer, Johann Lindner.

67. Reproduced by gracious permission of Her Majesty the Queen. O. C. L. Vangensten, A. Fonahn, & H. Hopstock (editors), *Quaderni d'anatomia,* Christiania, 1911-1916, V,6^V; K. Clark, *A catalogue of the drawings of Leonardo da Vinci in the collection of His Majesty at Windsor Castle,* Cambridge, 1935, 12603^R; C. D. O'Malley & J. B. de C. M. Saunders, *Leonardo da Vinci on the human body,* New York, Schumann, 1952, No. 142 on pp. 330–331.

68. See, J.P. McMurrich, *Leonardo da Vinci the anatomist (1452–1519),* Baltimore, Williams & Wilkins, 1930, pp. 204–209.

69. O'Malley & Saunders (*op. cit.* above, note 67), pp. 364–365.

70. *Philosophiae naturalis compendium,* Leipzig, M. Lother, 12 September 1499, F.91^V.

71. W. Le Fanu, "A primitive anatomy: Johann Peyligk's 'Compendiosa declaratio'", *Ann. Roy. Coll. Surg.,* 1962, 31:115–119. This article gives bibliographical and contents detail, as do: K. Sudhoff. *Die medizinische Facultät zu Leipzig im ersten Jahrhundert der Universität,* Heft 8 of *Studien zur Geschhte der Medizin,* Leipzig, J. A. Barth, 1909, pp. 113–121 (see Tafel VI to VIII); idem, "Ein unbekannter Druck von Johann Peyligks . . .", *Arch. Gesch. Med.,* 1916, 9:309–314; idem, "Der stöckelsche Nachdruck der Peyligkschen 'Compendiosa capitis physici declaratio' von 1510", *ibid.,* 1917, 10:251–254; Choulant-Frank (*op. cit.,* Chapt. 1, note 3), pp. 123-124.

72. *Compendiosa capitis physici declaratio . . .,* Leipzig, impressit Wolfgangus monacensis, 1516. This is a separate edition of the final chapter of the *Philosophiae naturalis compendium* (see note 70), as is the 1513 edition described by Le Fanu (*op. cit.* above, note 71).

73. *Op.cit.,* note 70, sig.Q6^V. These two were used by Magnus Hundt (1449–1519), also of Leipzig, in his *Anthropologia de hominis dignitate, natura, et proprietatibus, . . .,* Leipzig, Wolfgang Stocklin

1501: (a) is on F.23^R, and (b) on F.23^V. (=Sig.Liii^R and Liii^V). See, W. S., p. 203.

74. This was well described by A. Vesalius, *De humani corporis fabrica,* Basel, Oporinus, 1543, Book VII, Chapt. II (C. Singer, *Vesalius on the human brain,* London, Oxford University Press, 1952, pp. 51–56). Galen referred briefly to it in *De anatomicis administrationibus,* Book IX, Chapt. 4 (C. Singer, *Galen on anatomical procedures,* London, Oxford University Press, 1956, pp. 235–236).

75. J. Halle, *Katalog 62, 1928,* Item 562, pp. 134–136.

76. *Margarita philosophica,* Freiburg im Breisgau, J. Schott, 1503. There were 10 editions (1503 to 1583) and bibliographical details are in, J. Ferguson, "The *Margarita philosophica* of Gregorius Reisch. A bibliography", *Trans. Bibliograph. Soc.* (London), 1929, *10:*194–216.

77. Liber X, Trac.II, "De potentiis", fig. 18. It is described by Choulant-Frank *(op. cit.,* Chapt. 1, note 3), pp. 128–129.

78. Singer, 1956, *(op. cit.* above, note 74), p. 109.

79. See, "Raymond Lull", in, L. Thorndike, *op. cit.,* note 50 above, Vol. 2 (1923), pp. 862–873; and "Ramon Lull: doctor illuminate" in *Times Literary Supplement,* 29 June 1933, pp. 433–434. For his alchemy, see, Thorndike, "The Lullian alchemical collection" *(op. cit.* above), Vol. 4, 1934, pp. 3–64; for his art of memory, see, Yates *(op. cit.* above, note 58), "Lullism as an art of memory", pp. 173–198.

80. The figure is on F.cvi^V, the text being "De philosophiae naturali. Secunda pars".

81. *Ars memorativa,* Toulouse, J. Fabri, 1523, Liber I, on F.5^R. Also in 1520 edition (Paris, J. B. Ascensius or J. Bade), on F.IV^V, but we did not see it; this is said to be one of the rarest mnemonic works. It is reproduced in L. Volkmann, "Gulielmus Leporeus, *Ars memorativa,* Kopfschema", *Jahrbuch der Kunsthistorischen Sammlungen in Wien,* 1929, Abb. 172, and also by Magoun *(op. cit.* above, note 1).

82. Erlangen, Bibliothek Universitäts, Ms. 1463, F.67^V (courtesy of the Librarian). Reported by C. Ferckel ("Eine Bilderhandschrift v. J. 1524", *Mittheil. Gesch. Med. Naturw.,* 1913, *12:*278-281), but this illustration is not described.

83. *The noble experyence of the vertuous handy warke of surgeri . . .,* London, P. Treveris, 1525, on Sig.B.i^R. See, H. E. Sigerist, *Hieronymus Brunschwig and his work,* New York, Ben Abramson, 1946.

84. *Congestorium ortificiose memorie . . .,* Venice, G. de Rusconibus, 1520, "memorie, tractatus I, capitulum IV", Sig.B.I^V. Also in Venice, 1533 edition on F.12^V. Redrawn by Yates *(op. cit.* above, note 58), Fig. 9 on p. 256.

85. *Dialogo nel quale si ragiona del modo di accrescere et conservar la memoria,* Venice, G. B. Sessa, 1586, F.8^R. Probably also in editions of 1552, 1562, 1575, but these not seen. Same wood block as in Romberch, 1520 and 1533, and other plates plagiarized also.

86. *Thesaurus artificiosae memoriae,* Venice, A. Paduanius, 1579. The cut is on p. 138.

87. Bernhardi de Lavinheta, *Opera omnia quibus tradidit artis Raymundi Lulli compendiosam,* Coloniae, L. Zetzneri, 1612, p. 233. Illustrates section on "De generatione capitis . . .".

88. *Lunario, y pronostico perpetuo general . . .,* Alcala, n.p., 1614, pp. 124–125. The drawing in the 1601 (Madrid) edition differs in many respects and on the whole is less like the Reisch original, despite the fact that it is modelled on it.

89. *Utriusque cosmi maioris scilicet et minoris metaphysica . . . Tomus secundus . . . de supernaturali, naturali, praeternaturali et contranaturali microcosmi historia . . . .,* Oppenheim aere J. T. de Bry, Typis H. Galleri, Frankfort, E. Kempffer, 1619–1621.

90. This is abstracted from Fludd's account of his system which is in Tract. l, Sect. l, Lib. X, p. 217. See also, G. W. Corner, "Anatomists in search of the soul", *Ann. Med. Hist.,* 1919, *2:*1–7, see p. 5.

91. *Human physiology,* 5th edition, London, Longman, *et al.,* 1840, p. 370. It is attributed to "Dolce, 1562" and had already appeared with various stylistic emendations, in the *Phrenological Journal,* 1825, *2:* facing p. 387; in G. Combe, *A system of phrenology,* 3rd edition, Edinburgh, J. Anderson, 1830, p. 22; in, R. Dunglison, *Human physiology,* 3rd edition Philadelphia, Lea, Carey & Blanchard, 1838, Fig. 51 on p. 293; in R. W. Haskins, *History and progress of phrenology,* Buffalo, Steeple & Peck, 1839, p. 11, and other publications on phrenology. It was again redrawn and published by G. Redford, *Body and soul; or life, mind, and matter . . .,* London, J. Churchill, 1847, Plate II, fig. XIII; attributed to Dolce, 1575.

92. Pisa, University Library, Ms. Roncioni 99, F.2^R (courtesy of the Librarian). See, K. Sudhoff, "Weitere Beiträge zur Geschichte der Anatomie im Mittelalter . . . II . . . 5. Graphische Darstellungen innerer Körperorgane", *Arch. Gesch. Med.,* 1914, *7:*367–378, see p. 370 and Tafel XIV. Also reproduced by Herrlinger *(op. cit.,* Chapt. 1, note 1), Fig. 10 on p. 14.

93. Cambridge, Gonville & Caius College Ms. 190/223, F.6^R (courtesy of the Librarian). For a full description of manuscript, see, M. R. James, *A descriptive catalogue of the manuscripts in the Library of Gonville & Caius College,* Vol. I, Cambridge, University Press, 1907, pp. 218–219. Our figure is 9th in a series of ten "carefully but very unskillfully drawn". Colours are blue, red, green and dark red.

94. Oxford, Bodleian Library, Ms. Ashmole 399, F.22^V (courtesy of the Librarian). See, W. S., pp. 183–184, Figure 3. K. Sudhoff *(op. cit.*

above, note 92), p. 371, figure on this page merely mentions it and refers to W. S. above.

95. Sudhoff, *ibid.,* Tafel XV, 1.

96. C. Ferckel, "Diagramme der Sexualorgane in mittelalterlichen Handschriften", *Arch. Gesch. Med.,* 1917, *10*:225–263, see pp. 258–261 and Tafel XIII, 1 and 2.

97. Istanbul, Jeni gámi [Library of the New Mosque] 924 (courtesy of the Librarian).

98. M. Frank discussed eye drawings briefly in, "The schematic drawing of the eye in its historical development (fifteenth & sixteenth centuries)", *Contributions to medical and biological research dedicated to Sir William Osler . . .,* Vol. 2, New York, Hoeber, 1919, pp. 708–711.

99. "Weitere Beiträge zur Geschichte der Anatomie im Mittelalter. III. . . . 6. Augendurchschnittsbilder aus Abendland und Morgenland", *Arch. Gesch. Med.,* 1914, *8*:1–21, see pp. 12–16, & Tafel II.

100. "Die anatomischen Abbildungen vom Auge bei den Arabern" *Cbl. prakt. Augenheilk.,* 1904, *28*:292–296; he cited Soemmerring *De oculorum homina* but this could not be traced. Also, in, *Die arabischen Lehrbücher der Augenheilkunde. Ein Capital zur arabischen Literaturgeschichte,* Berlin, Königl. Akad. der Wissensch., 1905, pp. 77–79 (from *Abhandlung der Konigl. Preuss. Akad. der Wissensch.,* 1905, pp. 117); also, in J. Lippert & E. Mittwoch, in, *Die arabische Augenärzte nach den Quellen bearbeitet,* 2. Theil, Leipzig, Veit, 1905, pp. 161–164.

101. D. Diringer, *The illuminated book, its history and production,* London, Faber & Faber, 1958, p. 211.

102. British Museum, Ms. Sloane 981, F.68[R] (courtesy of the Librarian).

103. K. Sudhoff (*op. cit.* above, note 92), "(b) Text und Bild zum 'Liber de oculis, qui vocatur Salaracer id est secreta secretorum' des Macharias in einer Londoner Handschrift", pp. 3–6, Tafel 1, 2. For Zacharias, see, P. Pansier "La pratique de l'ophtalmologie dans le Moyen Age Latin" *Janus,* 1904, *9*:3–26, see pp. 9–10. For his text, see P. Pansier, "Mag-Zachariae Tractatus de passionibus oculorum . . . compiled *c.* 1143–1180", in, *Collectio ophthalmologica veterum auctorum,* Paris, J. B. Baillière, 1907; the figure is not reproduced.

104. Basel, Universität Öffentliche Bibliothek, Ms.F.IV.30, F.129[R] (courtesy of the Librarian).

105. K. Sudhoff, "Augenanatomiebilder im 15. und 16. Jahrhundert", in *Tradition und Naturbeobachtung,* Heft 1 of *Studien zur Geschichte der Medizin,* Leipzig, J. A. Barth, 1907, pp. 19–26.

106. For biography, see, D. L. Dovie, *Archbishop Pecham,* Oxford, Clarendon Press, 1952; and D. C. Lindberg, *John Pecham and the sci-ence of optics. "Perspectiva communis",* Madison, Wisc., University of Wisconsin Press, 1970, pp. 3–11.

107. Lindberg, *ibid.,* has published a text and translation. For excellent brief article, see, *idem,* "The 'Perspectiva communis' of John Pecham: its influence, sources, and content", *Arch. int. Hist. Sci.,* 1965, *18*:37–53.

108. Lindberg, *ibid.,* pp. 52–58.

109. Lindberg *(ibid.,* pp. 52–53) cites a personal communication from Bernard Rischoff.

110. A. Bednarski, in, "Die anatomischen Augenbilder in den Handschriften des Roger Bacon, Johann Peckham und Witelo", *Arch. Gesch. Med.,* 1931, *24*:60–78 reproduces this drawing (Fig. 6 on p. 66) and gives brief consideration to the Cell Doctrine (pp. 71–72). He does not discuss this or either of the two following drawings.

111. Vienna, Oesterreichische Nationalbibliothek, Ms. 5210, F.56[V] (courtesy of the Librarian). Figured by Bednarski, *ibid.,* Fig. 10 on p. 69.

112. Cracow, Biblioteka Jagiellonska, Ms. 1929 (Czechel). p. xiv (courtesy of the Librarian). Figured by Bednarski, *ibid.,* Fig. 7 on p. 66.

With the advent of Renaissance learning, the medieval Cell Doctrine began to lose ground. Although it was to persist into the 17th century by transmission through the writings of certain authors, the greater body of opinion gradually rejected it.

First, the true anatomy of the ventricular system, originally revealed by the Alexandrian anatomists and by Galen, was re-established and the crude medieval conceptual sketches were, therefore, no longer acceptable. It was shown concurrently that the ventricles contained a fluid, the cerebro-spinal fluid, and was thought unlikely that mental functions took place within it.

Anatomists now returned to the Ancient Greek concept of brain function (p. 3) whereby the animal spirits were produced either in the *rete mirabile* or in the substance of the brain and stored in the ventricles to be discharged thence by way of the hollow nerves.

This gradual transition was brought about by a group of men who stand between the medieval period and the Renaissance, men who having learned the old ways had begun to adopt the new. We have selected four of these pioneers: Leonardo da Vinci (1452–1519), Jacopo Berengario da Carpi (1457–1530), Andreas Vesalius (1514–1564), and Charles Estienne (1504–1564). They are representative of many more ardent investigators who were establishing modern anatomy in general, as well as advancing knowledge of the brain ventricles in particular. By their efforts they began a process of enlightenment which is continuing today in the study of anatomy and physiology. The outcome as far as the ventricular system is concerned is a vastly increased understanding of both form and function, although we are still far from total elucidation. For our present purposes, however, this story is irrelevant and need not be followed beyond this Transitional Period, other than linking it with the present by means of a modern illustration of the ventricular system.

FIGURE 67[1]

The best example of an individual who in his own lifetime attempted to reject the scholastic teachings of the Middle Ages in favour of the new Renaissance anatomy is that of Leonardo da Vinci. We have shown already how in 1490, or thereabouts, he was content to depict the brain according to accepted tradition (Figure 43). Sometime between 1504 and 1507, however, Leonardo carried out wax injections of the brain ventricles of the ox. It was the first time a cast of them had been prepared and much of their true shape was thus revealed. But even Leonardo was unable to break away completely from the all-pervading medieval lore and in the drawing, on the left, a lateral view of the ventricular system, he has placed these words on the ventricles: "imprensiva" (the perceptual centre) on the lateral, "sensus communis" on the third, and "memoria" on the fourth; again the third ventricle (second cell) had become the seat of the "sensus communis", rather than the first (cf. Figure 43). This is a remarkable example of the Transitional Period, medieval physiology superimposed upon Renaissance anatomy.[2] Leonardo, however, seemed to have no influence upon contemporary and subsequent anatomical studies.

A third sketch (not shown), another lateral view of the ventricles, allocates the sense of touch to the fourth ventricle, because it was considered that all the nerves of touch met there, at the top of the spinal cord.

FIGURE 68

About 20 years after Leonardo's wax experiments Berengario da Carpi was producing crude, yet much improved, anatomical illustrations in his *Isagoge breves* of 1522.[3] His reason was, ". . . so that the matters discussed may be better understood I have accommodated below such figures of the brain as I was able, in which some of the matters previously described can be understood, as

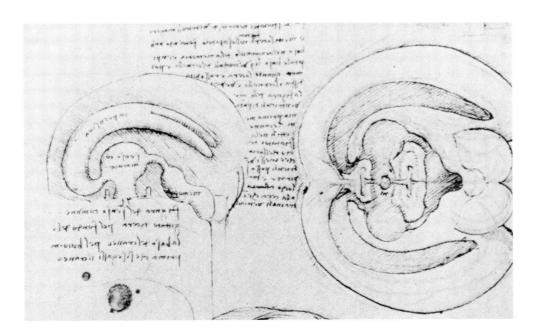

FIGURE 67

you see".[4] It seems strange to us to have to justify illustrating a text-book of anatomy.

Figure 68 is from the second edition of his *Isagoge breves,* 1523,[5] and shows the brain from above with at first one ventricle opened to show the "vermis", which is here applied to the choroid plexus whereas in the Dynamic Cell Doctrine it acted as a valve between cells one and two (see Figures 24, 25, 39, 48, 57). The lower view reveals both lateral ventricles ("anterior venter"), two veins in the mid-line, and the "embotum" which is either the opening into the aqueduct of Sylvius running between ventricles three and four or the hypothetical exit by way of the pituitary for ventricular wastes. Gone now are the medieval designations of the ventricles and in their place are anatomical terms. The pictorial representation of the Cell Doctrine had been removed from reputable text-books of anatomy for ever.

It had not, however, disappeared entirely. Berengario, like Leonardo, being a Renaissance man, though of medieval origin, is a good example of a transitionalist. Thus whilst expelling the Cell Doctrine from the illustrations of his treatise on anatomy, he still allowed a representation of it to appear on the title page of his book on fractures of the skull (Figure 35). Moreover, in the text of his *Isagoge* he accepted some of the Cell Doctrine, for he located all the mental functions in the lateral ventricles yet he believed that the other ventricles dealt with excretion, motion and sensation.[6] Like Leonardo he was unable to reject the Doctrine completely but he brought its destruction a little closer. In this regard Berengario can be compared with his contemporary, Dryander, who had both medieval (Figure 36) and Renaissance (Figure 81) illustrations in the same treatise.

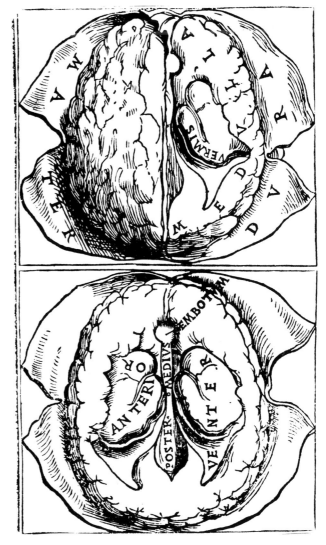

FIGURE 68

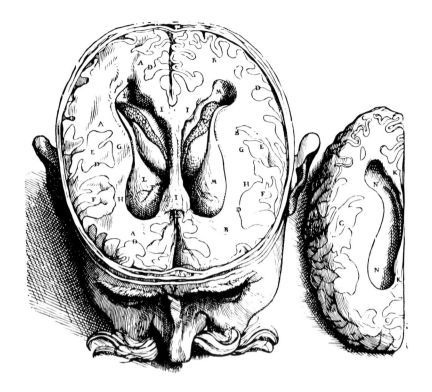

FIGURE 69

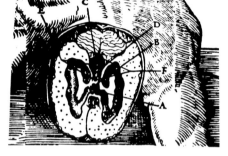

FIGURE 70

FIGURE 69

The greatest of the Renaissance anatomists,
Vesalius, is also a man of transition as regards brain
function.[7] In his remarkable book, the *De fabrica* of
1543,[8] he tells how he was taught the Cell
Doctrine and, although he described its basic
tenets, referring to Reisch's drawing (Figure 48), in
so doing, he was obviously casting doubt upon its
veracity.[9]

When he came to depict the ventricles, however,
he regarded them as purely anatomical structures
which, in keeping with the ancient Greek idea,
were the reservoirs of the animal spirits responsible
for sensory and motor activity of the body.[10]

The illustration on the left is a view of the brain
from above, as in Figure 68, and shows the lateral
ventricles and choroid plexuses. To the right is the
piece cut from the same cerebral hemisphere
showing the roof of its lateral ventricles.[11] These,
and other drawings of the brain, are, undoubtedly,
the best that had been published up to 1543.
There is considerable dispute as to the artists
responsible, but probably several were employed.
Thus Vesalius states, "[No longer] shall I have to
put up with the bad temper of artists and sculptors
[wood-block cutters] who made me more miser-
able than did the bodies I was dissecting"![12]

FIGURE 70

Our final figure of the Transitional Period is Charle[s]
Estienne[13] whose treatise of 1545, *De dissectione,*
is representative of the immediate pre-Vesalian
anatomy and illustrations; he began work on it in
1530 at the latest.[14] It has been described as "the
ugliest anatomical work we know".[15]

The wood-cut reproduced here is a small portio[n]
of one of the 62 full-page plates[16] and typifies
many of them. Although the background is
extensive and unnecessary, the anatomical detail is
minimal and inaccurate, and the style is mannerist[.]
As with other illustrations in this book, the view of
a horizontal section of the brain has been inserted
into a large plate. The key is as follows: A, fornix;
B, "vermis" (choroid plexus); C, pineal; D, vermis o[f]
cerebellum; E, glutia [= inferior corpora
quadrigemina or colliculi]; F, aqueduct of Sylvius.

As in the books by Berengario and Vesalius, the
artist was depicting anatomical structures as
accurately as possible, and although the
draughtsmanship was still quite crude, morpholog[y]
had been divorced entirely from function. It was n[o]
longer possible to illustrate a concept of function
without reference to a knowledge of anatomy.

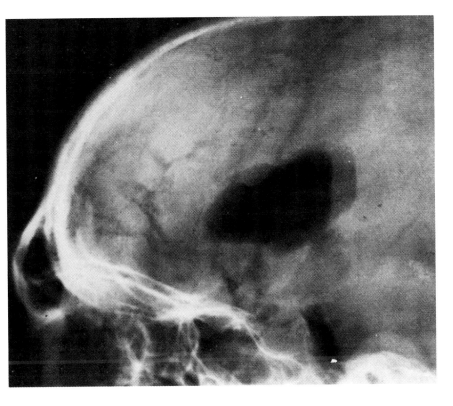

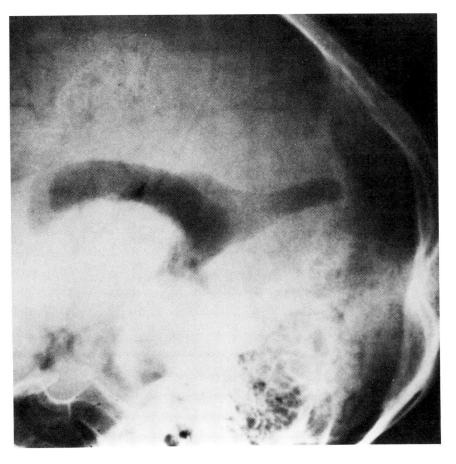

FIGURE 71

The Renaissance anatomists laid the foundations of modern anatomy. Building on the knowledge already established by the Ancient Greeks, they initiated a process of advancement which can be traced to the present.

The anatomy and physiology of the ventricular system is now known in some detail and special methods have been evolved of viewing it during life so that abnormalities may be detected and, hopefully, diagnosed and treated. This photo is a ventriculogram, carried out by replacing the fluid in the ventricles with air and taking a radiograph of the head.

FIGURE (A)

Normal ventriculogram—lateral view, brow up position to demonstrate the lateral horns of the lateral ventricle together with the anterior portion of the third ventricle.

FIGURE (B)

Lateral view with brow down position, demonstrates the posterior horns and portions of the temporal horns.

At this stage we can leave the brain ventricles which functionally have been regarded as reservoirs of animal spirits, mediators of mental functions, and the seat of the soul.[17] They are now known to be receptacles for cerebro-spinal fluid but the exact nature of its production and function is still not fully understood.

NOTES

1. *Quaderni,* V,7[R]; Clark 19127[R]; O'Malley & Saunders *(op. cit.* Chapt. 3, note 67) No. 147, pp. 340–341. (Reproduced by gracious permission of Her Majesty the Queen.)

2. See McMurrich *(op. cit.,* Chapt. 3, note 68); J. de Morsier, "Leonard et l'anatomie du cerveau humain", *Physis* (Florence), 1964, *6:*335–346; K. D. Keele, "Leonardo da Vinci's research on the central nervous system", in, L. Belloni (editor), *Per la storia della neurologia italiana, Studi e testi,* 6, Istituto di Storia della Medicina Universita degli Studi, Milano, 1963, pp. 15–30.

3. *Isagoge breves perlucide ac uberrime in anatomiam humani corporis,* Bologna, H. Hectoris, 1522. For English translation of the 1535 edition, see Lind *(op. cit.,* Chapt. 3, note 52).

4. *Ibid.,* F.55[R].

5. The second edition of 1523 has the same title and imprint as that of 1522. This figure is on F.56[R] but the 1522 edition does not have it.

6. Lind *(op. cit.,* Chapt. 3, note 52), pp. 144–145.

7. C. D. O'Malley, *Andreas Vesalius of Brussels 1514-1564,* Berkeley & Los Angeles, University of California Press, 1964.

8. *De humani corporis fabrica libri septem,* Basel, J. Oporinus, 1543, See H. Cushing, *A bio-bibliography of Andreas Vesalius,* 2nd edition, Hamden, Conn., Arcon, 1962.

9. *Ibid.,* p. 623. For translation see Clarke & O'Malley *(op. cit.,* Chapt. 2, note 15), pp. 468–469.

10. C. Singer, *Vesalius on the human brain . . .,* London, Oxford University Press, 1952, pp. 32–40. See also, M. Holl, "Vesals Anatomie des Gehirns", *Arch. Anat. Physiol. (Anat. Abt.),* 1915, pp. 115–192.

11. "Quarta septima libri figura" on p. 608 of *De fabrica* (1543); legend, p. 609. Reproduced in Singer *(op. cit.* above, note 10), pp. 94–95 and in J. B. de M. Saunders & C. D. O'Malley, *The illustrations of Andreas Vesalius of Brussels . . .,* Cleveland & New York. World Publishing Co., 1950, pp. 190–191. For a critical appraisal of the illustrations in general, see Herrlinger *(op. cit.,* Chap. 1, note 1), pp. 103–120.

12. O'Malley *(op. cit.* above, note 7), p. 124. See his detailed discussion, pp. 124–130.

13. His latinized name is Carolus Stephanus. The name of Estienne de la Rivière (Stephanus Riverius) must be included with that of Estienne. See Herrlinger *(op. cit.,* Chapt. 1, note 1), p. 87.

14. *De dissectione partium corporis humani libri tres . . .,* Paris, S. Colinaeus, 1545. See K. F. Russell, "The *De dissectione* of Charles Estienne", *Australian & New Zealand Journal of Surgery,* 1952, *22:*146–148; Choulant-Frank *(op. cit.,* Chapt. 1, note 3) pp. 152–155; Herrlinger *(op. cit.,* Chapt. 1, note 1), pp. 87–101.

15. C. Singer & C. Rabin, *A prelude to modern science, being a discussion of the history, sources and circumstances of the 'Tabulae anatomicae sex' of Vesalius,* Cambridge, University Press, 1946, p. xix.

16. In Liber II, p. 242. Reproduced by Singer *(op. cit.* above, note 10), p. 136.

17. Soemmerring's contribution to functional localization in the brain will be dealt with later—see Figure 109. Suffice it to say that in his book of 1796, *Über das Organ der Seele,* he proposed the fluid of the ventricles as the seat of the soul.

Another traditional concept which suffered from the Renaissance was the *rete mirabile* (see pp. 3–6). This network of blood vessels of unknown function which lies at the base of the brain in ungulates is never present in man, monkey or rodent. Galen, having described it in the pig and ox, incorporated it into his system of brain function so that medieval physicians assumed its presence in the human body (see Figures 1, 2). Throughout the Middle Ages and later its reality went unchallenged even by those dissecting human bodies, such as Mondino dei Luzzi (*c.* 1275–1326),[1] Leonardo da Vinci (Figure 72), and Ryff (Figure 74). Some Renaissance anatomists did, however, successfully challenge its existence in man. In 1521, and again a year later, Berengario da Carpi unequivocally denied its presence,[2] as also did Vesalius (Figure 75), who had earlier accepted it (Figure 73). Nevertheless, the *rete* still figured occasionally in 17th century textbooks (Figures 76 and 77). The blood vessels of the human brain can now be readily visualized by means of an angiogram outlining its vascularity but not the *rete* (Figure 78).

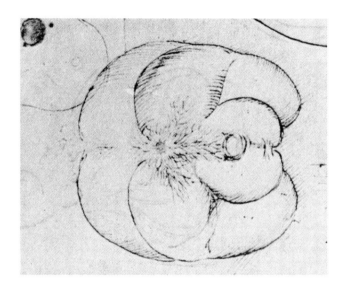

FIGURE 72

FIGURE 72 [3]
The folio of Leonardo da Vinci's drawings containing Figure 67 also has a crude outline of the base of a brain. Instead of the arterial Circle of Willis, a mass of fine vessels is drawn, the *rete mirabile*. McMurrich has suggested that this is the brain of an ox[4] but it may well be that Leonardo imposed the Ancient Greek concept of animal brain function on the human. He had done this already with the brain (Figure 43) and there are other examples in his sketches.

✣ARTERIA MAGNA, AOPTH, הנכיב HAORTI EX SI-
NISTRO CORDIS SINV ORIENS, ET VITALEM SPIRITVM TOTI CORPORI DEFERENS, NATV.
RALEMQVE CALOREM PER CONTRACTIONEM ET DILATATIONEM TEMPERANS.

A *Plexus choriformis in cerebri anterioribus ventriculis ex arterys & venis constitutum.*

B *Plexus reticuleris ad cerebri basim, Rete mirabile, in quo vitalis spiritus ad animale preparatur.*

C *Post aures, & ad tempora, & faciem arterie.*

D *Ad linguam, laryngem & fauces.*

E *Arterie καρόπιδις id est soporarie, Apopletice, Subetice, ביתרד דםיל benirdamim.*

F *Ad transuersos vertebrarum ceruicis processus ad cerebrum vsque excurrentes.*

G *Ad pectoris os & mamillas, que cū illis que in rectis musculis sunt, communicantur.*

H *Ad humeri musculos & gibba scapularis.*

I *Ad supercostales musculos & mamillas.*

K *Sub axillari vena in brachium excurrit.*

L *Ad cubiti articulum vtrimque vna.*

M *In interna parte manus, & ramulus ad partem exteriorem pollicis.*

N *Ad superiores thoracis costas.*

O *Diuisio maxima, cuius maior ramus ad inferiorem corporis partem diffunditur, à quo mox in singulos costas propagines diuaricantur.*

P *Vena caua in dextrum cordis sinum aperta.*

Q *Arteria venalis in sinistrum sinum aerem ex pulmonibus deferens.*

R *Vena arterialis ex dextro sinu sanguinem pulmonibus communicans.*

S *Septi transuersi arterie satis insignes.*

T *In licenis sinū, pro visceris ratione maxime.*

V *Ad iecoris cauum, & bilis vesicam.*

X *Ad ventriculum, & omentum.*

Y *In mesenterium par te superiori.*

A *Ad renes, Emulgentes dictæ, venis ipsis minores.*

B *Arterie seminales: vtrimque vna.*

C *Per mesenterium ad intestina vsque diffusa.*

D *Ad lumborum vertebras, musculos abdominis transuersos & obliquos.*

F *Ad foramina ossis sacri, quas nōnulli pro venis hemorrhoidibus male demonstrare solent.*

G *Ad vesicā, in viris ad penē, in mulieribus ad vuluefundum et collum.*

H *Arterie per quas foetui spiritus in vtero cōmunicatur, que interdum in maiores truncos implantate conspiciuntur.*

I *Ad rectos abdominis musculos, cum pectoris arterys coeuntes, per quas vtero cum mamillis communio est.*

K *Ad coxendicis articulum, & femoris exteriorem regionem.*

L *In poplite bifurcatio in alto latens.*

M *Ad interiorem pedis partem letitans.*

N *Exteriorem pedis partem (licet profunda) perreptans, à quibus minimi rami in pedis superiorem partem excurrunt, remulum tamen manifestum ad exteriora pollicis diffundunt.*

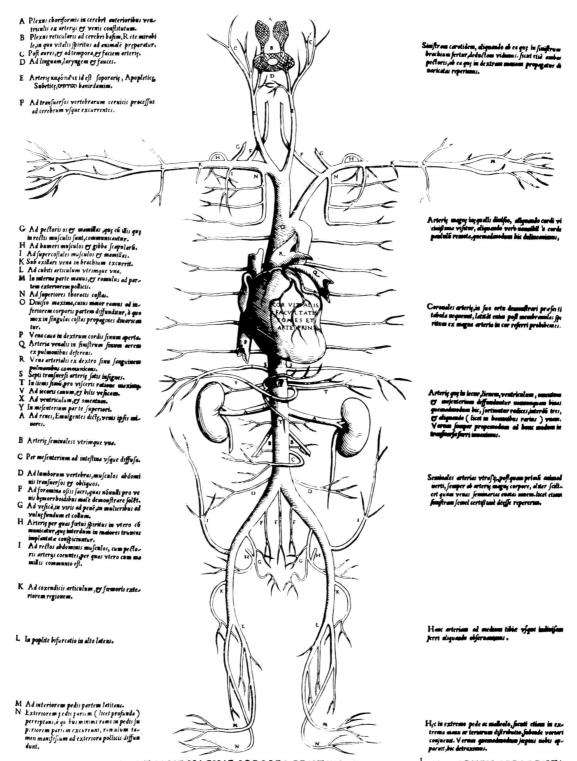

Sinistram carotidem, aliquando ab ea que in sinistrum brachium fertur, deductam vidimus, sicut etiā ambæ pectoris, ab ea que in dextram manum propagatur di uaricatas reperimus.

Arterie magne inequalis diuisio, aliquando cordi vi cinissima visitur, aliquando verò nonnihil à corde paululū remota, quemadmodum hic delineauimus,

Coronales arterie, in suo ortu demonstrari præsenti tabula nequeunt, latitāt enim post membranulas spiritum ex magna arteria in cor referri prohibentes.

Arterie que in iecur, lienem, ventriculum, omentum & mesenterium diffunduntur communquam binas quemadmodum hic, sortiuntur radices, interdū tres, & aliquando (licet in bonominibus rarius) vnam. Verum semper propemodum ad hunc modum in transuersis ferri inuenimus.

Seminales arterias vtrasque, postquam primū animad uerti, semper ab arterys magne corpore, alter scili cet quam venas seminarias enatas inueni. licet etiam sinistram semel certissimè deesse repererim.

Hanc arteriam ad medium tibie vsque indiuisam ferri aliquando obseruauimus.

Hæc in extremo pede ac malleolo, secuti etiam in extrema manu ac terarum distributio, subinde variari coniecant. Verum quemadmodum sepius nobis apparuit, hic detraximus.

NOTATV DIGNAE ARTERIAE MAGNAE SOBOLES CENTVM ET QVADRAGINTA SEPTEM APPARENT·

FIGURE 73

FIGURE 73

The writings of Vesalius are also characteristic of the transition from the old beliefs to the new experimental learning. The *rete mirabile* can, for example, be traced by looking at his two works: the *Tabulae anatomicae sex* of 1538 (this figure) and the *De fabrica* of 1543 (Figure 75).

This drawing is from the third plate of the *Tabulae sex* which depicts the arteries.[5] A is the choroid plexus *of* the lateral ventricles and B is the *rete mirabile,* formed from the carotid arteries, EE. There is no doubt that Vesalius accepted its existence at this time, as had Magnus Hundt in 1501 (Figure 32), Nicolas Massa in 1536, Johann Dryander in 1537 (Figure 36), and Charles Estienne c. 1538. However, Berengario da Carpi, to his credit, had in 1522 denied its presence in man: "I have never seen this *rete*", he stated.[6] Realdus Columbus (1516–1559), professor of anatomy at Rome and an important pre-Harveian investigator of the pulmonary blood transit, also came close to discrediting it. He did not name it, but instead used the term "reticular" when describing the choroid plexuses.[7]

FIGURE 74

Despite the fact that the plates of Vesalius' *Tabulae sex* may now seem crude, yet in 1538 they were the best available; hence they were soon plagiarized. Walter Hermann Ryff (*fl.* 1539) of Strassburg and Mainz was one of the first to do so. In 1541 he published his *Anatomi*, another important pre-Vesalian anatomical landmark,[8] wherein there is a similar drawing to the above, produced by superimposing Vesalius' plate of the arterial system (Figure 73) on the outline of a seated figure, retaining the same lettering. Our illustration is from Ryff's fugitive folio sheets of the same year, 1541,[9] which differs from that in his *Anatomi* only as regards the shading of the configuration in the cranium.

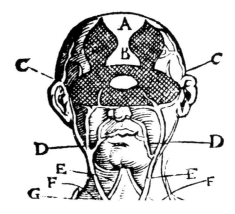

FIGURE 74

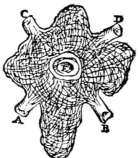

FIGURE 75

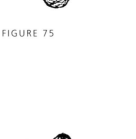

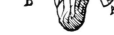

FIGURE 76

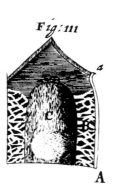

FIGURE 77

FIGURE 75
In the five years between the *Tabulae sex* (1538) and the *De fabrica* (1543), Vesalius became convinced that the *rete mirabile* did not exist in man and was astonished at his own credulity that had led him to accept what manifestly was not there.[10] His recantation in the text of the *De fabrica* was quite frank, yet he still included a drawing of the *rete,* stating that it was fashioned according to Galen's description.[11] He was thus illustrating a concept and not a human entity although he made it clear that he understood the difference in the *rete* between animals and man; he was in fact probably paying homage to the great weight of tradition whereby the writings of Galen were acknowledged with acclaim.

FIGURE 76
After Vesalius the *rete mirabile* as a human structure came gradually to be rejected. It was, however, still referred to in the 17th century and thus Robert Fludd (see Figures 38, 57) had Vesalius' representation of it redrawn in 1623.[12] He, likewise, reproduced many of Vesalius' plates of the brain. Jean Riolan *fils* (1580–1657) of Paris was another defender of lost causes, an unswerving Galenist in the changing world of the 17th century. Having opposed Harvey's circulation of the blood, it is not surprising that he perpetuated the myth of the *rete.* He accepted it in 1626[13] and, despite the contrary evidence accumulating around him, continued to do so in 1650.[14]

FIGURE 77
Even as late as 1664 Thomas Willis found it necessary to discuss the *rete mirabile* in his renowned book on the brain.[15] He was, of course, dealing primarily with comparative anatomy and, in contrasting man with beasts, stated that the *rete* was thought by some to be present occasionally in man. Its occurrence in the human he considered indicated subnormality ("slender wit and unmoved disposition") because of the person's affinity with beasts.

In this drawing of the *rete* in a calf,[16] the pituitary gland (C) is viewed from above with an artery (A) lateral to it. The *rete,* (B) appears between them. He used injection techniques to demonstrate it.

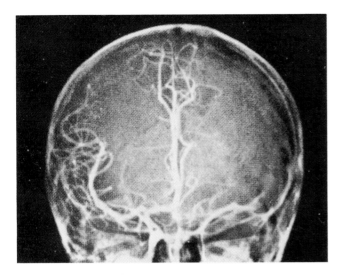

FIGURE 78A

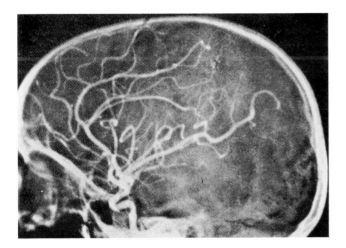

FIGURE 78B

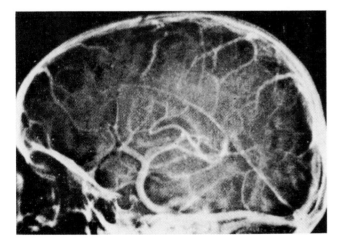

FIGURE 78C

FIGURE 78

Although the dispute over the *rete mirabile,* especially its functional rôle in animals, and its possible presence in man, continued,[17] there are no further illustrations of it. Its function even today has not been explained adequately. Gradually the detailed anatomy of the arterial and venous systems of the human brain was elucidated, in health and disease. It thus became increasingly clear that the vascular network at the base of the brain does not exist in man. The most recent method of displaying the cerebral and cranial vasculature is the angiogram, examples of which are shown here. Radio-opaque dye injected into the internal carotid artery can demonstrate the arterial, (A & B) and the venous phase (C) of the cerebral circulation, but not a *rete mirabile.*

NOTES

1. Clarke & O'Malley (*op. cit.*, Chapt. 2, note 15), pp. 763–764.

2. *Ibid.*, pp. 764–766.

3. *Quaderni, V*, 7^R; Clark 1912 7^R; O'Malley & Saunders No. 147. (Reproduced by gracious permission of her Majesty the Queen.) This has been reproduced on many occasions, for example by W. C. Gibson "The early history of localization in the nervous system", in, P. J. Vinken & C. W. Bruyn, *Handbook of clinical neurology*, Vol. 2, *Localization in clinical neurology*, Amsterdam, North-Holland Publishing Co., 1969, pp. 4–14.

4. McMurrich (*op. cit.*, Chapt. 3, note 68), p. 205.

5. Singer & Rabin (*op. cit.*, Chapt. 4, note 15), pp. xliii–xlv and 14–15.

6. *Isagogae breves*, Bologna, H. Hectoris, 1522, F.56^V.

7. *De re anatomica libri xv*, Venice, N. Bevilacqua, 1559, Lib. VIII, p. 191.

8. *Anatomi des allerfürtrefflichsten, höchsten und adelichsten gschöpffs aller Creaturen . . . Das ist des menschen . . . warhafftige beschreibung oder Anatomi . . .*, Strassburg, [B. Beck], 1541, p. xlv. See, K. F. Russell, "Walter Hermann Ryff and his anatomy", *Australian and New Zealand Journal of Surgery*, 1952, 22:66–69; H. Cushing, *A bio-bibliography of Andreas Vesalius*, New York, Schumann, 1943, pp. 22–23, Cushing II. 9, Fig 20 A. See also, C. Singer, "Brain dissection before Vesalius", *J. Hist. Med.*, 1956, 11:261–274.

9. *Tabulae decem . . . omnium humani corporis partium descriptio seu ut vocant Anatomia*, Strassburg, 1541, Fol. D. See Cushing (1943) (*op. cit.* above, note 8), Cushing II.-11, p. 24; our figure is reproduced in Fig. 20, B.

10. Clarke & O'Malley (*op. cit.*, Chapt. 2, note 15), pp. 767–769.

11. *De humani corporis fabrica*, Basel, Oporinus, 1543, "Decima septimi libri septimi figura" on p. 621. Reproduced in Singer (*op. cit.*, Chapt. 4, note 10), pp. 116–117. Vesalius' denial of the *rete mirabile* is in the *De fabrica* (1543) at III, 14, p. 352.

12. *Anatomiae amphitheatrum effigie triplici . . . Sectionis primae portio tertia de anatomia triplici . . .*, Frankfort, [E. Kempfer] for J. T. de Bry, 1623, Tab. VII on p. 168. The key is as in Vesalius' original.

13. *Anthropographia et osteologia*, Paris, D. Moreau, 1626, pp. 389–390. See also, *Les oeuvres anatomiques . . .*, Vol. 1, Paris, D. Moreau, 1629, pp. 588–590.

14. *Opera anatomica vetera*, Paris, 1650, pp. 261–262.

15. Willis, *Cerebri anatome . . .*, London, J. Martyn and J. Allestry, 1664 (Octavo), Caput VIII, pp. 53–57. See W. Feindel, *Thomas Willis. The anatomy of the brain and nerves*, Vol. 2, Montreal, McGill University Press, 1965, pp. 77, 84–87 of the S. Pordage translation into English of 1681.

16. *Ibid.* (1664), Fig. III on plate facing p. 56.

17. See, for example, H. Ridley, *The anatomy of the brain . . .*, London, S. Smith & B. Walford, 1695, Chapt. VIII "Of the rete mirabile", pp. 64–70.

It is paradoxical that the most obvious part of the brain and one of the most important from the functional point of view should have been mostly ignored until the beginning of the 19th century. This is its external surface, the cerebral gyri with their surrounding sulci and their covering mantle of cortex. Before the 17th century, attention was directed exclusively to the inside of the brain, in particular to the ventricles, the cerebral cortex being regarded as functionless. As little was known about it there seemed no need to depict the convolutions of the brain with any accuracy. Had not Erasistratus of Alexandria stated in the third century B.C. that the appearances of the gyri were comparable to coils of small intestine? A later observer, with a more culinary bent compared the cerebral convolutions to a plate of macaroni.[1] Thus it was thought that there was no precise anatomical pattern or determinable functional organization, a misconception that survived until the first few decades of the 19th century. Once again, the influence of Galen was crucial; in addition to highlighting the ventricular system and brain substance at the expense of the convolutions, he denied that the latter had any association with psychic activity, mental capacity, or the evolutionary scale.

It is known now that the cerebral cortex is a highly complex functional structure in man, and as it is intended to trace the emergence of this concept of cortical localization of function up to the present day, we must first examine the history of the cerebral convolutions before Thomas Willis's notable contribution in the middle of the 17th century.

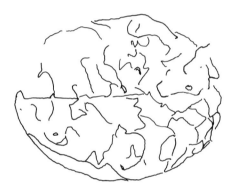

FIGURE 79

FIGURE 79
The appearance of the cerebral convolutions was first described by the Ancient Egyptians,[2] but the earliest pictorial representation so far discovered seems to be that seen already in Figure 22, dating from 1345. This pencil sketch seen here from the same leaf of Leonardo da Vinci's notebooks as Figures 67 & 72, dated between 1504 and 1507 is less vague. A convolutional pattern can be detected with certainty[3] and by the identification of certain gyri it has been suggested that the brain is that of an ox, seen from above.[4] This then is the first certain drawing of the cerebral convolutions, although probably not those of man.

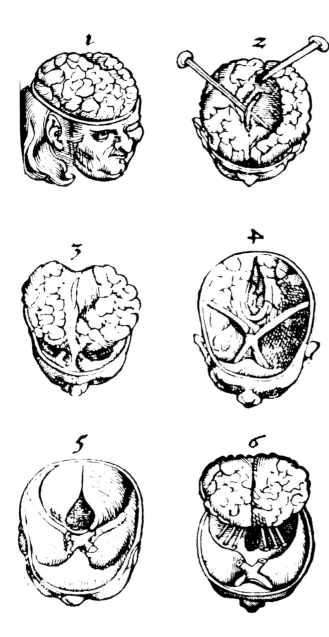

FIGURE 80

FIGURE 80 (LEFT)
The first printed illustrations of the brain appeared in a popular treatise on medicine, *Spiegl der Arztny,* written by a Dutch physician, Lorenz Fries or Lorent Friesz (d. 1531) living in Alsace, and published in Strassburg in 1519.[5] These small figures surround a body opened to reveal thoracic and abdominal viscera, and the plate, which is entitled *Anatomia corporis humani,* is dated 1517; it is based on a dissection carried out by Dr. Wendelin Hock von Brackenau at Strassburg and is in keeping with the anatomy of Mondino (1275–1326). It was published first by Johann Schott of Strassburg in 1517 as an anatomical fugitive sheet in a book by Hans von Gersdorf (b. c. 1455), *Feldbuch der Wundtartzney* [1527?].[6] The drawings of the brain showing the stages of brain dissection are quite crude and the cortex is most unnaturally represented. There is no key or legend.[7]

FIGURE 81 (OPPOSITE TOP LEFT)
Johann Eichmann (Dryander), as a purveyor of scholastic, medieval anatomy, has already been encountered (Figure 36). He was essentially a transitional figure for in his small book of 1537[8] he also published a series of good illustrations of the brain revealing in sequence the progressive stages of a dissection. The artist is unknown but the influence on Dryander of his predecessors, especially Berengario and Fries, is detectable and, in turn, his influence on Vesalius can also be traced.[9]

The drawing is from the 1536 edition of the *Anatomia* which does not contain the schematic head shown in Figure 36.[10] The meninges (B, B) have been pulled aside to reveal the cerebral convolutions, D, C. There is no gyral pattern and the appearances are unlife-like.

FIGURE 82 (OPPOSITE TOP RIGHT)
As with most other organs and systems, the best brain illustrations produced thus far appeared in the *De fabrica* of Vesalius in 1543. This, of course, is not to under-rate the importance of pre-Vesalian anatomists, some of whom we have already encountered.[11]
This head[12] is one of a series which, like Dryander's (Figure 81), demonstrates a sequence of proce-dures in the dissection of the brain. Veins and their sinuses are shown and the meninges are retracted. As with the companion drawings, Vesalius was more concerned to identify structures other than

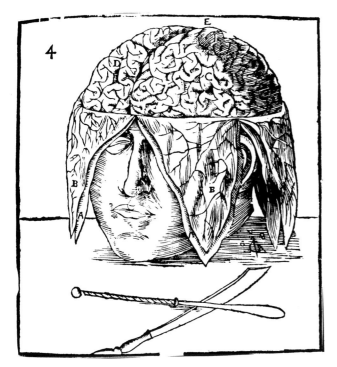

FIGURE 81

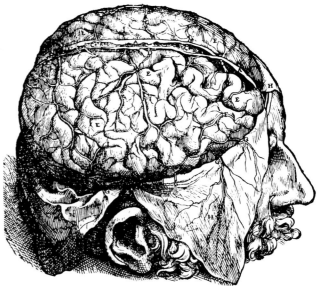

FIGURE 82

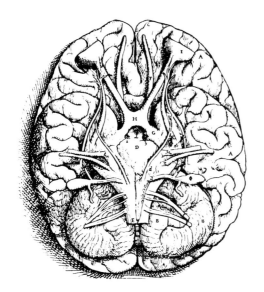

FIGURE 83

the convolutions, which are barely mentioned in the legends, and dealt with only briefly in the text.[13] He agreed, however, that they appeared like coils of small gut or like clouds drawn by schoolboys, having no standard pattern.

FIGURE 83
This was the first time a view of the base of the brain had been presented.[14] It is still relatively crude and the brain stem in particular is unlife-like. The cranial nerves are classified according to Galen,[15] but show much confusion. As in Figure 82, the artist seems to have gone out of his way to make the cerebral convolutions look like small intestines.

FIGURE 84
This drawing of the cerebral convolutions from the *De dissectione* (1545)[16] of Charles Estienne and Estienne de la Rivière (see Figure 70) is even less life-like than Vesalius' (Figures 82, 83); they really do have the appearance of a plate of macaroni! A, B, dura mater: C, pia mater through which the cerebral substance can be seen. The gyri are not mentioned.

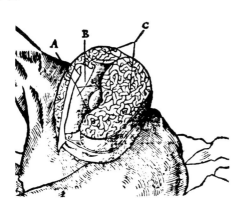

FIGURE 84

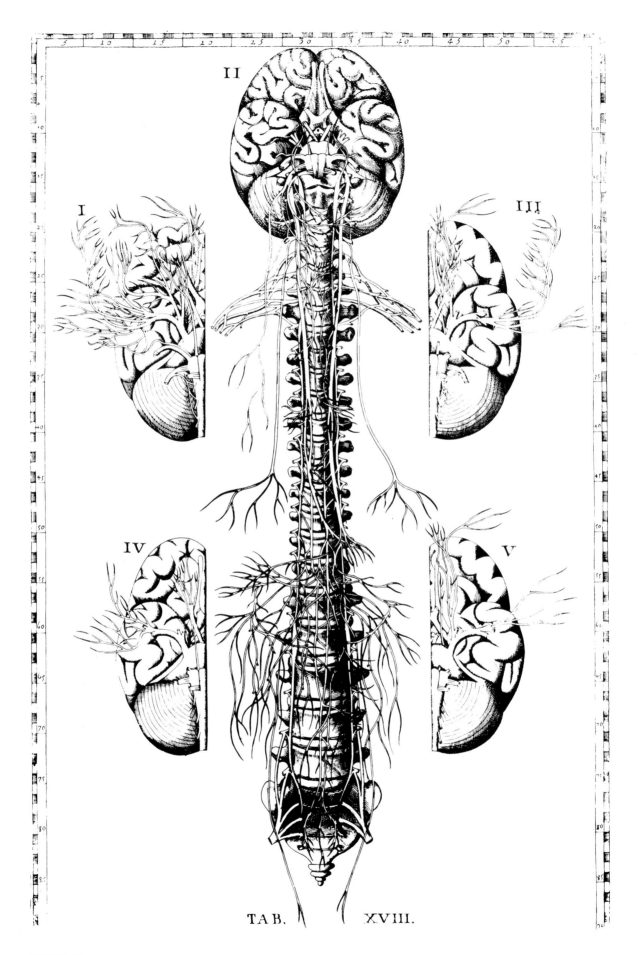

TAB. XVIII.

FIGURE 85

FIGURE 85 (OPPOSITE)

In 1552 Bartholommeo Eustachio (1520–1574),[17] a contemporary of Vesalius, and after whom the Eustachian tube is named, had assembled a series of copperplate engravings.[18] They were not published, however, until 1714 as *Tabulae anatomicae*.[19] This is Tab. XVIII[20] showing the sympathetic nervous system and regarded as the best of the collection.[21] It was still in use in 1817, when it appeared in the *Encyclopaedia Britannica*.[22] Again the gyri are like intestines, especially those depicted in III and V. Nevertheless Eustachius' illustrations in general are remarkable. Unlike Vesalius, he was not copying from nature but was composing standard anatomical figures made up from many observations. The geodetic-like scales on three sides of each plate intensify "the artistic tension between pose and frame, nature and mathematics"[23] and between life and geometry.

FIGURE 86 (TOP RIGHT)

After Vesalius' view of the base of the brain (Figure 83) and that of Eustachius (Figure 85), another, by Constanzo Varolio (1543–1575),[24] was published in 1573 without his permission.[25] He initiated a new method of dissecting the brain, which was to begin with the base rather than the convexity as all anatomists before him had done. The convolutions as depicted, however, reveal little fidelity to life.

Varolio is credited with the first adequate representation of the pons (*h* in Figure 86), "which I call the pons cerebelli", as he stated. It is still known today as the "pons Varolii" but this drawing of it is not as good as that of Eustachius (Figure 85) prepared 20 years earlier, although not published until 1714.

FIGURE 87 (TOP LEFT)

In 1583 a German surgeon-oculist, Georg Bartisch (1535–1607?)[26] published the first book in the German vernacular on surgery of the eye.[27] It contains many woodcuts, two of which have superimposed flaps, a technique frequently used in the 16th century.[28] The one that interests us deals with the head and by means of 5 flaps reveals structures at various levels in it.[29] Figure 87 shows the level at which the cerebral convolutions are encountered but they are crudely drawn. The illustration is, in fact, intended to demonstrate cerebral veins and sinuses.

By means of this book Bartisch revolutionized ophthalmic surgery, although, being a man of his times he could not divest himself completely of myth, legend, and superstition. Nevertheless, he did for ophthalmology what Vesalius had done for general anatomy.

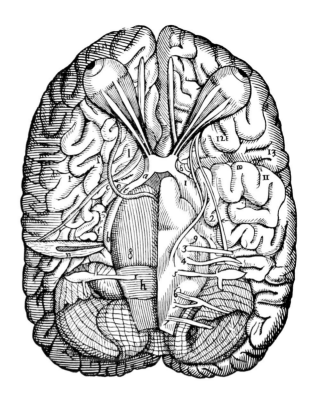

FIGURE 86

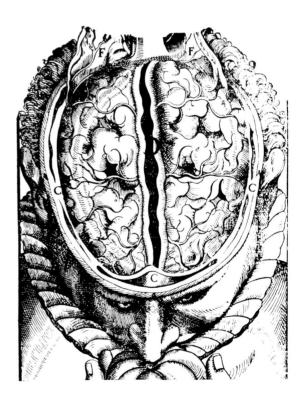

FIGURE 87

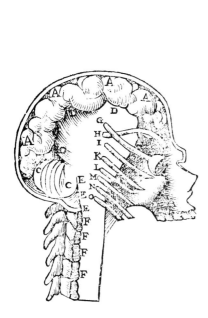

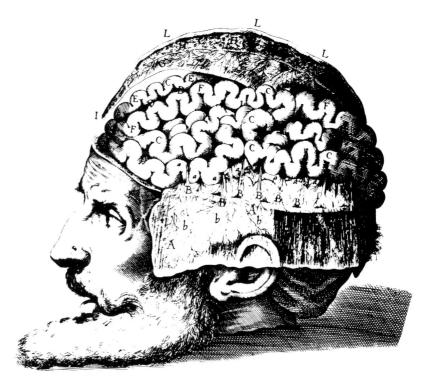

FIGURE 88

FIGURE 89

FIGURE 88

In view of the functional importance that was eventually to be attached to the cerebral cortex, it is of interest to know when it was distinguished from the medullary white substance of the hemisphere. As in the case of the cerebral convolutions one might have expected this to have been made early in the history of anatomy, if only for the reason that the distinction is so apparent, or rather it is patently obvious to us. But again it was function that determined the amount of attention paid to a structure. If the latter was thought to be functionless, it followed that its morphology was of little importance. Such was the position regarding the grey and white matter and although differences had been noted already, a clear distinction between them was not made until 1586.

Archangelo Piccolomini (c. 1526–1586) of Rome[30] made this differentiation and Figure 88 is from his book of 1586.[31] It is extremely inaccurate and almost stylized. The convolutions are most unnatural, and the artist seems to have depicted them like clouds, as Vesalius suggested (Figure 82); it is known that he influenced Piccolomini, and this similarity is part of the confirmatory evidence. Vesalius, for his part, could hardly have been impressed by the illustrations of his follower. In

fact, it is difficult to understand how, after Vesalius' shining example, draughtsmen could slip back into inaccuracy and crudity. But although there was a gradual improvement in anatomical illustrations after Vesalius and up to modern times, there were also relapses and Piccolomini's was by no means the last.

FIGURE 89

This provides another excellent example of how an anatomical structure can be drawn according to a preconceived idea rather than in keeping with its morphological appearances revealed by direct inspection. It is as though the anatomist informed his artist that cerebral convolutions look like coils of small gut, whereupon the latter went off and drew them with this in mind and without having looked at the brain itself. One glance would surely have convinced him of his transgression. Nevertheless, the anatomist accepted the drawing for publication which is even more difficult to understand.

The anatomist here was Giulo Casserio (1561–1616), pupil and successor of Fabricius ab Aquapendente in the chair of anatomy at Padua. He claimed his drawings "excel in nicety, clearness, and finally in workmanship and pains all that have

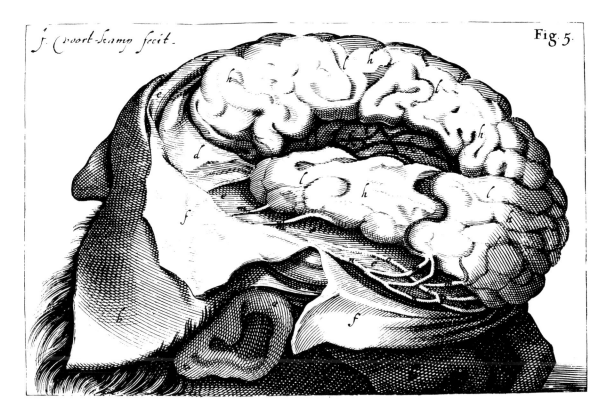

FIGURE 90

hitherto been published".[32] However, he died
before they were printed, and a book composed of
most of his copperplates, with a text by Adrian van
der Spiegel (Spigelius, 1578–1625), was edited by
Daniel Rindfleisch of Breslau (Bucretius, c. 1600–
1631) in 1627.[33] Of all these early representations,
this is one that looks most like coils of small bowel.

FIGURE 90
From 1641 until the 19th century only one part of
the surface of the cerebral hemispheres had been
given a name; this was the fissure of Sylvius after
Franciscus de le Boë (1614–1672)[34] by the famous
Danish anatomist, Caspar Bartholin (1585–1629),
in his popular book *Institutiones anatomicae* of
1641, subsequently published by his equally
illustrious son Thomas (1616–1680).[35] He included
this illustration, showing the usual shapeless gyri; it
is to be noted, however, that the insula (kk) is
figured for the first time. Sylvius did not describe
the fissure himself until 1663.[36]

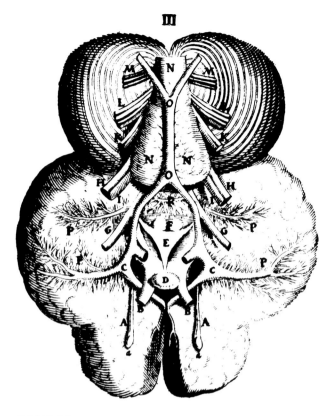

FIGURE 91

The arterial circle at the base of the brain named after Willis, is clearly outlined and is complete except for the anterior communicating artery. This is seventeen years before Willis's description (see Figure 96).[41]

FIGURE 91
One of the most popular textbooks of anatomy in the 17th century was first published in 1641 by Johann Vesling (1598–1649), professor of anatomy and surgery in Padua. In 1647 an illustrated edition the *Syntagma anatomicum*[37] came out and was widely circulated and translated; an English version by Nicholas Culpeper was published in 1653 containing plates and legends similar to the 1647 Latin edition.[38] Moreover, his illustrations were frequently re-engraved and copied into many subsequent manuals of anatomy.[39]

It is surprising, therefore, that these copperprints are, on the whole, inferior and lacking in artistic quality. Figure 91 shows that the cerebral convolutions obviously are of little functional significance to the author and have been merely shaded in lightly.[40] They are not even mentioned in the text or legend. Here, as in other drawings of the brain, the gyri have a vague similarity to clouds, a comparison first proposed by Vesalius (Figure 82) and also seen in Figure 88. It is of interest to note that ppppp are "small branches of arteries called the *rete mirabile*". The old concept (see Chapter 5) had disappeared but the term was still being used by Vesling to denominate terminal branches of the middle cerebral and perforating arteries.

NOTES

1. A. Ecker, *On the convolutions of the human brain,* London, Smith, Elder & Co., 1873, p. 3.

2. J. H. Breasted, I, *The Edwin Smith surgical papyrus . . .,* Chicago, University of Chicago Press, 1930, Case 6 on pp. 165–166. This dates from the Pyramid Age (*c.* 3000–2500 B.C.). See Clarke & O'Malley *(op. cit.,* Chapt. 2, note 15), pp. 383–384.

3. McMurrich *(op. cit.,* Chapt. 3, note 68), p. 205.

4. O'Malley & Saunders *(op. cit.,* Chapt. 3, note 67), p. 340, fig. 3.

5. *Spiegl der Arztny . . .,* Strassburg, J. Grieninger, 1519. The figure is between F.VI[V] and XIII[R].

6. L. Crummer, "Early anatomical fugitive sheets", *Ann. Med. Hist.,* 1923, *5*:189–209. This corresponds to his Type II(b).

7. See, Choulant-Frank *(op. cit.,* Chapt. 1, note 3), pp. 130–135. They are reproduced by Singer *(op. cit.,* Chapt. 4, note 10), p. 127.

8. *Anatomiae, hoc est, corporis humani dissectionis pars prior . . .,* Marburg, E. Cervicornus, 1537.

9. Herrlinger *(op. cit.,* Chapt. 1, note 1), pp. 84–85. See also, Choulant-Frank *(op. cit.,* Chapt. 1, note 3), pp. 148–149. See also, Singer *(op. cit.,* Chapt. 5, note 8); E. Turner, "Les planches anatomiques de J. Dryander et de G. H. Ryff", *Gaz. hebd. Méd. Chir.,* 1876, *33*:785–791, 817–823.

10. *Anatomia capitis humani,* Marburg, E. Cervicornus, 1536, Figure 4.

11. See Herrlinger *(op. cit.,* Chapt. 1., note 1, pp. 60 ff.) who is referring to illustrations, and G. Rath ("Pre-Vesalian anatomy in the light of modern research", *Bull. Hist. Med.,* 1961, *35*:142–148) who deals with the texts.

12. *De fabrica,* p. 606, "secunda septimi libri figura"; legend pp. 606–607. Reproduced by Saunders & O'Malley *(op. cit.,* Chapt. 4, note 11), Plate 67 on pp. 188–189; and by Singer *(op. cit.,* Chapt. 4, note 10), pp. 90–91.

13. Clarke & O'Malley *(op. cit.,* Chapt. 2, note 15), pp. 385–387.

14. *De fabrica*, p. 318, "prior duarum figura novem . . ."; legend, p. 320. Reproduced by Saunders & O'Malley, *ibid.*, Plate 48, pp. 144–145; and by Singer, *ibid.*, p. 123.

15. T. Beck, "Die Galenischen Hirnnerven in moderner Beleuchtung", *Arch. Gesch. Med.*, 1909, *3*:110–114. See also, C. D. O'Malley, "Gabriele Falloppia's account of the cranial nerves", *Sudhoffs Arch.*, Beiheft 7, 1966, pp. 132–137; and Singer, *ibid.*, p. 76.

16. In Liber II, p. 239.

17. G. Bilancioni, *Bartolomeo Eustachi*, Florence, Istituto Micrografico Italiano, 1913.

18. Herrlinger (*op. cit.*, Chapt. 1, note 1), pp. 132–138.

19. Eustachius, *Tabulae anatomicae clarissimi viri . . .*, Rome, F. Gonzaga, 1714. Edited by J. M. Lancisi.

20. Facing p. 45; legend is on pp. 45–47. In the 1744 edition published in Leyden outline sketches and commentaries were provided by Bernhard Siegfried Albinus (1697–1770).

21. C. Singer, *The evolution of anatomy . . .*, London, Paul, Trench & Trubner, 1925, p. 138.

22. Plate XXXI in Section on Anatomy.

23. Herrlinger (*op. cit.*, Chapt. 1, note 1), p. 132.

24. M. Medici, *Compendio storico della scuola anatomica di Bologna*, Volpe & Sassi, 1857, pp. 84–98.

25. This was a letter to Hieronymus Mercurialis, *De nervis opticis nonnullisq.; . . .*, Padua, P & A. Meitti, 1573, "Figura prima" on F.17^V, legend, Ff.17^R-18^V. "Fig. II" on F.19^R is different, but the convolutional arrangement is much the same. A copy of this essay is attached to the commoner *Anatomiae . . . libri IIII*, Frankfurt, Wechel & Fischer, 1591; the two drawings of the base of the brain differ slightly from those of the 1573 edition. See Clarke & O'Malley (*op. cit.*, Chapt. 2, note 15), pp. 634–635.

26. P. Tower, "Notes on the life and work of George Bartisch", *A.M.A. Arch. Ophthalmol.*, 1956, *56*:57–70; *Augendienst. The service of the eyes. George Bartisch 1535-1607*, Masnon (Barcelona), Laboratorios del Norte de España, S. A., 1962, p. 81.

27. Bartisch, *Ophthalmoduleia* [in Greek script]. *Das ist Augendienst . . .*, Dresden, M. Stöckel, 1583.

28. F. W. Faust, "Anatomical flap illustration. XVI to XX Century", *Marquette Med. Rev.*, 1956, *21*:151-158; L. Crummer, "A checklist of anatomical books illustrated with cuts with superimposed flaps", *Bull. Med. Lib. Assoc.*, 1932, *20*:131-139.

29. *Op. cit.* above, note 27. The legend to the woodcut is on F.5^V-6^R.

30. F. Pierro, *Archangelo Piccolomini Ferrarese (1525–1586) e la sua importanza nell' anatomia postVesaliana*, Ferrara, Universitá degli Studi di Ferrara, 1965 (*Quaderni di Storia della Scienza e della Medicina*, VI).

31. *Anatomicae praelectiones . . . explicantes mirificam corporis humani fabricam . . .*, Rome, B. Bonfadinus, 1586, p. 265. Translation of text in, Clarke & O'Malley (*op. cit.*, Chapt. 2, note 15), pp. 387–388.

32. Choulant-Frank (*op. cit.*, Chapt. 1, note 3), p. 224. Casserio is discussed on pp. 223–228.

33. *Tabulae anatomicae LXXIIX . . . D. Bucretius XX . . .*, Venice, E. Deuchinum, 1627. Figure 86 is in Liber X, and is Tab. II, fig. 2 on F.87^R; legend on F.86^V, Casserio's plates were also published in Spigelius', *De humani corporis fabrica libri decem*, Venice, E. Deuchinum, 1627.

34. Baker, *op. cit.*, Chapt. 7, note 14.

35. *Institutiones anatomicae . . . ab auctoris filio Thoma Bartholino*, Leyden, F. Hack, 1641, p. 262.

36. "Disputationum medicarum", in, *Opera medica*, Geneva, Tournes, 1681, IV, ix, 7, pp. 43–44, the first edition of which was Leyden, 1663.

37. *Syntagma anatomicum . . .*, Padua, P. Frambottus, 1647. The illustrated 1641 edition was Frankfurt, J. Beye.

38. *The anatomy of the body of man . . .*, Englished by Nich. Culpeper, London, P. Cole, 1653; from the 1647 Latin edition. There were Latin editions or reprintings in 1649, 1651 (twice), 1659, 1666, 1677, 1696 and translations into Dutch (1652) and German (1676, 1688).

39. Choulant-Frank (*op. cit.*, Chapt. 1, note 3), p. 243.

40. Figure 91 is Tabula III, Cap. XIV, III, facing p. 194.

41. A. Meyer & R. Hierons, "Observations on the history of the 'Circle of Willis'," *Med. Hist.*, 1962, *6*:119-130.

7

17TH CENTURY CONCEPTS OF BRAIN FUNCTION: DESCARTES AND WILLIS

By the 17th century, theories of brain function such as the medieval Cell Doctrine (Chapter 3) and the concept of the *rete mirabile* (Chapter 5) received hardly any support. Nevertheless, in the first half of the century, attention was still focussed on the ventricular system which, according to Ancient Greek tradition, was the site of production and storage of the essential animal or psychic spirits. The cerebral cortex continued to be almost entirely neglected.

In the middle of the century, however, a revolution in the appreciation of brain function came about when Franciscus de le Boë (or Sylvius) and Thomas Willis separately proposed that the cortex of the brain had some specific functions. This shift of interest away from the ventricles was accentuated by Willis who indicated other parts of the brain substance as areas of functional significance. It is at this stage in the evolution of theories of brain function that our story moves into the beginning of the modern era; indeed Sir Charles Symonds[1] has stressed Willis's importance in attempting to explain the functional significance of parts of the brain, particularly the vascular circle around the base of the brain which still bears his name. But Willis's unique contribution should be considered in relation to another outstanding 17th century figure, René Descartes. It is probably true to state that Willis's notions have now assumed a greater importance in the history of neuro-anatomy and neurophysiology whereas Descartes' ideas have permeated the history of philosophy and psychology. Finally the work of Nicolaus Steno (1638–1686) must be mentioned. In a lecture on the brain delivered in Paris in 1665, and published four years later, Steno displayed a healthy scepticism. His work was a useful counterblast to the overspeculative theories of his predecessors, and in the field of localization of brain functions he set forth fair and objective criticism of the work of Descartes and Willis.

FIGURE 92

Since Classical Antiquity, the ventricular system of the brain had been the focus of attention and the writings of Descartes[2] reveal that the ventricles together with the pineal body continued to be of paramount functional significance. He maintained that the pineal was the seat of the soul and the governing centre of the human body, whose functions he explained purely in mechanical terms. The pineal controlled the flow of animal spirits in the ventricles, whereas the cerebral cortex, which is scarcely mentioned in his writing, played no part in his theory.[3] It is, therefore, curious that Descartes' famous book, *De homine* (1662) should, judged by contemporary standards, have such a good drawing of the gyri, as this.[4]

The brain is viewed from behind, revealing the occipital lobes of the cerebral hemispheres with the cerebellum above and in the middle the pineal is visible. In the human brain, however, the latter is too deeply placed to be seen and considerable manipulation and artistic licence has obviously been used. But, what is of greater interest is the realistic depiction of the cerebral and cerebellar convolutions. This is the most accurate representation encountered so far, which evokes a double paradox; first, that this drawing should be presented by an author who has no interest in the brain surface, and secondly, the fact that it is more accurate than the illustrations of Thomas Willis (Figures 96–98) who believed in the prime importance of cortical function.

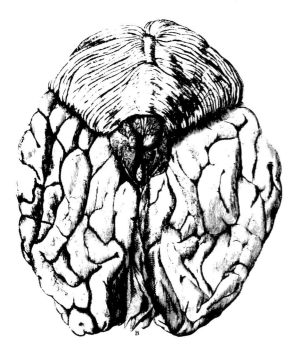

FIGURE 92

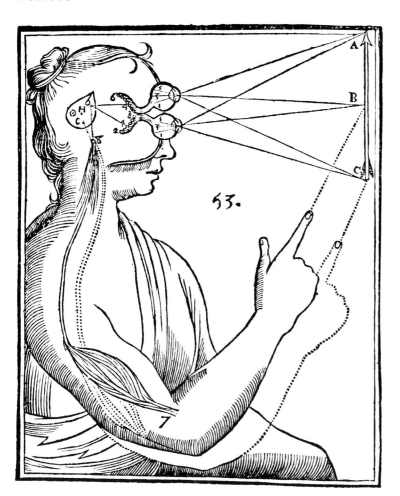

FIGURE 93

FIGURE 93
Many of the drawings in Descartes' book, *De homine* (1662) and its French version of 1664, are diagrammatic in form. This one[5] demonstrates his mechanistic theory of brain function. Light from the object (ABC) enters the eyes and forms visual images (135) on the retina which is connected to the walls of the ventricle by hollow tubes representing the optic nerve. The circular open ends of the tubes can be seen and 246 is the incoming or sensory stimulus. From the tubes the message goes through the ventricles by way of the animal spirits and reaches the pear-shaped pineal (H) which initiates the motor stimulus. Thus animal spirits from the ventricles are sent by way of the opening 8 into the nerve to the arm muscle which it inflates, producing motion. This, of course, is the basis of the reflex, and the modern theory of reflex action begins with Descartes' primitive concept of afferent and efferent components.[6]

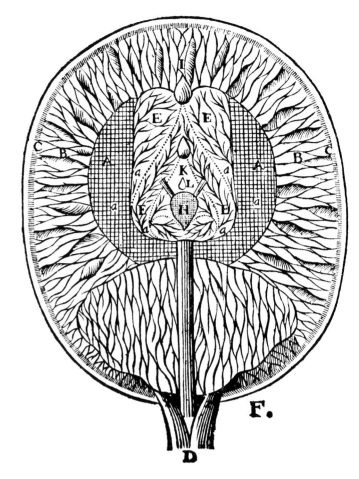

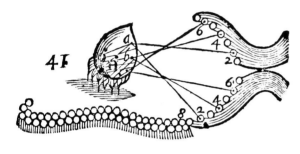

FIGURE 94

FIGURE 94
This shows the nerve tubes' openings in the walls of the ventricles and connections being made with the pineal (H).[7]

FIGURE 95

FIGURE 95
Also in *De homine* is this curious diagram[8] reminiscent of the medieval schematic drawings seen earlier (Chapter 3). The central area (EEEE) represents the ventricles. The pineal is at H, and ventricular wastes can be drained off into the nose by way of I or through the pituitary into the posterior nasopharynx through K and L. The criss-cross area AA represents a cross section of nerve tube openings on the ventricular wall and peripherally to this the areas CB and BC show the nerves running towards the ventricles. The nerves are thus presented in two planes, transversely and longitudinally. This is the simplest representation of Descartes' notion of brain function.

His remarkable ingenuity and originality were unfortunately based on pure speculation and incorrect anatomical observations. These factual errors caused the Danish anatomist Nicolaus Steno[9] to attack Descartes in a lecture given in Paris in 1665 and published four years later.[10] More stringent criticisms, derived trom the accumulation of increasingly accurate anatomical knowledge, led to the downfall of Descartes' concepts.[11] Nevertheless, his text did provide, particularly in his vague notion of the reflex, a useful and provocative model of nervous function. As Crombie has pointed out,[12] Descartes' mechanistic hypotheses, as applied to the senses, raised questions that could be answered in his own time and stimulated new researches into animal life, the complexity and value of which gradually become apparent.

Thomas Willis[13] is one of the most important figures since Galen in the history of brain function. Like Galen, he placed the functional centre of the brain in its substance and not in the ventricles. Willis, however, had a forerunner: Franciscus de le Boë or Sylvius (1614–1672)[14] who in 1660 suggested that the animal or psychic spirits, instead of being produced in the *rete mirabile* or in the ventricles, were secreted from the cerebral and cerebellar cortex.[15] Thus, for the first time, the grey matter was allocated a specific function and Willis, in his *Cerebri anatome* (1664)[16] accepted this idea and extended it to include other parts of the brain substance.

Like other devout seventeenth-century neuro-anatomists, Willis was sensitive about the attitude of the Church. When dedicating his *Cerebri Anatome* (1664) to the Archbishop of Canterbury he mentioned that the study of nature had long been regarded "as a certain schoolhouse and mystery of Atheism", although he carefully explained that he was prepared to look into the secrets of nature with the same reverence as he looked into his Bible.[17] In order to solve this dilemma between science and religion, Willis modified Gassendi's theory. The latter had claimed that animals must have souls since they showed evidence of memory, reason and other psychological traits common to man. Willis attributed these characteristics to the corporeal soul, or as he termed it, the "soul of brutes". He postulated that in man the corporeal soul was controlled by the rational soul; thus by attributing man's higher functions to an immortal rational soul he put God in his rightful place beyond the realm of the scalpel, scepticism or speculation of the anatomist. This concept of twin souls allowed Willis to speculate on a highly controversial aspect of psychiatry and neurology which had hitherto been regarded as coming partly within the theologians' sphere.[18] Thus Willis felt able to localize the three mental functions which had hitherto been relegated to the ventricles (Chapter 3): the corpus striatum receiving all in-coming sensation became the seat of the "sensus communis"; imagination was located in the corpus callosum (here Willis meant all cerebral white matter between basal

ganglia and cortex);[19] and the cerebral cortex was the seat of memory. Whereas the cerebrum controlled voluntary motor activity, the cerebellum was concerned with vital and involuntary actions[20] but this further localization is beyond the scope of this book.

Willis's theory was of the utmost significance; its widespread influence extended for more than a hundred years until Albrecht von Haller (1708–1777), opposing the cerebral localization doctrine,[21] gradually undermined it. Nevertheless, the force of Willis's arguments were implemented by the relative excellence of the accompanying illustrations.

FIGURE 96
Although in this illustration, Willis's drawing of the surface of the brain was not of a high standard, other details of structures at the base of the brain were accurately depicted. Indeed, Steno substantiates this opinion when he wrote in his essay (see p. 76) "the best figures of the brain up to the present are those presented to us by Willis", although he went on to state that they were by no means perfect.[22] Figure 96[23] is probably the most famous 17th century brain illustration. It was drawn, together with others of Willis's plates, by Christopher Wren, and depicts elegantly the complete circle of Willis (cf. Figure 91) and the cranial nerves.[24] Willis acknowledges his indebtedness to

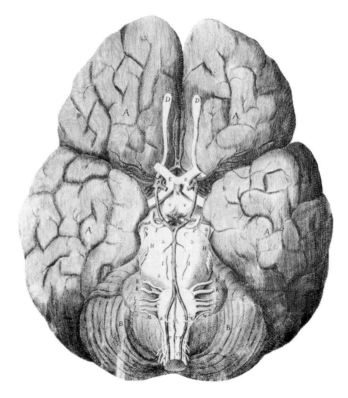

FIGURE 96

Wren, who was "frequently present at our Dissection, to confer and reason out the use of the Parts". ". . . Dr Wren, on account of his singular humanity, wherewith he abounds," wrote Willis, "was pleased to delineate with his own most skilful hands many figures of the Brain and Skull so that the work could be more exact."[25–26]

The cerebral convolutions receive much less adequate treatment, however, but it could be argued that this is because they are merely a background to the basal structures, which the artist wished to high-light. The gyri are sketched in with equal vagueness in the rest of Willis's illustrations of the human brain. Blood vessels emerging from gyri are shown.

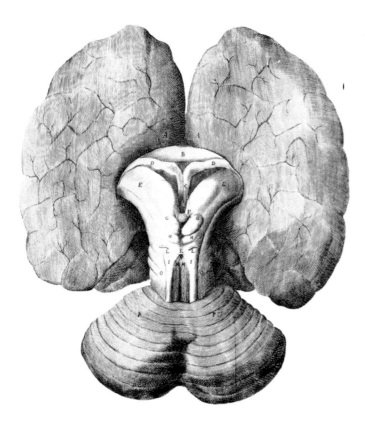

FIGURE 97

FIGURE 97

The fact that some of Willis's plates are of sheep brains was overlooked by Grünthal.[27] Figure 97,[28] however, depicts a human brain seen from behind, and is similar to that of Descartes (Figure 92); Willis may have decided to illustrate this aspect of the brain in response to Descartes' teachings. The convolutions are drawn even less precisely than in Figure 96; the cerebellar folia are stylized and perhaps the draughtsman intended the cerebral gyri to be similar. Below is the cerebellum with the brain stem in the centre. As with Descartes' plate (Figure 92) considerable artistic licence must be allowed. B, corpus callosum; C, fornix with limbs, DD; EE, peduncles; F, pineal; G, H quadrigeminal bodies; LL, 4th cranial nerves.

Steno criticized this drawing and pointed out errors which we would accept.[29]

FIGURE 98

Willis put an end to ventricular localization of brain function and proposed three areas in the brain itself: the corpus striatum, corpus callosum, and the cerebral cortex. These mediated "sensus communis", imagination, and memory, respectively. This plate is from Willis's *De anima brutorum* of 1672[30] showing the basal structures cut coronally. The main structures are: BBBB, corpus callosum; C, fornix; D, I, corpus striatum; K, thalamus; N, pineal; LPOO, quadrigeminal bodies. Interestingly enough, in none of Willis's plates was the cerebral cortex depicted in section and here the convolutions have the same flat and lifeless appearance as in his other drawings (Figures 96, 97).[31]

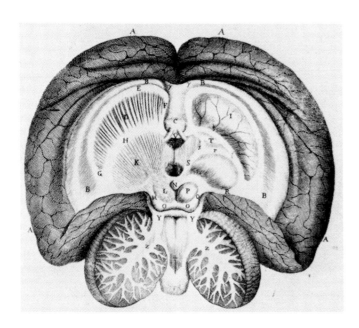

FIGURE 98

NOTES

1. C.P. Symond's, "The Circle of Willis", *Brit. Med. J.,* 1955, *i*:119–124.

2. C. Adam, *Descartes: sa vie et son oeuvre*, Paris, Boivin, 1937.

3. A. Souques, "Descartes et l'anatomo-physiologie du système nerveux", *Rev.neurol.,* 1938, *70*:221–245.

4. *De homine*, Leyden, Leffen & Moyardus, 1662, Fol. 118, Fig. LIII.

5. *L'homme de René Descartes . . .,* Paris, N. Le Gras, 1664, Fig. 53 on p. 79.

6. Clarke & O'Malley (*op. cit,* Chapt. 2, note 15), pp. 329–333.

7. *Op. cit.* above, note 5, Fig. 4, on p.78.

8. *Ibid.,* unnumbered figure on p. 62.

9. See G. Scherz (editor), "Nicolaus Steno and his Indice", *Acta Historica Scientiarum Naturalium ex Medicinalium,* 1958, Vol. 15. Also, G. Scherz (editor) *Steno and brain research in the seventeenth century,* in, *Analecta Medico-Historica,* 1968, Vol. 3.

10. *Discours de Monsieur Stenon, sur l'anatomie du cerveau à messieurs de l'Assemblée, qui se fait chez Monsieur Thevenot,* Paris, R. De Ninville, 1669, pp. 12–22. See, *Nicolaus Steno's Lecture on the anatomy of the brain,* Copenhagen, A. Busck, 1965 which has a facsimile copy of the discourse and translations, not entirely reliable, into English and German.

11. G. Jefferson, "René Descartes on thc localisation of the soul", *Irish J. Med. Sci.,* 1949, No. 285, pp.691–706.

12. A.C. Crombie, "The mechanistic hypothesis and the scientific study of vision: some optical ideas as a background to the invention of the microscope", *Proc. Roy. Microscop. Soc.,* 1967, Vol. 2, Part 1, pp. 3–112, see p.83.

13. Dr. Dewhurst published *Thomas Willis's Oxford lectures,* Oxford, Sandford, 1980 and *Willis's Oxford Casebook* (1650–52), *ibid.*, 1981, but, regrettably, his promised, definitive biography of Willis did not appear.

14. F. Baker, "The two Sylviuses. An historical study", *Bull. Johns Hopkins Hosp.,* 1909, *20*:329–339.

15. Sylvius, "Disputationum medicarum IV, de spirituum animalium in cerebro, cerebelloque confectione, per nervos distributione, atque usu vario", Reply to G. Ypelaer, 4th February 1660, in, *Disputationum medicarum,* Amsterdam, J. van den Bergh, 1663, para. 29 on pp. 52–53.

16. Willis, *Cerebri anatome . . .,* London, J. Martyn & J. Allestry, 1664. There is both a quarto and octavo issue of this date. Here the octavo has been used throughout, because it is more readily available. See Caput X.

17. *Ibid.,* p.3 of "Epistola dedicatoria".

18. More fully discussed by K. Dewhurst in, *Thomas Willis as a physician,* Los Angeles, William Andrews Clark Library, 1964.

19. E. Clarke, "Brain anatomy before Steno", in, G. Scherz (*op. cit.,* note 9 above [1968]), pp. 27–34.

20. M. Neuburger, *Die historische Entwicklung der experimentellen Gehirn- und Rückenmarksphysiologie vor Flourens,* Stuttgart, F. Enke, 1897. English transl., Johns Hopkins University Press, 1981, see pp. 21–45.

21. *Ibid.,* pp. 113–152.

22. *Op. cit.* above, note 10, p.23.

23. *Op. cit.* above, note 16, Fig. 1a, facing p. 13 in the copy used.

24. See W.C. Gibson, "The bio-medical pursuits of Christopher Wren", *Med. Hist.,* 1970, *14*:331–341.

25. *Op. cit.* above, note 16, p[6] of "Praefatio".

26. "Dr Wren hath drawn most excellent schemes of the brain, and the several parts of it, according to the doctor's [Willis] design and the next week he will have finished the scheme of the eighth pair of nerves. . . .", *The works of the Hon. Robert Boyle,* editor, T. Birch, London, J. & F. Rivington, Vol. 6, 1772, p.467.

27. *Op. cit.,* Chapt.1, note 14.

28. *Op. cit.* above, note 16, Fig. III, facing p. 26 in the copy used.

29. *Op. cit.* above, note 10, pp. 23–24. Steno's criticisms have been discussed by K. Dewhurst, "Willis and Steno", in, Scherz, (*op. cit.* above, note 9[1968]), pp. 43–48.

30. *De anima brutorum,* London, R. Davis, 1672, Tabula VIII, facing p. 80 in the copy used.

31. Willis's work on the basal ganglia is discussed in an excellent article by F. Schiller "The vicissitudes of the basal ganglia (Further landmarks in cerebral nomenclature)", *Bull. Hist. Med.,* 1967, *41*:515–538.

17TH CENTURY ORIENTAL
CONCEPTS OF
BRAIN FUNCTION

8

While Western theories of brain function were undergoing revolutionary changes, the East still clung to traditional concepts. This contrast can be illustrated by three drawings, two from the Near East and one from China, each transmitting ideas of Antiquity or of the Middle Ages, although copied in the 16th or 17th centuries. They provide a ready means of comparing occidental and oriental notions of brain function in the 17th century.

FIGURE 99[1]

This bizarre diagrammatic representation of the brain is unique, as we have been unable to trace any comparable manuscript or printed material from either Eastern or Western sources. It appears in a Persian text, *Tashrīḥ i Mansūrī* of an illustrated anatomical treatise written by Manṣur bin Muḥammad, etc.,[2] of which there are several copies, some with inscriptions as in Figure 99, and others without.[3] The original was composed about 1400 A.D., later copies being made in the 17th, 18th, and 19th centuries (1623–1841). The majority come from the second half of the 17th century and may be compared chronologically with the writings of Descartes, Willis and Steno in Chapter 7. Our specimen (Figure 99) was also prepared in the 17th century. The fact that its date of origin cannot be more precisely determined is only of slight consequence, as it is included primarily as an example of the lengthy period of survival of an oriental text and its illustrations. Thus in the East such medieval drawings were still acceptable, when in 17th century Europe they had been generally superseded. The influence of the medieval Islamic Empire had long waned and

medicine was to change little in the Near East until relatively recent times.

The figure demonstrates the nervous system and belongs to the Alexandrian Series of medieval anatomical drawings of the osseous, muscular, venous, and arterial systems (the *Fünfbilderserie* of Sudhoff), a tradition which most likely originated in Alexandria (p.3), but possibly in China (pp.82–83).

The drawing of the head is unparalleled in all Eastern and Western sources. The writing on the left states, "Figure of head [in] inverted [position] for the sake of the dissection". Both the cranial cavity and the face are contained in the circle: the former is in the lower half and the latter in the upper. In the cranium, there is a central square named in other manuscripts as "centre of brain". Running caudally is presumably the brain stem, connecting with the spinal cord which is named; the terms "posterior blood vessels" and "single nerve of the 7th pair" (hypoglossal in our nomenclature) also appear on it, but the precise relations of these structures are difficult to determine. The remainder of the writing identifies central structures, and from before backwards beginning beside the left eye, includes the cranial nerves: first (optic), third (trigeminal), and sixth (our ninth to eleventh).

There is no suggestion here of the ventricular system or of the *rete mirabile,* and cerebral functions are not discussed. This is the only medieval illustration of the brain which directs attention to the function of structures other than the ventricles, in this instance the cranial nerves. The oriental art form is in similar style to that of Figures 62 and 100.

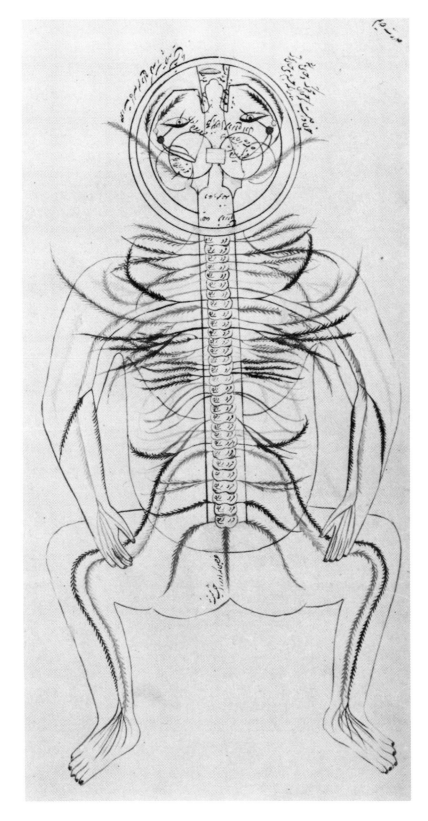

FIGURE 99

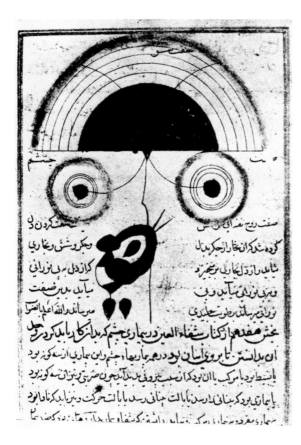

FIGURE 100

FIGURE 100[4]

This oriental eye-brain diagram has been reproduced on several occasions. It is similar to Figure 62
but is included here rather than in Chapter 3 as it
does not depict fully the Cell Doctrine. Like Figure
99 it is unique amongst Islamic manuscripts.[5]
Persian in origin, it was written in 1690 by Baward,
about whom little is known. It promulgates the
teaching of Ḥunain ibn Isḥaq or Joannitus (809–
873), one of the most prominent physicians of
Baghdad. The text describes how sensation and
motion are mediated by a spirit arising from the
liver, lungs and heart, (below the eyes,) which
enters the optic nerves (visual spirit) seen running
to the brain and crossing (optic chiasma). It also
reaches the brain (psychic spirit), which is covered
by the traditional layers of pia mater, dura mater,
bone, pericranium, and skin. The anterior cell is
probably the triangular black area lying between
the optic pathways as in Figure 62. In it the spirit is
"clarified, refined, purified, and cleansed"; its
function is to transmit sensation and movement to
all sensory organs and limbs by way of the hollow
nerves "for the nerves are but a part of the brain,

as the branches are but a part of the tree".

Here the author is subscribing to the Ancient
Greek concept of brain function (p. 5) then still
widely accepted in the West as well as in the East.
This diagrammatic depiction of the notion,
characteristic of Islamic anatomical illustrations,
would not, however, have been acceptable in the
West in 1690 (see Figures 62, 99).

FIGURE 101 (OPPOSITE)
The evolution of Western anatomy in Classical
Antiquity and in the Middle Ages is said to have
been closely paralleled in China.[6] It is often
thought that the Chinese had only scanty anatomical knowledge but in the 7th to 9th centuries it has
been described as "rather advanced"[7] and may
have been the source of the famous Alexandrian
Series of anatomical illustration which proliferated
in medieval Europe (see p. 3). Thereafter, however,
it remained relatively static until modern times.

Thus the drawing in Figure 101 is transmitting a
very old tradition although it was printed as late as
1682 by Andreas Cleyer (1615–1690),[8] surgeon to
the Dutch East Indies Company, who[9] is alleged to
have plagiarized it from Michael Bohm (1612–
1659).[10] Cleyer was one of the first Europeans
whose publications acquainted the West with
Oriental medicine in general and of Chinese in
particular.[11] His book deals mainly with the pulse,
which was a cardinal feature of Chinese medicine.
The leaf shaped brain cannot be compared with
other illustrations and its odd shape suggests that
it was functionally unimportant. Some reproductions have "the sea of the marrow" written on the
drawings of the brain.

Like the Ancient Egyptians and Hebrews,
together with Aristotle and his followers, the
Chinese considered the heart to be "the monarch
of the whole body";[12] the brain was of less
functional significance and only worthy of
schematic representation in an anatomical
drawing. The "brain" is connected by a tube, to
the organ of generation; as one author stated,
"The head is the sea of the brain — [marrow], the
brains are in the head. It extends from the top of
the head to the tail bone . . .".[13] Little or nothing
can be found in Chinese writing on the structure of
the brain and even Hübotter who dealt with
Chinese anatomy did not discuss it.[14]

Relationships between brain substance, bone
marrow, and semen were commonly made by the
Chinese and also by the Ancient Greeks. Thus Plato
postulated a life substance or marrow (of which

the seed was a part) from which the brain and bone-marrow were formed.[15] The association is natural enough as they share a number of common features. But whereas the Greeks advanced their ideas, discarding this notion, the Chinese did not, so that it was still current in 1700. They had derived it from Taoism; "the brain is the ocean into which the marrow runs", the marrow having been prepared in the testes.[16] In an anthology of Taoist works, the *Sing-ming kuei-che* of about 1622, the human body is said to be divided into three regions. The first is the head from whence the spirits originate. The brain is termed the "sea of bone-marrow" which together with the testes, produces the seminal essences. The middle region is the spine which is the canal linking the brain with the genitalia. The lower region is the seat of sexual activity, represented by the kidneys. By means of this system the Taoists considered that the basic instincts could be ruled by the brain. Thus, pressure on the urethra at the moment of ejaculation (*coitus reservatus*), according to them, sent the sperm back up the spinal cord to rejuvenate and revivify the upper parts of the body and, in particular, to nourish the brain.[17]

Another way of achieving longevity was the breathing techniques of the Taoists which also involved the brain. By means of air (identified with spirit and the gods), the individual could make intimate physical contact with the heavens and thereby gain the immortality of the gods. Air had to be directed through the body including the centre of the head, thought to represent the brain ventricles.[18] If this is so a further interesting parallel with Western medieval notions of brain function can be made. In the brain, the air concocted with the essence to exert a restorative effect. The rejuvenating qualities contained within the brains of certain long-lived monkeys has also been reported.[19] These and other ideas concerning brain function which are quite alien and mostly incomprehensible to us, are part of the traditional cosmology still part of present-day "native" Chinese medicine. It is as though the teachings of Galen or the medieval Cell Doctrine continued to be disseminated and used in modern Western communities; it is, at the same time, of considerable interest to observe the recent popularity of acupuncture in the West, an outstanding component of ancient Chinese medicine. A detailed study of the rôle of the brain in Chinese thought has yet to be made.

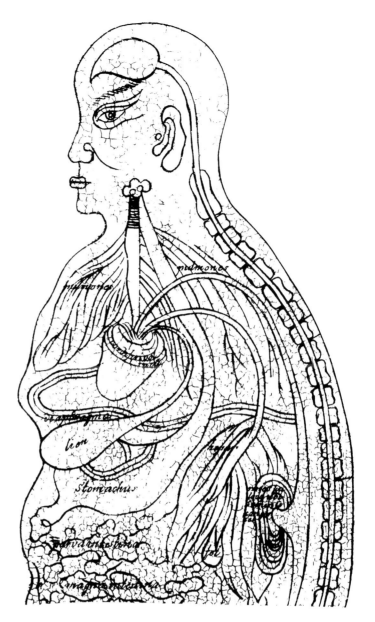

FIGURE 101

NOTES

1. Wellcome Historical Medical Library, Ms. OP.32427, (From the original Ms. in the Wellcome Library, by courtesy of the Trustees). It has not yet been dated precisely or examined in detail. See K. Sudhoff, "5. Eine anatomische Sechsbilderserie in zwei persischen Handschriften", in, *Ein Beitrag zur Geschichte der Anatomie der anatomischen Graphik...*, Heft 4 of *Studien zur Geschichte der Medizin*, Leipzig, J.A. Barth, 1908, pp. 52–72. See also E. Seidel & K. Sudhoff, "Drei weitere anatomische Fünfbilderserien aus Abendland und Morgenland", *Arch. Gesch. Med.*, 1909, 3:165–187. The figure is also reproduced by Choulant-Frank (*op.cit.*, Chapt. 1, note 3), p. 63. See note 3 below.

2. A. Fonahn, *Zur Quellenkunde der persischen Medizin*, Leipzig, J. A. Barth, 1920, pp.3–4.

3. There are at least 10 illustrated copies of the *Tashrīḥ i Mansūrī* known (C.E. Storey, *Persian literature. A bio-bibliographical survey*, Vol. II, Part 2, E. Medicine, London, Royal Asiatic Society of Great Britain & Ireland, 1971 (p. iv, 193–346), item 384(2) on pp. 226–227). The more important ones are:

(1) *India office Library*, Persian Ms.2296. Dated 5 December 1672. See, Sudhoff (1908) (*op. cit.* above, note 1), pp. 52, 53–66 and Tafel XI; and E. Seidel, "Zur den Legenden der persischen anatomischen Bildserie", *Arch. Gesch. Med.*, 1910, 3:347–348.

(2) *British Museum*, Add. Ms.23556, F.485^V. Dated 1684. No legends on drawing. See Seidel & Sudhoff (*op. cit.* above, note 1), pp. l67–169.

(3) Oxford, *Bodleian Library*, Ms.1576 (Fraser 201). Dated 13 February 1722. No legends on drawing. See, Seidel (*op.cit.* above, note 3(1)): and Sudhoff (1908) (*op. cit.* above, note 1), pp. 66–72 and Tafel XVI(2).

(4) *Bibliothèque Nationale*, Persian Ms. 1555 (Schefer, p.239), F.13^V. Date? See Seidel & Sudhoff (*op. cit.* above, note 1), pp. 169–185.

There are also printed editions: Delhi, 1848 and 1868; Lahore, 1878, 1889, 1895.

4. Persian Ms., p. 17. It seems to have belonged to Max Meyerhof but its present whereabouts has not been discovered. The best account of it is by M. Meyerhof & C. Prüfer, "Die Lehre vom Sehen bei Ḥunain b. Isḥāq", *Arch. Gesch. Med.*, 1912, 6:21–33. See also, *idem* "Die Augen-anatomie des Hunain b. Ishaq," *ibid.*, 1910, 4:163–190, which deals with the structure and function of the brain and nerves in greater detail.

5. Meyerhof & Prüfer (1912), *op. cit.*, note 4, above.

6. J. Needham, *Science and civilisation in China*, Vol.1, *Introductory orientation*, Cambridge, University Press, 1954, pp. 150–151.

7. J. Needham, "The Chinese contribution to science and technology", in, *Clerks, craftsmen in China and the West*, Cambridge, University Press, 1970, p. 78.

8. *Dictionaire des sciences médicales. Biographie médicale*, Vol.3, Paris, Panckoucke, 1821, pp. 286–287.

9. *Specimen medicinae Sinicae...* Edidit A. Cleyer, Frankfort, J.P. Zubrodt, 1682. Figure 101 is the first plate and it and the others are described by Choulant-Frank (*op. cit.*, Chapt. 1, note 3), pp. 362–369.

10. Apparently Cleyer was never in China, but visited Japan, 1682–1683. Bohm published *Clavis medicae ad Sinarum doctrinum et pulsibus*, Norimberg, 1686, which Cleyer had plagiarized in 1682. See, *Histoire de la médecine en Extrême Orient*, Paris, Fondation Singer-Polignac, 1959, Item 57 on p. 47.

11. P. Huard & M. Wong, *Chinese medicine*, London, Weidenfeld & Nicolson, 1968, pp. 122–131.

12. Choulant-Frank (*op. cit.*, Chapt. 1, note 3), p. 368.

13. W.R. Morse, *Chinese medicine (Clio medica)*, New York, P.B. Hoeber, 1934, p. 88. This is from the anonymous *Secrets of the pulse*, composed 907–960 A.D. and published in French (1735) and later in English. The last edition seems to have been 1891. Slightly different version in, W.R. Morse, "A memorandum on the Chinese procedure of acupuncture", *J. West. China Border Res. Soc.*, n.d. 5:153–216, see p. 196.

14. F. Hübotter, *Die Chinesische Medizin zur Beginn des XX. Jahrhunderts und ihr historischer Entwicklungsgang*, Leipzig, B. Schindler, 1929. Likewise, K.C. Wong, & Wu Lien-Teh, *History of Chinese medicine*, Tientsin, Tientsin Press, 1932 in their large book quickly dismissed it; they reproduced Figure 101 in Figure 6, facing p. 10. See also, I. Veith, "Non-Western concepts of psychic function", in, Poynter (*op. cit.*, Chapt. 2 note 18), pp. 29–42. See also E.T. Hsieh "A review of ancient Chinese anatomy", *Anat. Rec.* 1920–1921, 20:97–127.

15. F.M. Cornford, *Plato's cosmology. The Timaeus, translated with a running commentary*, London, Routledge & K. Paul, 1937, 73c–73d on pp. 293–294. See also, Clarke & O'Malley (*op. cit.*, Chapt. 2, note 15), pp. 7–9.

16. Morse (1934, *op. cit.* above, note 13), p. 76.

17. J. Needham, *Science and civilisation in China*, Vol.2, *History of scientific thought*, Cambridge, University Press, 1956, pp. 149–150. See also, G.J. Gruman, *A history of ideas about the prolongation of life. The evolution of prolongevity hypotheses to 1800*, in, *Trans. Amer. Philosoph. Soc.*, 1966, Vol. 56, Part 9, see pp. 45–47.

18. Gruman, *ibid.*, pp. 39–42

19. *Ibid.*, p. 54

It might have been expected that Willis's introduction of the concept of cortical function would have provided an impetus to elucidating other aspects of brain function. But, on the whole, progress was slow. There were advances in techniques of illustrating, with the introduction of increasingly refined and accurate reproductions of the cerebral surface so that by the end of the 18th century drawings were vastly improved, though still not entirely life-like, and from a morphological point of view, often quite crude. From the mid-17th century to the end of the 18th little or no investigation of the convolutions was carried out and so the idea of a definite pattern with named gyri and sulci had yet to be established.

An important scientific advance in the second half of the 17th century was the application of the microscope in relating the structure and function of the cerebral cortex. The three individuals who tackled this problem arrived at different conclusions: Marcello Malpighi (1628–1694) thought the cortex was made up of "glands"; Frederick Ruysch (1638–1731) of blood vessels; and Anton van Leeuwenhoek (1632–1723) of "globules". It transpired eventually that although each erred they all, nevertheless, stimulated much research. It is not intended to present an illustrated history of the histology of the cerebral cortex for this fascinating story is sufficiently detailed and important enough to constitute a separate volume.

Steno's essay of 1665 which presents an excellent review of brain anatomy and physiology in the mid-17th century has already been referred to (p. 76). He attacked in particular the speculations of Descartes and Willis as well as the continuing adherence to tradition. Finally he called for a programme of research which makes good sense today. Unfortunately he did not carry it out himself

and few after him were inspired to do so. There were, therefore, no revolutionary advances in brain anatomy or function in the second half of the 17th century or during all of the 18th.

The gradual improvement in drawings of the cerebral convolutions as the 19th century is approached will be appreciated in the following series.

FIGURE 102
Steno (p. 74) warrants special attention on account of his excellent essay (1665)[1] and illustrations.[2] The latter are as good as any yet published, and Figure 102 shows one of the first accurate sagittal sections of the brain. Admittedly the medial surface of the cerebrum had been crudely drawn by, amongst others, Dryander in 1537.[3] Even so, Steno's illustration is by no means perfect by present day standards. The convolutions still look somewhat cloudlike (cf. Vesalius, Figure 82) and the massa intermedia of the third ventricle seems larger than that of the human brain, although it often varies in size.[4]

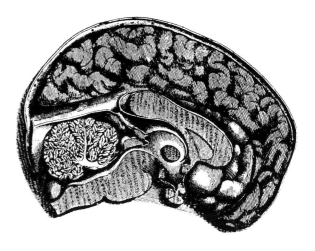

FIGURE 102

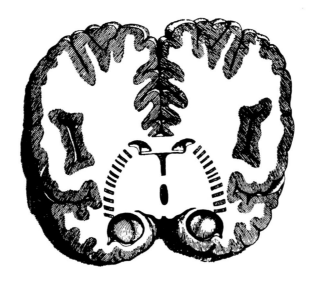

FIGURE 103

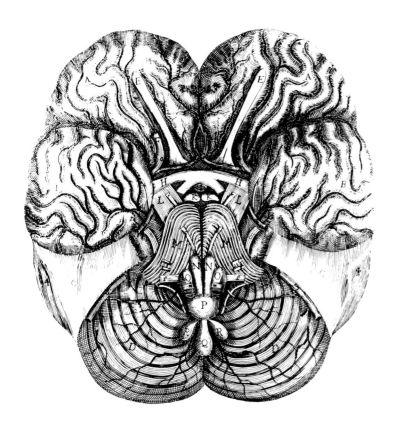

FIGURE 104

FIGURE 103

Another notable feature in Steno's plates is the depiction of the cerebral cortex, seen here cut coronally. This seems to be the first reasonable drawing of it. On the other hand, his representation of the corpus striatum is almost schematic and inferior to that of Willis (Figure 98).

FIGURE 104

In his research protocol of 1665 (p. 74) Steno had suggested an investigation of the cerebral white matter which had been begun by Thomas Willis. However, Raymond de Vieussens of Montpellier (1644–1716)[5] is remembered particularly for his labours in this field.

His investigations were the best that had been carried out, and his name is still occasionally associated with the "centrum ovale" and with the "anterior medullary velum" (Vieussens' valve). In 1685 he published a large book on the anatomy and physiology of the brain, *Neurographia universalis*, wherein the cerebral convolutions and cortex received scanty attention.[6] Figure 104[7] shows the base of the brain with unlife-like convolutions together with many aberrations of the brain stem and associated structures. AA and BB refer to the "anterior and posterior lobes of the brain", but the gyri are not indicated.

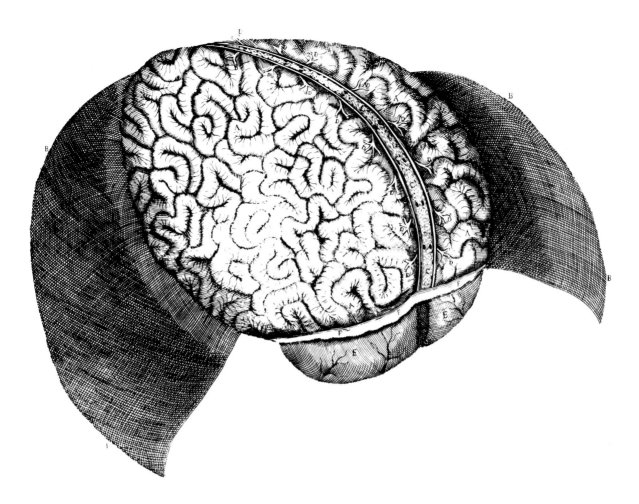

FIGURE 105

FIGURE 105
The surface of the cerebral hemispheres is drawn
thus,[8] the dura mater having been folded back
(BBBB) and the sagittal sinus (CCC) opened. The
convolutions (AAAA) are styled "circumvolutions of
the intestines", and are traversed by arteries and
veins. Vieussens described briefly the cerebral
cortex,[9] but omitted any account of the gyri. On
the whole, his plates are inferior to those of Willis
and they certainly lack the artistic quality of
Vesalius's.

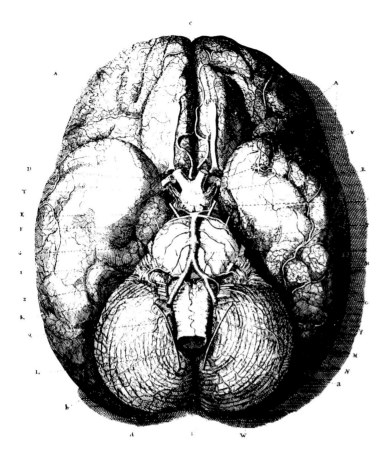

FIGURE 106

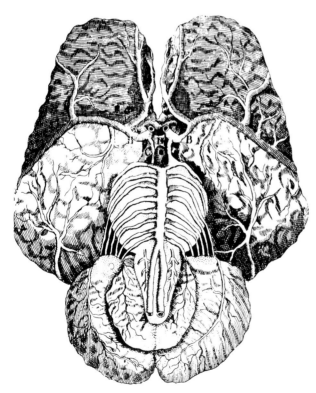

FIGURE 107

FIGURE 106

In the second half of the 17th century new
techniques were developed to supplement the
traditional methods of dissection. One was the
microscope which, soon after the middle of the
century, was applied to biological problems,[10] in an
attempt to elucidate the function and basic
constituents of animal and human organs. The
early instruments were crude and, as there was no
staining, sectioning or other histological methods
available, the results of this research were not on
the whole spectacular, except for those of two
pioneers, Malpighi[11] and Leeuwenhoek.[12] They
both examined the cerebral cortex and Malpighi[13]
regarded it as being made up of "glands" which
subsequently have been shown to be an artefact;[14]
Leeuwenhoek in 1684,[15] on the other hand,
thought it was composed of "globules", which
likewise have turned out to be an artefact.[16]

Frederick Ruysch[17] of Amsterdam developed
Willis's technique of blood-vessel injection for the
examination of the brain[18] and in 1699 concluded
that the cerebral cortex consisted of blood vessels
only. In Figure 106 the vascularity of the cortex is
emphasized, but the convolutions have been
sketched in with the usual vagueness.[19]

It was now widely accepted that the cortex
produced the animal spirits, as Sylvius and Willis
had contended (p. 77), and Malpighi,
Leeuwenhoek and Ruysch all thought that the
basic component they had identified, whether
"gland", "globule", or blood vessel, was concerned with its production. Although they all erred,
their functional concepts survived through the 18th
century and were only rejected when the neurone
was discovered in the 1830's.[20]

FIGURE 107

At any stage in history, regression as well as
advancement is taking place. This has happened
frequently during the development of brain
illustration. Thus while some illustrations exhibited
an increasing degree of artistic quality, others were
wretchedly poor anatomically and lacking in artistic
merit. This is true of René-Jacques Croissant de
Garengeot (1688–1759),[21] a famous Parisian
surgeon and anatomist whose anatomical treatise
was published in 1733.[22] Although he qualified his
title, "with original figures drawn from cadavers",
yet the plates, as is obvious from Figure 107, are
exceedingly crude. The convolutions are no better
than those depicted by Vesling 75 years earlier
(Figure 91) and are surpassed by several 16th-
century illustrators (Chapter 6).

FIGURE 108

We now pass from the crude to the mature, in the work of a contemporary of Garengeot, Giovanni Domenico Santorini (1681–1737) of Venice.[23] An exact and meticulous dissector, Santorini made many discoveries, only some of them appearing in his main work published thirty years after his death. Figure 108 is from Santorini's *Anatomici . . .* of 1775[24] and like others has been drawn with a light crayon which does not impair anatomical detail. They are not realistic anatomically, as the gyri, for example, are imperfectly depicted but they are probably the most elegant artistic production yet studied. They have a graduated border with explicatory outlines like those of Eustachius (Figure 85). They were drawn by Giovanni Battista Piazzetto (1682–1754), and Florentia Marcella engraved the plates, under Santorini's personal direction. We agree with Choulant-Frank's statement that "The work belongs to the best of its time . . . not only as regards the dissections and illustrations, but also as to the very elaborate commentary".[25]

FIGURE 109 (FOLLOWING PAGE)

The 18th century closed without any notable changes in concepts of brain function. Animal spirits had been replaced by an equally hypothetical substance, the "nerve fluid", prepared in the brain and circulated in hollow nerves to effect motion and sensation.[26] But the basic principles were much the same as those of Willis and to a lesser degree of the Ancient Greeks. But, the advent of "animal electricity" in the closing decades of the 18th century portended revolutionary changes in the understanding of nervous tissue and brain function.[27]

Meanwhile Samuel Thomas Soemmerring (1755–1830), the most famous German anatomist in the second half of the 18th century,[28] who introduced our present classification of the cranial nerves,[29] regressed to the medieval theory of ventricular function when he contended in 1796 that fluid in the brain ventricles could be animated and was the immediate organ of the soul, the "sensorium commune". Like Descartes he thought nerves ended in the ventricular walls and were activated and united by the ventricular fluid. Among his critics were Goethe, and Kant who challenged any attempt to localize the soul. Soemmerring's argument, combined with 19th-century materialism, eventually dispelled this idea which had originated in the 6th and 5th centuries

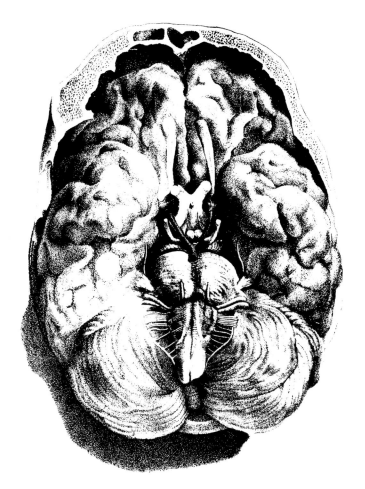

FIGURE 108

B.C. (p. 5). It must, therefore be one of the longest surviving aspects of biological thought.

Soemmerring published his sensational theory in *Über der Organ der Seele,* of 1796[30] wherein appears this excellent sagittal view of the brain, showing the ventricular system as the repository of the soul.[31] He is noted for the clarity and accuracy of his anatomical illustrations for, like his teacher, Bernhard Siegfried Albinus (1697–1770), he followed nature as closely as possible. This drawing is one of Soemmerring's best illustrations, being the work of a gifted artist, Christian Koeck, trained by Soemmerring, and engraved by Ludwig Schmidt, whom Soemmerring carefully directed. Gratiolet (see Figure 130) writing about 60 years later thought that it could still be profitably consulted.[32] He was referring in particular to the gyri which are well depicted and correspond closely to a modern drawing or photograph. They are not yet named, for this was to be the task of Gratiolet

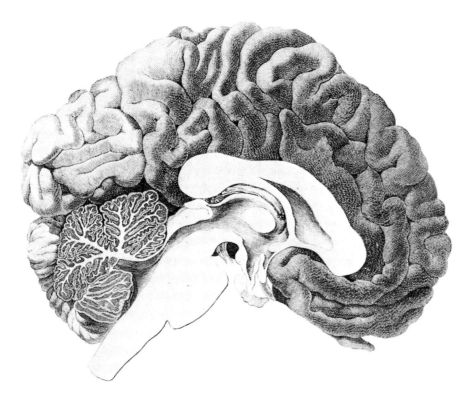

FIGURE 109

and others in the 19th century (pp. 107–113). Soemmerring admitted that the sulci and gyri, despite their seeming variability in different individuals, have great constancy and analogy to one another.[33] Riese has claimed this illustration as "the first correct picture of the mesial aspect of the cerebral hemispheres" and "a masterpiece of observation and reproduction".[34] As he pointed out, modern techniques do not always exceed the level of accuracy and beauty achieved by earlier anatomists and their draughtsmen. Clearly Soemmerring's plates are an important contribution to art and anatomy, and Choulant-Frank has contended that, together with the Italian anatomist-surgeon Antonio Scarpa (1752–1832),[35] Soemmerring introduced a new epoch of anatomical illustrations "in respect to more exact representation, artistically conceived".[36] Like Bernhardus Siegfried Albinus (1697–1770), he endeavoured to depict structures as they are during life, and not as they appear in death. This is one of the reasons why his influence on anatomy and on anatomical illustrations was felt for so long.

FIGURE 110 (OPPOSITE TOP)
Pierre Gratiolet, one of the 19th-century pioneers in the scientific investigations of the cerebral convolutions (Figures 130, 131), named Soemmerring and the eminent French anatomist and physician, Felix Vicq d'Azyr (1748–1794) as the first, after Willis and Malpighi, to advance this field of study.[37]

Vicq d'Azyr, whose name is still associated with the mammillo-thalamic tract,[38] was, like his contemporary Soemmerring, imbued with a desire to depict nature as it really is.[39] In this spirit he tackled the anatomy of the brain,[40] describing in detail the fissure of Sylvius (Figure 90)[41] and frequently mentioning the convolutions although he was more concerned with their size than pattern.[42] In this paper of 1781, Vicq d'Azyr dealt more with deeper structures than with the surface and Figure 110 is, therefore, taken from his book of 1786, *Traité d'anatomie*.[43] Despite his good intentions and the legend stating that: "This drawing represents the convolutions of the brain as they appear in the natural state after the dura mater has been elevated", this elegant plate still gives the impression of coils of small intestine. He did, however, begin to differentiate gyri by grouping them into anterior, middle, posterior and inferior and by describing the pre- and post-central convolutions.

FIGURE 111 (BELOW)
Eleven years after the death of Vicq d'Azyr, a
collected edition of his works appeared containing
this drawing of the brain.[44] Although there is some
conformation to nature as in Figure 110 the
convolutions still look like coils of intestine.
Whether Vicq d'Azyr himself would have allowed
this plate to be published cannot be determined
but it does show that the old Erasistratian analogy
(p. 60) seems to have persisted until 1805 at least.

Unlike his predecessors, Vicq d'Azyr examined
the cerebral surface carefully instead of ignoring it.
He enumerated anterior (1, 2), middle (3, 3, 4) and
posterior (7, 7, 7) lobes of the cerebrum which
Haller preferred to term frontal, parietal and
occipital regions respectively.[45] Vicq d'Azyr also
described some of the lobes' constituent convolutions: "convolution that follows the corpus
callosum" (20, 24, 26, 27); "the convolution that
follows this one" (18, 22, 9, 9, 19); etc. Artistically
this plate is inferior to that of Soemmerring (Figure
109), executed 9 years earlier, but from the
anatomical point of view it was an important
advance directly stimulating the researches of the
French anatomists who will be discussed in
Chapter 11.

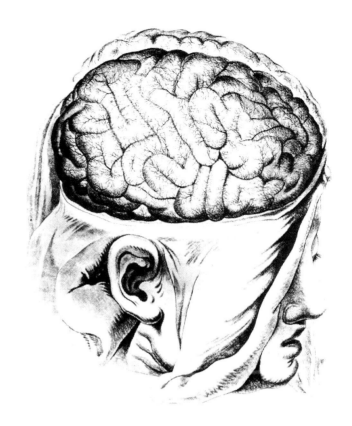

FIGURE 110

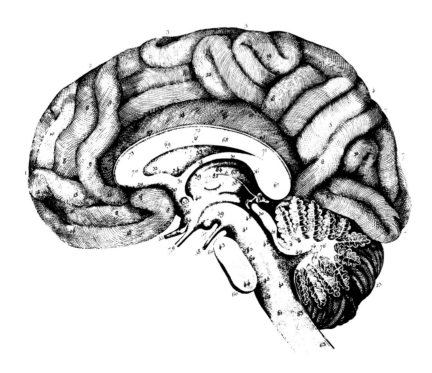

FIGURE 111

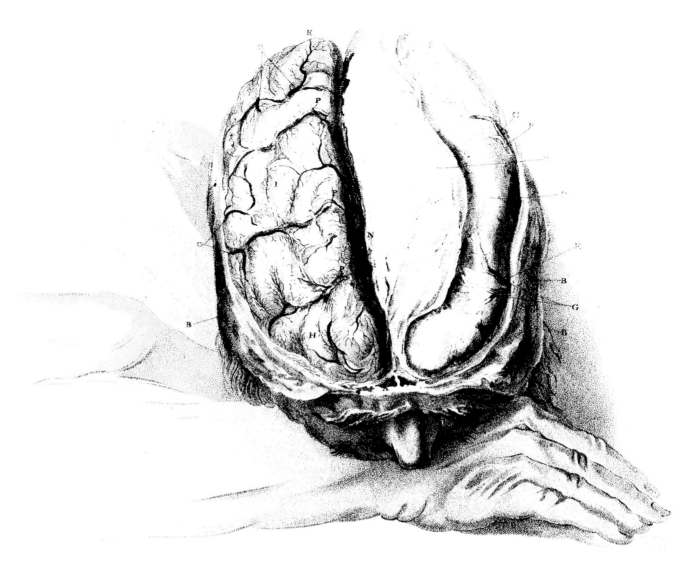

FIGURE 112

FIGURE 112
Charles Bell (1774–1842),[46] the famous British
anatomist and surgeon, at about the same time
was content to accept the three divisions of the
brain. In his lengthy legend to this plate he did not
make any special comments on the gyri.[47] The
importance of this plate is as an accurate portrayal
of the cerebral gyri drawn by Bell himself and
engraved by T. Medland.

Together with those of Soemmerring and Vicq
d'Azyr it characterizes the pre-scientific era of the
anatomical investigation of the cerebral convolutions. Anatomists tended to depict structure as
faithfully as they could but were not primarily
concerned with a scientific attack on the problem
for they were not approaching function by way of
morphology. This was to be their role during the
later decades of the 19th century.

NOTES

1. Steno (*op. cit.,* Chapt. 7, note 10); See, Clarke & O'Malley (*op. cit.,* Chapt. 2, note 15), pp. 823–825.

2. Steno, (*op. cit.,* note 1 above). Figure 102 is from the first plate, Figure 103 from the third. There are no legends and each drawing has an outline figure but no naming of structures.

3. *Op. cit.,* Chapt. 6, note 8, Figure [6].

4. F. Morel, "La massa intermedia ou commissure grise", *Acta Anat.,* 1947/48, *4:*203–207.

5. C. E. Kellett, "The life and works of Raymond de Vieussens", *Ann. Med. Hist.,* 1942, *4*(3rd ser.):31–54. Clarke & O'Malley (*op. cit.,* Chapt. 2, note 15), pp. 585–590.

6. *Neurographia universalis . . .,* Lyons, J. Certe, 1685. The first edition, if it can be designated thus, was published in 1684 and is identical with that of 1685. It is, however, very rare.

7. *Ibid.,* Tabula V, facing p. 37.

8. *Ibid.,* Tabula II, facing p. 11.

9. *Ibid.,* pp. 54–55.

10. S. Bradbury, *The evolution of the microscope,* Oxford, Pergamon Press, 1967; E. Clarke & J. G. Bearn, "A seventeenth century microscope", *Med. Biol. Ill.,* 1967, *17:*74–80.

11. A. B. Adelmann, "The life and works of Marcello Malpighi", in, *Marcello Malpighi and the evolution of embryology,* Vol. 1, Ithaca, N.Y., Cornell University Press, 1966, pp. 3–727.

12. C. Dobell, *Antony van Leeuwenhoek and his "little animals",* London, Staples Press, 1932.

13. *De viscerum structura exercitatio anatomica,* Bologna, J. Monti, 1666, "De cerebri cortice", pp. 50–72. See, Clarke & O'Malley (*op. cit.,* Chapt. 2, note 15), pp. 416–418.

14. L. Belloni, "I trattati di M. Malpighi sulla struttura della lingua e della cute", *Physis* (Florence), 1965, *7:*431–475; E. Clarke & J. G. Bearn, "The brain 'glands' of Malpighi elucidated by practical history", *J. Hist. Med.,* 1968, *23:*309–330.

15. "De structura cerebri diversorum animalium: etc.," in, *Opera omnia, seu arcana naturae,* Vol. 1, Leyden, Langerak, 1722, pp. 29–41. A letter written on 25 July 1684 to the Royal Society of London, abstracted in *Phil. Trans.,* 1685, *15:*883–895. See, Clarke & O'Malley (*op. cit.,* Chapt. 2, note 15), pp. 418–420.

16. The nature of Leeuwenhoek's "globules" has not yet been elucidated but they certainly were not cells. J. R. Baker has discussed this problem and the "globule theory" in general in "The Cell-theory: a restatement, history, and critique, Part I", *Q. J. Microscop. Science,* 1948, *89:*103–125, see pp. 114–121.

17. A. T. Hazen, "Johnson's life of Frederick Ruysch", *Bull. Hist. Med.,* 1939, *7:*324–334.

18. See, Willis (*op. cit.,* Chapt. 5, note 15) and Figure 77. See also, F. J. Cole, "The history of anatomical injections", in, C. Singer (editor), *Studies in the history and method of science,* Vol. 2, Oxford, Clarendon Press, 1921, pp. 285–343.

19. *Frederici Ruyschii responsio ad expertissimum virum Mich. Ernestum Ettmullerum . . . de corticali cerebri substantia . . .,* in, *Opera omnia anatomico-medico-chirugica,* Vol. I, Amsterdam, Jansson-Waesberg, 1737. The letter is dated 21 August 1699. Table 13 is Figure 102. See, Clarke & O'Malley (*op. cit.,* Chapt. 2, note 15), pp. 420–421.

20. C. G. Ehrenberg in 1833 and G. G. Valentin in 1836. See, Clarke & O'Malley (*op. cit.,* Chapt. 2, note 15), pp. 421–423.

21. J. E. Dezeimeris, *Dictionnaire historique de la médecine ancienne et moderne,* Vol. II, 2, Paris, Béchet Jeune, 1835, pp. 486–488.

22. *Splanchnologie, ou l'anatomie des visceres . . .,* 2nd. edition, Paris, C. Osmont, 1742. Figure 107 is "Tab:XIX.p:387". The illustrations are the same in all the editions and translations.

23. Choulant-Frank (*op. cit.,* Chapt. 1, note 3), pp. 262–264.

24. *Septemdecem tabulae quas nunc primum edit atque explicat . . .,* Parma, ex regia typographia, 1775, Tab. II which follows p. 30.

25. Choulant-Frank (*op. cit.,* Chapt. 1, note 3), p. 264.

26. E. Clarke, "The doctrine of the hollow nerve in the seventeenth and eighteenth centuries", in, L. G. Stevenson & R. P. Multhauf (editors), *Medicine, science and culture. Historical essays in honor of Owsei Temkin,* Baltimore, Md., Johns Hopkins Press, 1968, pp. 123–141.

27. L. Galvani published his, *De viribus electricitatis in motu musculari commentarius* in 1791 (*Bononien. Sci. Art. Instit. Acad.,* 1791, *7:*363–418; see Clarke & O'Malley [*op. cit.,* Chapt. 2, note 15], pp. 178–183). With it electrophysiology became a potent force in the elucidation of nerve function. See, M. A. B. Brazier, "The evolution of concepts relating to the electrical activity of the nervous system, 1600–1800", in Poynter (*op. cit.,* Chapt. 2, note 17), pp. 191–222; and, G. C. Pupilli & E. Fadiga, "The origins of electrophysiology", *J. World History,* 1963, *7:*547–589.

28. See Choulant-Frank (*op. cit.,* Chapt. 1, note 3), pp. 301–311; I. Döllinger, *Gedächtnissrede auf Samuel Thomas von Soemmerring . . . 25 August 1830,* Munich, A. Weber, 1830; "Biography of Sömmerring", *Lancet,* 1830, *ii:*243; T. H. Bast, "The life and work of Samuel Thomas von Sömmerring", *Ann. Med. Hist.,* 1924, *6:*369–386.

29. *De basi encephali et originibus nervorum cranio egredientium libri quinque,* Göttingen, A. Vandenhoeck, 1778.

30. *Über das Organ der Seele,* Königsberg, F. Nicolovius, 1796. W. Riese has analyzed this book carefully, in, "The 150th anniversary of S. T. Soemmerring's *Organ of the soul.* The reaction of his contemporaries and its significance today". *Bull. Hist. Med.,* 1946, *20:*310–321.

31. Tab. I; legend, pp. 76–79.

32. L. P. Gratiolet, *Mémoires sur les plis cérébraux de l'homme et des primates,* Paris, A. Bertrand, 1854, p. 7.

33. *Vom Hirn und Rückenmark,* Mainz, P. A. Winkopp, 1788, p. 65.

34. Riese (*op. cit.* above, note 30), p. 312, where he reproduces Soemmerring's Tab. I (our Figure 109).

35. See Choulant-Frank (*op. cit.,* Chapt. 1, note 3), pp. 298–300.

36. *Ibid.,* pp. 38–39.

37. Gratiolet (*op. cit.* above, note 32), pp. 6–7.

38. Clarke & O'Malley (*op. cit.,* Chapt. 2, note 15), p. 592.

39. J. L. Moreau, "Discours sur la vie et les ouvrages de Vicq d'Azyr", in, *Oeuvres de Vicq d'Azyr,* Vol. 1, Paris, L. Duprat-Duverger, 1805, pp. 1–88; [Anonymous], "Biographical sketch of Vicq D'Azyr", *Edinburgh Med. Surg. J.,* 1807, *3:*185–191; R. Spillman, "Felix Vicq d'Azyr", *J. Nerv. Ment. Dis.,* 1941, *94:*428–444.

40. "Recherches sur la structure du cerveau, du cervelet, de la moelle alongée, de la moelle épinière; & sur l'origine des nerfs de l'homme & des animaux", *Hist. Acad. roy. Sci.,* 1781, pp. 495–622. Published in 1784.

41. *Ibid.,* pp. 505–506.

42. Clarke & O'Malley (*op. cit.,* Chapt. 2, note 15), p. 391.

43. *Traité d'anatomie et de physiologie avec des planches coloriées représentant au naturel les divers organes de l'homme et des animaux,* Vol. 1, Paris, F. A. Didot l'aîné, 1786, Planche III.

44. *Oeuvres. Recueillies et publ. avec des cotes et un discours sur sa vie et ses ouvrages, par Jacq L. Moreau,* Paris, 1805. Figure III is from *Planches pour les oeuvres de Vicq d'Azyr,* Paris, L. Duprat-Duverger, 1805, Planche

XXII, Figure 1 (legend, pp. 141–144).

45. C. Bell, *The anatomy of the brain, explained in a series of engravings,* London, Longman, *et al.,* 1802, p. 4.

46. G. Gordon-Taylor & E. W. Walls, *Sir Charles Bell. His life and times,* Edinburgh & London. E. & S. Livingstone. 1958.

47. *Op. cit.* above, note 45, Plate 1.

At the beginning of the 19th century the slowly increasing interest in the cerebral gyri rapidly gathered momentum as the so-called "science" of cranioscopy or phrenology developed. Introduced in the 1790's by an anatomist, Franz Joseph Gall (1758–1828), who was aided in its dissemination by his pupil Johann Caspar Spurzheim (1776–1832),[1] it postulated that the brain was the organ of the mind with mental and moral faculties located in specific areas of its surface so that a surfeit or deficiency of each could be detected by examining the cranium. They and their followers, therefore, carefully divided the head into precisely defined compartments, each with its own specific function. This naturally directed attention to the surface of the cerebral hemispheres and thus to the convolutions. It also represents a milestone in the history of brain function for it raised a vitally important question. Could particular activities be mediated by the cerebral cortex, and localized to specific regions? Thus from both a morphological and functional point of view phrenology was an exceedingly significant stimulus.

Moreover, it is also of interest to the general historian, for, like the contemporary cult of mesmerism, it pervaded all strata of early 19th century society.[2] It harmonized with the "free thought" movement, and with the general tendency of Romantic criticism to concentrate on the analysis of character. Thus phrenology might be regarded historically as a radio-active marker in the complex metabolism of early Victorian society.[3]

But phrenology was not entirely new. It represented, in fact, a variation of physiognomy, "the art of judging character and disposition from the features of the face or the form and lineament of the body generally",[4] which had been popular in various forms for centuries. Gall began his studies in 1792 and gradually built up a system largely based on flimsy evidence, unscientifically and naively selected and interpreted.[5] Phrenology was widely popular in medical, scientific, and lay communities until the 1830's when it began to lose favour. There was, however, a revival with the scientific discovery of cortical localization (Chapter 12) in 1870 but it was never again accepted in medical and scientific circles. It became a means of assessing character and of forecasting the future; in this form it still has some limited vogue.[6]

Gall's sincerity and concern for the advancement of science cannot be doubted. He and his relatively modest system, however, were swamped by a number of vociferous and over-enthusiastic followers such as Spurzheim (Figure 116), George Combe (Figure 117) and later in the century, the Fowlers (Figure 121). They all seem to have had two features in common, prolixity and a towering forehead, indicative, according to their system, of intellectual prowess! Without doubt it was in no small measure due to their misplaced and misdirected zeal that phrenology fell into disrepute, although as a science it could not in any event have survived.

As phrenology evolved, variations were introduced by its more outstanding exponents. These are of interest to the historian of psychology but for our purpose they are of little consequence. We are concerned with phrenology as a seminal force driving individuals to look more closely at the cerebral convolutions and to consider with greater cogency the possibility of localizing function within the covering cortex. For this reason the following illustrations have not all been fully elucidated in irrelevent detail.

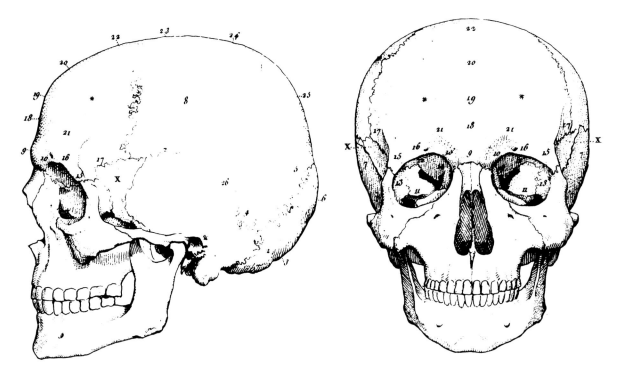

FIGURE 113

FIGURE 113

Basically Gall, as well as being an outstanding anatomist, was interested in the physiology of the brain, or "psycho-physiology" as we may style it. He regarded the brain as being not only the organ of the soul but also the repository of all moral and intellectual faculties, of all feelings and tendencies, despite the fact that almost everyone else postulated other locations, such as the thorax or abdomen for the passions and mania. This alone was a vitally important advance.

Gall named 27 mental faculties or qualities, and sited them in gyral areas called "organs" or "centres". Figure 113 is from an anonymous French work of 1803 which has been selected on this account as one of the earliest discussions of his doctrine.[7]

At this time there were only 26 "organs" and their exact confines had not yet been determined. The numbers have not been elucidated because the qualities they represent differ somewhat from those in Gall's authoritative account of the scheme (Figures 114–115). As will be seen, the doctrine of phrenology, as well as manifesting considerable variation, became increasingly complex as new "organs" were discovered and old ones subdivided.

FIGURES 114–115 (OPPOSITE)

In his great work of 1810–1819, helped by Spurzheim with the first two of four volumes, Gall published these drawings of the localization of the "organs" on the skull.[8] It is curious that each is indicated by a bump, for in some individuals there could be a deficiency of a quality and so a depression rather than an elevation would be present. The numbered "organs" do not yet have strict boundaries, but there is more evidence of localization than in Figure 113, reminiscent of the types of pictures of the Cell Doctrine (Chapter 3); Figures 114, 115 are midway between Figure 113 (1803) and Figure 116 (1825), and the Roman numerals, which are also used in Figures 123–125 and also as the Arabic ones in Figure 113, refer to the organs' qualities. They are as follows:

A. Organs common to men & animals:
1. Instinct of reproduction 2. Love of offspring
3. Friendship 4. Self-defence & courage
5. Carnivorous instinct, tendency to murder
6. Cunning, cleverness 7. Ownership, covetousness, tendency to steal 8. Pride, arrogance, haughtiness, love of authority 9. Vanity, ambition, love of glory 10. Caution, forethought 11. Memory of things and facts, educability 12. Sense of places and space 13. Memory and sense of people

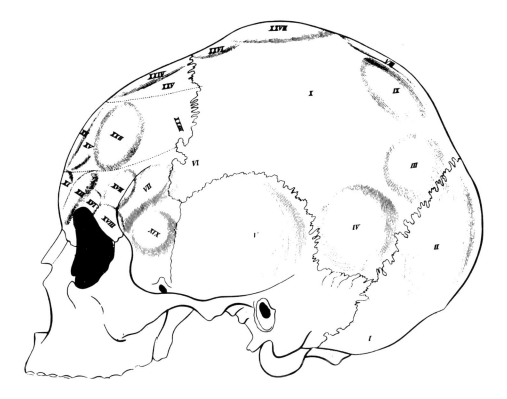

FIGURE 114

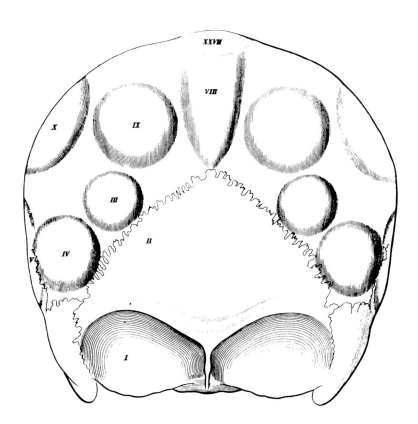

FIGURE 115

14. Memory of words 15. Sense of language and speech 16. Sense of colour 17. Sense of sound, music 18. Sense of numbers, mathematics 19. Sense of mechanics, architecture.

   B. Organs in humans alone

20. Wisdom 21. Sense of metaphysics 22. Satire, witticism 23. Poetical talent 24. Kindness, compassion, morality 25. Mimicry 26. Religion

27. Firmness of purpose, obstinacy, constancy.

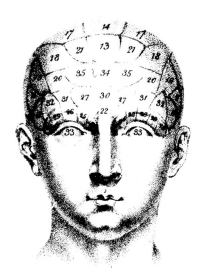

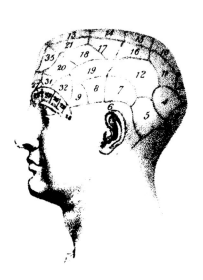

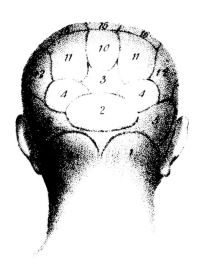

FIGURE 116

FIGURE 116

Of the two, Gall was the originator of phrenology and a skilled anatomist, whereas Spurzheim although an able dissector of the brain did more to publicize and, for a time, to promote the discipline. He travelled widely to spread the gospel and died in harness during a lecture tour of the U.S.A. However, he modified the system by adding another eight organs, and his schema became more popular than Gall's original.

This drawing is from a book published by Spurzheim in 1825[9] and the numbers again refer to the "powers and organs of the mind". Their listing is unnecessarily detailed for our purposes.

FIGURE 117 (OPPOSITE TOP)

One of the most articulate exponents of phrenology in Britain was George Combe (1788–1858) of Edinburgh, a lawyer by profession but a psychologist-phrenologist, philosopher and liberal reformer by inclination.[10] He published extensively and his *System of phrenology* was widely distributed. This drawing is taken from the second edition.[11] As can be seen, there were 33 organs in Combe's system, with some minor alterations in their location as compared with Spurzheim's; he divided them into propensities, sentiments and intellect. This lack of consistency between those practising phrenology (of which there are many examples), merely testifies to the uncertain and shifting basis upon which the structure was built and necessarily casts doubt upon the whole edifice. There were almost as many varieties as there were of the medieval Cell Doctrine (Chapter 3) with which the phrenologists identified themselves, possibly in order to acquire respectability and historical continuity, by adopting a time-honoured lineage which also served to support their theory of functional brain localization (see Figure 58).

FIGURE 118 (OPPOSITE BOTTOM)

As will be seen in the next chapter, Gall in 1810 by placing the numbers of his organs directly on the convolutions of the brain as well as on areas mapped on the surface of the cranium brought together our two main themes: localization of brain function and the morphological arrangement of the cerebral gyri. We have finally arrived at a theory of localized function of the cerebral convolutions. Dr. N. J. Ottin, at one time a professor in the University of Paris, did much the same as Gall, except that his numbering was more extensive.[12] He followed more or less the scheme of Gall (Figures 114–115).

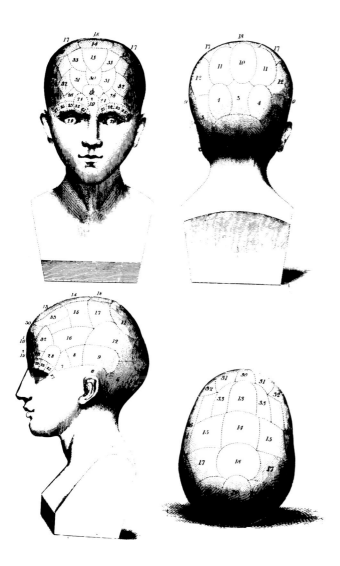

FIGURE 117

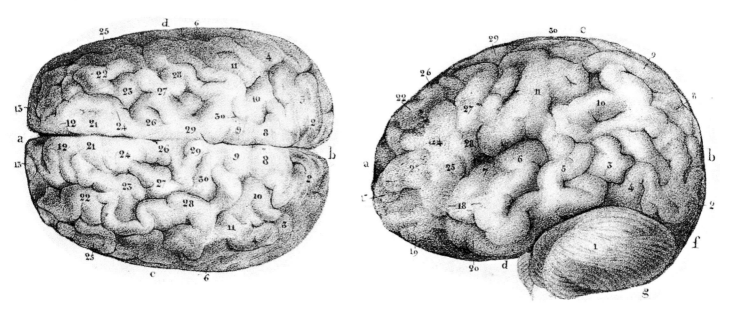

FIGURE 118

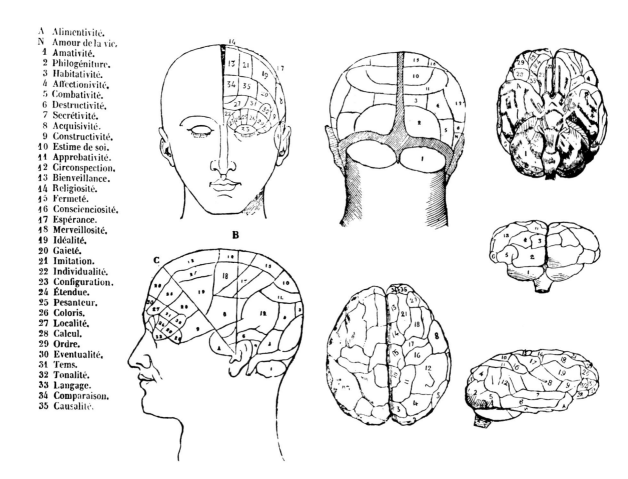

A   Alimentivité.
N   Amour de la vie.
 1 Amativité.
 2 Philogéniture.
 3 Habitativité.
 4 Affectionivité.
 5 Combativité.
 6 Destructivité.
 7 Secrétivité.
 8 Acquisivité.
 9 Constructivité.
10 Estime de soi.
11 Approbativité.
12 Circonspection.
13 Bienveillance.
14 Religiosité.
15 Fermeté.
16 Conscienciosité.
17 Espérance.
18 Merveillosité.
19 Idéalité.
20 Gaieté.
21 Imitation.
22 Individualité.
23 Configuration.
24 Étendue.
25 Pesanteur.
26 Coloris.
27 Localité.
28 Calcul.
29 Ordre.
30 Eventualité.
31 Tems.
32 Tonalité.
33 Langage.
34 Comparaison.
35 Causalité.

FIGURE 119

FIGURE 119

The next step was to mark on an outline of the brain itself the precise boundaries of the organs, rather than delineating them on the surface of the cranium, and numbering gyral areas imprecisely. This was done in 1836 by another French phrenologist, T. Thoré who seems to have been as obscure as Ottin.[13] He extended the Spurzheim 35-organ scheme (Figure 116) by adding two more.

At this stage a direct link may be discerned with the early 20th-century researchers into cyto-architechtonics who were also attempting to relate function to structure, by associating physiological data, derived from cortical stimulation and ablation, with cortical cytology. They too prepared diagrams (Figures 138–146), but all that the two groups had in common was that both subscribed to a notion of localized cortical function and both prepared maps to illustrate it. There, similarities cease. The phrenologists had arrived at a modern notion by an unorthodox route, based on false hypotheses.

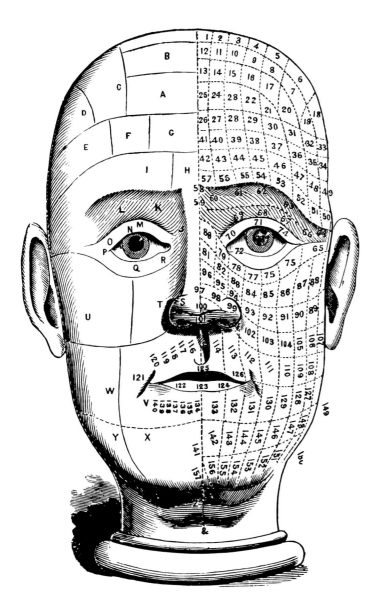

FIGURE 120

FIGURE 120

In the development of any new doctrine there are those whose enthusiasm and compulsion lead them to extremes. Such was the case with physiognomy and phrenology, as also with cortical localization (Figure 141). J. W. Redfield, M.D., of New York City was the author of the most elaborate system of physiognomy ever conceived.[14] By involving the head as well as the face, he linked it with phrenology: indeed it has been stated, erroneously, that physiognomy was founded on physiology and phrenology.[15]

This is functional localization gone mad! There are no fewer than 160 numbered, and a convenient 26 alphabetically labelled faculties; into Z are squeezed "Economy, Submission, Subserviency, etc. Independence & Firmness". The qualities vary from "65A. wave motion" to "149. Republicanism", the latter having as immediate neighbours "148. Faithful Love" and "149A. Responsibility"!

FIGURE 121

This pictorial method of demonstrating the phrenological "organs" instead of numbering them was common in the 19th century and later. It appeared first in an American phrenological periodical, published in New York between 1870 and 1911 and originated with the Fowlers, a family of ardent and commercially-minded phrenologists practising in New York and London.

FIGURE 122 (OPPOSITE)

Phrenological busts executed in china or in other media were as popular as diagrams and charts for teaching purposes. This is the most familiar, advertized in 1916 as "Fowler's new phrenological bust . . . with upwards of 100 divisions". Here is another example of the over-enthusiastic phrenologist's refinements (cf. Figure 120). The maker's "blurb" mentions that "newly discovered organs are added, and the old organs have been sub-divided to indicate the various phases of action which many of them assume. It is a perfect model, beautiful as a work of art, and is undoubtedly the latest contribution to phrenological science and the most complete bust ever published".[16] In 1916 they cost half a sovereign but now a diligent searcher may be fortunate to get one for £100. A bust of similar vintage, displaying orthodox anatomy would probably be unsaleable. Such is the attraction of the bizarre and unorthodox!

Gall had stumbled upon a theory of brain function that was to prove of the greatest significance. But though pioneering the concept of convolutional, and even cortical localization, he had clearly done so for the wrong reasons. The contribution of the phrenologists has been aptly summarized by Edwin G. Boring, "The theory of Gall and Spurzheim is, however, an instance of a theory which, while essentially wrong, was just enough right to further scientific thought". Phrenology helped to move ideas concerning the mind "away from the concept of the unsubstantial Cartesian soul to the concept of the more material nerve function", and in so doing "was wrong only in detail and in respect of the enthusiasm of its supporters".[17]

NOTES

1. See, E.H. Ackerknecht & H.V. Vallois, *Franz Joseph Gall, inventor of phrenology and his collection,* Madison, Wisconsin, University of Wisconsin Medical School, 1956 (*Wisconsin Studies in Medical History,* No. 1); A. Carmichael, *A memoir of the life and philosophy of Spurzheim,* Dublin, W.F. Wakeman, 1833.

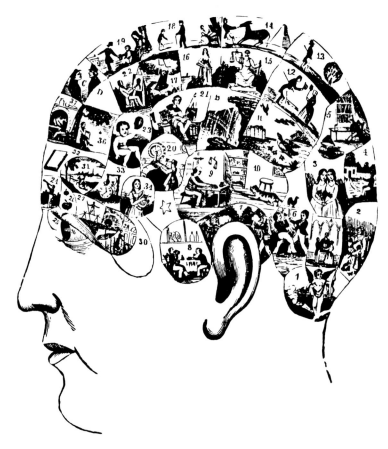

FIGURE 121

2. O. Temkin, "Gall and the phrenological movement", *Bull. Hist. Med.,* 1947,21:275–321.

3. J.D. Davies has traced its history in the U.S.A. (*Phrenology, fad or science. A 19th-century American crusade,* New Haven, Yale University Press, 1955) and G. Lanteri-Laura deals with France (pp. 145–163) in a broader history (*Histoire de la phrenologie. L'homme et son cerveau selon F.J. Gall,* Paris, Presses Universitaires de France, 1970). For a history of it in Britain, see R. J. Cooter, *The cultural meaning of popular science. Phrenology* (1985) in "Additional Bibliography".

4. *The shorter Oxford English dictionary,* 3rd edition, Oxford, Clarendon Press, 1955.

5. His beliefs are embodied in the great work, *Anatomie et physiologie du système nerveux en général, et du cerveau en particulier . . .,* Paris, F. Schoell, *et al.,* 1810–1819, 4 vols. & Atlas; Spurzheim was his co-author for the first two volumes only. The second edition, by Gall alone, was entitled, *Sur les fonctions du cerveau . . .,* Paris, J.B. Baillière, 1825, 6 vols.; it was an altered and extended version of the first but the Atlas was not republished.

6. There is an excellent survey of phrenology and its rôle in the 1900's by Miss Frances Hedderly F.B.F.S., who was a former President and Secretary of the British Phrenological Society, Inc. before its liquidation in 1967: *Phrenology. A study of mind,* London, L.N. Fowler, 1970.

7. [Anonymous] *Exposition de la doctrine physiognomique du Docteur Gall, ou nouvelle théorie du cerveau, consideré comme le siège des facultés intellectuelles et morales,* Paris, Henrichs, [1803].

8. *Op. cit.* above, note 5.

9. *Phrenology, or, the doctrine of the mind; and of the relations between its manifestations and the body,* 3rd edition, London, C. Knight, 1825, frontispiece.

10. C. Gibbon, *The life of George Combe, author of "The constitution of man",* London, Macmillan, 1878, 2 vols.; the book referred to in the title was a very popular work based on the doctrines of phrenology. See also, A. A. Walsh, "George Combe: a portrait of a heretofore generally unknown behaviorist", *J. Hist. Behavioral Sciences,* 1971, 7:269–278.

11. *A system of phrenology,* 2nd edition, Edinburgh, J. Anderson, 1825, frontispiece.

12. *Précis analytique et raisonné du système du Dr Gall . . .,* 5th edition, Paris, Crochard,1834, Pl. 6.

13. T. Thoré, *Dictionnaire du phrénologie, et de physiognomonie . . .,* Paris, Librairie Usuelle, 1836; first diagram, which precedes p. 1.

14. This is described by Samuel R. Wells, in, *New physiognomy, or, signs of character, as manifested through temperament and external forms,* New York, Fowler & Wells, 1894, pp.54–68 (first published, 1866). Figure 120 is on p. 60.

15. *Ibid.,* p. xxv.

16. Found, for example, with the advertisements following U. Buchanan, *The mind's attainment. A study of laws and methods for obtaining individual happiness, success and power through the silent force of thought,* London, L.N. Fowler, 1916, p. [xxiii].

17. E.G. Boring, *A history of experimental psychology,* 2nd edition, New York. Appleton-Century-Crofts, 1957, pp.57–58.

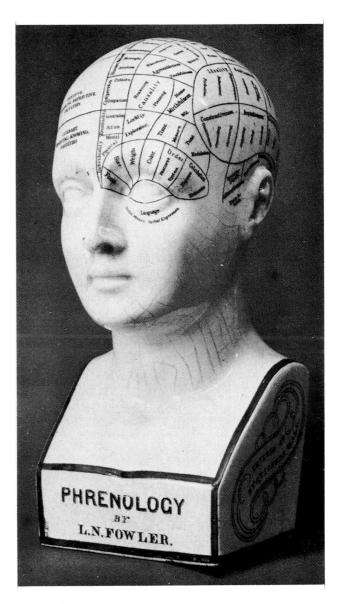

FIGURE 122

THE SCIENTIFIC INVESTIGATION
OF THE CEREBRAL CONVOLUTIONS
IN THE 19TH CENTURY

The early 19th century was a remarkable period for several reasons. Political convulsions and social reform provided a background which fostered revolutionary changes in medicine. Anatomical interpretation of disease, the roots of modern medicine, was well-established in France, where basic medical sciences were also developing rapidly and soon the Germans were to join and surpass their neighbours.

Our story is part of this widespread upheaval. As already noted (pp. 89–91), the late 18th-century anatomists were beginning to depict the cerebral gyri with scrupulous care and artistic talent, even though there seemed little reason, from a functional point of view for such minute attention. At the same time Gall's cranioscopy came into being, and what had previously been an activity, purposeless other than to satisfy anatomical perfection, was transformed into an urgent and meaningful desire to know more about the convolutions and sulci. This coincided with the rapidly developing macroscopical, embryological, and comparative anatomy at the beginning of the 19th century.

This tripartite basis for further research led, by the middle of the century, to transmuting the chaos of the cerebral convolutions into an orderly gyral pattern in man and animals. In the 19th century the cerebral convolutions were often described as "enteroid processes", a reference to their similarity to the intestines, suggested by Erasistratus of Alexandria.[1] This term was first used by M. V. G. Malacarne (1744–1876) and by his pupil Rolando (Figure 129).

FIGURES 123–125
When Gall's system of phrenology (or "cranioscopy" as he preferred to call it) is examined, particularly in respect of the evidence he accumulated to support his theoretical assertions (pp. 95–98), his true contribution to scientific knowledge *per se* appears to be slight or even negligible. When viewed, however, in historical perspective his discoveries in neuro-anatomy, for which he has been rightfully acclaimed, were considerable.[2] Unfortunately they have been overshadowed by the stigma of phrenology, the cult of cranial bumps. His system gave him virtually a proprietary interest in the anatomy of the surface of the brain and he regarded convolutions as peripheral expansions of white matter "fibres". He interpreted them as "the sites where instincts, sentiments, likes, talents, and in general the moral and intellectual forces are exercised".[3]

His drawings of the gyri and sulci shown here (Figures 123–125) are both faithful to nature and of artistic merit;[4] they were reproduced repeatedly throughout the 19th century. The Roman numerals on the convolutions indicate the location of the moral and intellectual qualities, the "organs" of his phrenological system; they are the same as in Figures 114 and 115. As mentioned earlier this arrangement manifests a fascinating convergence of the two notions which we have traced through several centuries: the morphology of the gyri and the precise localization of function in the brain. Gall had found the correct answer by using incorrect data (p. 95).

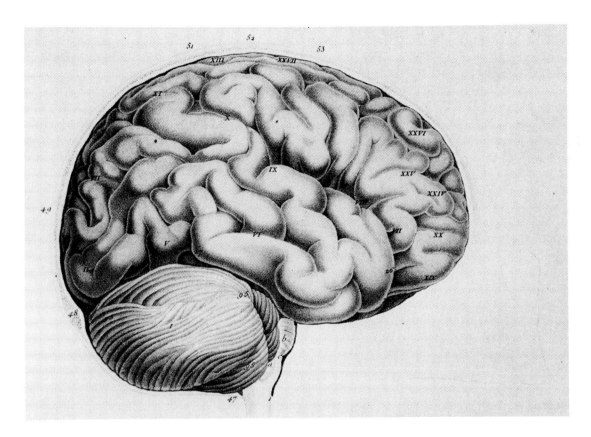

FIGURE 123

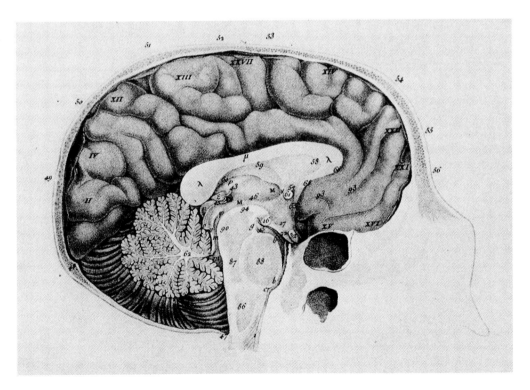

FIGURE 124

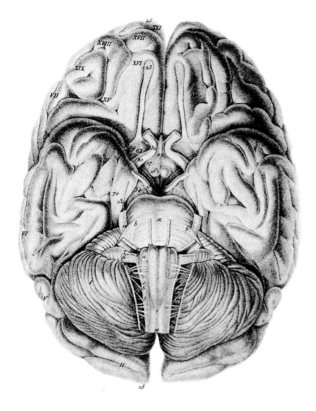

FIGURE 125

It is paradoxical that he and his followers, despite the fact that they were so committed to the brain's surface as far as function is concerned, made no attempt to study the convolutions in any detail. Nevertheless, they stimulated other anatomists to do so.

FIGURE 126 (BELOW)
Concurrent with the macroscopical investigations of cerebral convolutions in the first half of the 19th century was embryological research, with the same object of imposing a sense of order on this confused field of enquiry. The most important contributor was the German anatomist, Friedrich Tiedemann (1781–1861)[5] who reported his findings in 1816.[6] He carefully examined foetal brains of various ages, both human and animal, in order to piece together the evolution of the cerebral surface. He was able to observe a definite order of development so that chaos was eventually replaced by an evolutional pattern of maturation. Moreover, the importance of the sulci, hitherto neglected, became evident. Figure 126 shows the brain of a 27 week old human foetus: o, p, and q are posterior, middle, and anterior lobes, and tttt are commencing gyri.[7]

As well as contributing to the embryological aspects of convolutions, Tiedemann also studied comparative anatomy.[8] Here, as with the embryonic brain, the sulci as well as the gyri were seen to be important and for the first time they became of equal, if not of greater, significance.

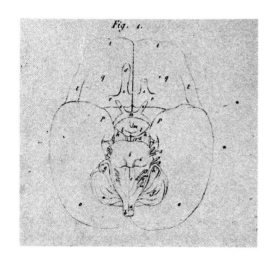
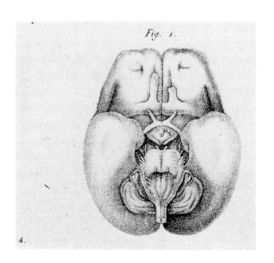

FIGURE 126

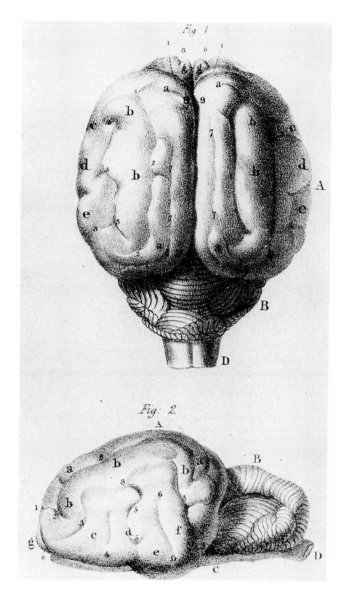

FIGURE 127

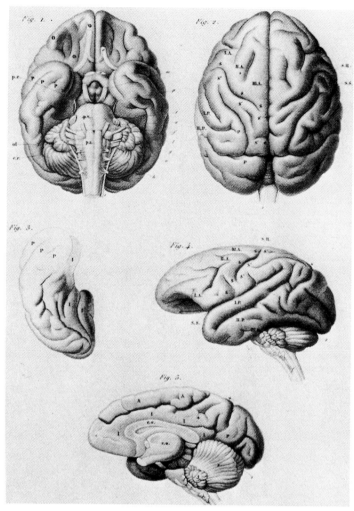

FIGURE 128

FIGURE 127

The comparison of the human and animal brain
began with Willis (see p. 74) and Gall and
Spurzheim emphasized the importance of
comparative studies, especially of the cerebral
convolutions. This was borne out by Tiedemann
(Figure 126) and also by the famous English
anatomist and zoologist, Robert Owen (1804–
1892)[9] who in 1835 reported on the convolutional
pattern of the cheetah's brain.[10] He could
demonstrate consistencies in "primary" or
"principal" gyri and sulci, whereas the "secondary" were less symmetrical; the differentiation
between the two was based on evolutionary
evidence, that is, on the order of their appearance.[11] It is a measure of the times that Owen
enlisted the help of a phrenologist to elucidate
function in the gyri he had delineated![12]

Letters relate to gyri and numbers to sulci. a, b, c,
d, e, are principal or primary convolutions; 7 is a
secondary fissure or sulcus and others are also
indicated by means of digits.

FIGURE 128

The French anatomist and psychiatrist, François
Leuret (1797–1851),[13] extended Owen's work and
examined mammals other than cats.[14] Figure 128
depicts the brain of the baboon.[15] His examinations, together with other considerations, led him
to conclude that variations in the convolutional
patterns between species represent an index of
differentiation. When listing animals in the order of
complexity of their convolutional patterns, Leuret
also arranged them according to intelligence,
thereby attempting a direct correlation between
convolutions and intellect.

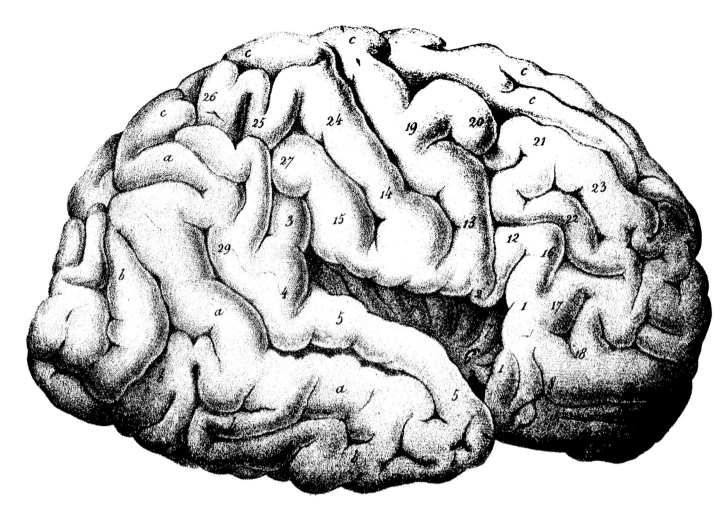

FIGURE 129

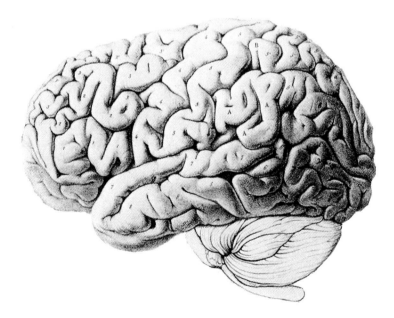

FIGURE 130

FIGURE 129 (OPPOSITE TOP)
Meanwhile considerable advances had been made
by macroscopical study of the convolutions. The
fissure of Sylvius was the first sulcus to be
identified and named (Figure 90). The island of Reil
or insula, clearly depicted by Bartholin (Figure 90)
in 1641, was described in detail by Johann
Christian Reil (1759–1813) in 1809.[16] They were
the first two landmarks to which was added in
1831 the fissure of Rolando.[17] Figure 129 shows it
clearly, together with other sulci and the gyri on
the lateral surface. The numbering relates to
phrenological "organs" so we can assume Rolando
had not advanced in his ideas of function.
Nevertheless he forecast correctly the discovery of
regularity in shapes and sizes of the gyri. It was
Rolando who used the term "enteroid processes",
as had his teacher (p. 104).

FIGURE 130 (OPPOSITE BOTTOM)
Louis Pierre Gratiolet (1815–1865),[18] the colleague
of Leuret in Paris, is the most renowned of the
French anatomists who investigated the cerebral
gyri and sulci. By comparative studies he distinguished primary from secondary gyri, in accordance with their chronological appearance in
evolutionary sequence. He introduced a system of
nomenclature, which proved to be a simple but
significant advance; until a structure has been
named it has no anatomical entity and tends to be
ignored or forgotten. Gratiolet used the terms,
"frontal", "temporal", "parietal" and "occipital"
lobes introduced by Arnold in 1838,[1] and defined
their limits. He published first in 1854,[19] and Figure
130 shows the high standard that pictorial
representation of gyri had reached. The legend
gives the convolutions names, several of which are
still used.[20]

FIGURE 131 (ABOVE RIGHT)
Another excellent plate of the cerebral convolutions is from the second volume of *Anatomie
comparée* (1857) in which Gratiolet summarized
his views.[21] It was prepared under the direction of
Leuret who, however, died six years before its
publication.[22] Again there is precise labelling of gyri
and sulci.

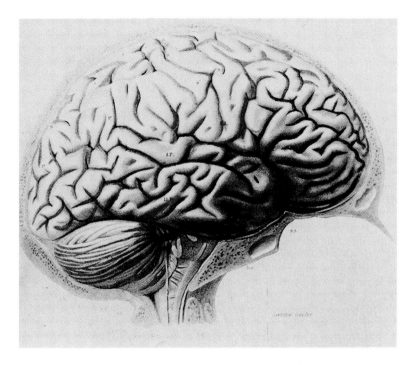

FIGURE 131

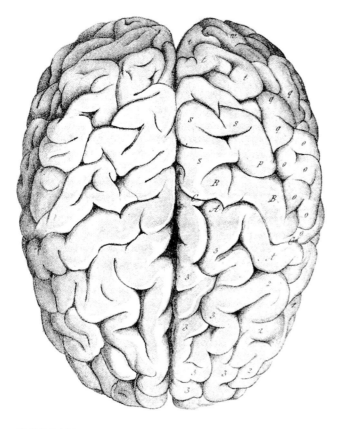

FIGURE 132

FIGURE 132 (LEFT)

The technological revolution of the 19th century brought forth the photographer who replaced the artist as the middle man between the anatomist and his reader. The camera recorded with utmost faithfulness and could, if used legitimately, neither conceal, distort, misinterpret, nor indulge in artistic licence. It was indeed the ultimate in precisional reproduction.

This is the first lithograph photograph of the brain by a little-known anatomist, Emil Huschke (1797–1858) of Jena.[23] It appeared in 1854[24] and was the first step towards direct photography of the brain. The title of Huschke's book is a reminder of earlier centuries when the cerebral location of the soul was debated (p. 3), and race and ethics were also discussed. In addition, Huschke contributed to gyral morphology by naming the "fusiform" and "lingual" convolutions.

FIGURE 133 (OPPOSITE)

The final phase in the process of unravelling, defining, tracing and naming the cerebral convolutions was carried out by a Scot and a German. The former, William Turner (1832–1916) Professor of Anatomy in the University of Edinburgh,[25] published his researches in 1866.[26] He redefined the limits of the cerebral lobes, and generally supplemented Gratiolet's detailed studies by, for example, establishing the fissure of Rolando as the posterior limit of the frontal lobe. Figure 133 illustrates some of his work.[27] Darwinian evolutionary theory must now be considered in relation to the correlation between the gyral patterns of animals and man with intelligence, a problem which is still unresolved.[28]

FIGURE 134 (FOLLOWING PAGE)

The German anatomist was Alexander Ecker (1876–1887) of Freiburg,[29] who, with obsessional exactitude gave an even more detailed account than Turner of the gyri and sulci. His little book of 1869[30] greatly contributed to the dissemination of his ideas which became better known than Turner's there was an English translation in 1873.[31] In Figure 134 the main sulci and gyri are named; "F" is for frontal, "T" temporal, etc.[32]

As might be expected, increased knowledge of form turned investigators' thoughts to functional problems. Now that the gyri and sulci had been

FIG. 1.

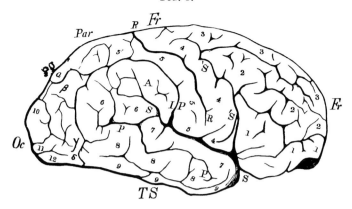

Note of Explanation to FIG. 1.—This and the succeeding outline figures are drawn from nature, with the help of the camera lucida, from the brain of a Scotchman, aged 23 :—Fig. 1. A profile view.—Fr., Fr., frontal lobe. Par., parietal lobe. Oc., occipital lobe. T. S., temporo-sphenoidal lobe. S. S., horizontal ; and ʻS. ʻS., ascending limb of the Sylvian fissure. R., R., fissure of Rolando. I. P., intra-parietal ; and P. P., parallel fissures. 1, 1, 1, inferior ; 2, 2, 2, middle ; and 3, 3, 3, superior frontal gyri. 4, 4, ascending frontal ; and 5, 5, 5, ascending parietal gyri. 5', outer part of postero-parietal lobule. 6, 6, angular gyrus. 7, 7, superior ; 8, 8, 8, middle ; and 9, 9, 9, inferior temporo-sphenoidal gyri. 10, superior ; 11, middle ; and 12, inferior occipital gyri. A., supra-marginal lobule. α, β, γ, δ, first, second, third, and fourth annectent gyri.

FIG. 2.

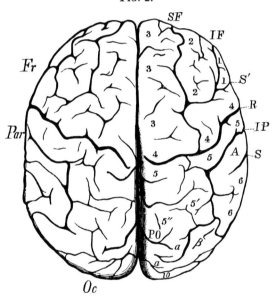

FIG. 2.—Vertex view of the Brain represented in Fig. 1. The same letters and numerals indicate the same parts. In addition, note PO, the parieto-occipital fissure, the external part of which, unshaded, is continuous with the internal part represented in shadow. SF, supero-frontal, and IF, infero-frontal fissure.

FIGURE 133

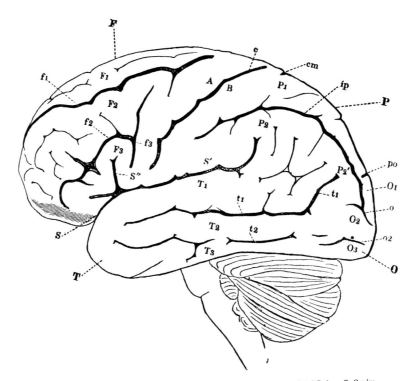

FIG. 1.—LATERAL VIEW OF THE BRAIN.   F. Frontal Lobe. P. Parietal Lobe. O. Occipital Lobe. T. Temporo-Sphenoidal Lobe.   S. Fissure of Sylvius. S′ horizontal, S″ ascending ramus of the same.   c. Sulcus Centralis. A. Anterior, B Posterior Central Convolution. F_1 Superior, F_2 Middle, F_3 Inferior Frontal Convolutions. f_1 Superior, f_2 Inferior Frontal Sulcus. f_3 Sulcus Praecentralis. P_1 Superior Parietal Lobule. P_2 Inferior Parietal Lobule, viz. P_2 Gyrus Supramarginalis, P_2′ Gyrus Angularis.   ip. Sulcus Interparietalis.   cm. Termination of the Calloso-marginal Fissure. O_1 First, O_2 Second, O_3 Third, Occipital Convolutions.   po. Parieto-occipital Fissure.   o. Sulcus Occipitalis transversus. o_2 Sulcus Occipitalis longitudinalis inferior. T_1 First, T_2 Second, T_3 Third, Temporo-Sphenoidal Convolutions. t_1 First, t_2 Second, Temporo-sphenoidal Fissures.

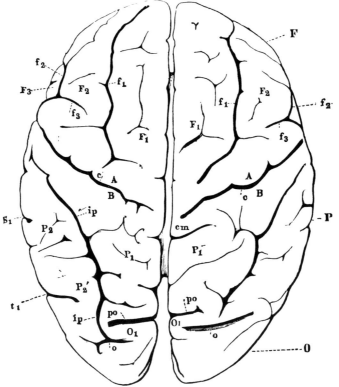

FIG. 2.—VIEW OF THE BRAIN FROM ABOVE.   F. Frontal Lobe. P. Parietal Lobe. O. Occipital Lobe. S_1 End of the horizontal ramus of the Fissure of Sylvius.   c. Central Fissure. A. Anterior, B. Posterior Central Convolution. F_1 Superior, F_2 Middle, F_3 Inferior Frontal Convolution. f_1 Superior, f_2 Inferior Frontal Sulcus. f_3 Sulcus Praecentralis. P_1 Superior Parietal Lobule. P_2 Inferior Parietal Lobule, viz., P_2 Gyrus Supramarginalis, P_2′ Gyrus Angularis.   ip. Interparietal Fissure. cm. Calloso-marginal Fissure.   po. Parieto-occipital Fissure. t_1 Superior Temporo-sphenoidal Fissure. O_1 First Occipital Convolution.   o. Sulcus Occipitalis transversus.

FIGURE 134

accurately delineated and named, what did they do? While the final phases in the elucidation of the anatomy of the cerebral convolutions was being enacted during the 1860's the stage was set for the emergence of new concepts concerning functional localization which will be discussed in the next chapter. Before doing so the history of the convolutions up to the present day must be very briefly mentioned.

FIGURE 135

Photography and other techniques of depicting and recording have largely replaced the artist, although in special circumstances his help is invaluable. The monumental collections of photographs of brain sections made by Luys should be mentioned here although they do not deal with surface characteristics.[33] This photograph is of the brain of Sir William Osler, physician and medical historian, who died in 1919.[34]

FIGURE 136

This shows the cerebral surface as seen during life through a craniotomy.[35] The bone-flap has been turned back and the dura mater opened to reveal the gyri, sulci and associated blood vessels. Many will agree that there *is* a faint resemblance to the abdominal contents of an animal with its tight-packed coils of ileum, which brings us back full circle to Erasistratus in the third century B.C.

A number of problems concerning the morphology of the cerebral convolutions still remain: their mode of production; the specificity of their arrangement in individuals, their phylogeny and function and, in particular, their possible correlation with intelligence.

It may well be that interest has lagged somewhat in this area of research as attention is more often focussed on more exciting and dynamic problems needing sophisticated machines and techniques for their elucidation.

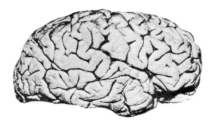

FIGURE 135

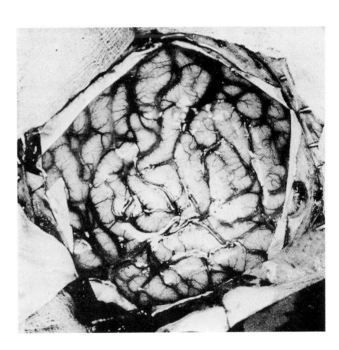

FIGURE 136

NOTES

1. For an excellent survey, see, F. Schiller, "The rise of the 'enteroid processes' in the 19th century. Some landmarks in cerebral nomenclature", *Bull. Hist. Med.,* 1965, *39*:326–338. Friedrich Arnold *(Bemerkungen über den Bau des Hirns und Rückenmarks . . .,* Zürich, S. Höhr, 1838, pp. 51–52) gave the names "frontal", "parietal", etc. to the lobes, whereas Haller applied them to imprecise regions (see, Figure 111). See also, A. Meyer, *Historical aspects of cerebral anatomy,* London, Oxford University Press, 1971, pp. 121–153 for an authoritative history of the gyri.

2. McD. Critchley, "Neurology's debt to F. J. Gall (1758–1828)", *Brit. med. J.,* 1965, *ii*:775–781.

3. F. J. Gall & G. Spurzheim, *Recherches sur le système nerveux en général, et sur celui du cerveau en particulier; Mémoire présenté à l'Institut de France le 14 mars 1808 . . .,* Paris, 1811.

4. F. J. Gall & G. Spurzheim, *Anatomie et physiologie du système nerveux en général, et du cerveau en particulier*, Paris. F. Schoell, *et al.*, 1810–1819. These illustrations are from the *Atlas* which is usually at the end of Vol. 1: Plates IV, VIII, and XI.

5. P. Flourens, "Éloge historique de Frédéric Tiedemann", *Recueils des éloges historiques,* Paris, Garnier Frères, 1862, pp. 251–295; K. Licktelg, *Die Verdienste des Heidelberger Professors Friedrich Tiedemann um die Entwicklung der Heilkunde,* in, Heft 9 of *Dusseldorfer Arbeit. Gesch. Med.,* 1939.

6. F. Tiedemann, *Anatomie und Bildungsgeschichte des Gehirns im Foetus des Menschen . . .,* Nürnberg, Stein, 1816. See, Clarke & O'Malley *(op. cit.,* Chapt. 2, note 15), pp. 395–397.

7. F. Tiedemann, *op. cit.,* note 6 above, Taf. V, Fig. 1.

8. *Icones cerebri simirium,* Heidelberg, Mohr & Winter, 1821.

9. R. Owen, *The life of Richard Owen,* London, J. Murray, 1894, 2 vols.; N. Rupke, *Robert Owen,* New Haven, Yale University Press, 1994.

10. "On the anatomy of the cheetah, *Felix jubata,* Schreb", *Trans. Zool. Soc. London,* 1835, 1:129–136. Figure 127 is from Plate XX, Fig. 1, superior view of the brain of the Cheetah.

11. Clarke & O'Malley *(op. cit.,* Chapt. 2, note 15), pp. 397–399.

12. *Op. cit.* above, note 10, pp. 135–136, note 3.

13. R. Semelaigne, *Les pionniers de la psychiatrie française avant et après Pinel,* Vol. 1, Paris, J. B. Baillière, 1930, pp. 214–226.

14. *Anatomie comparée du système nerveux considéré dans ses rapports avec l'intelligence,* Paris, J. B. Baillière, 1839. This is Vol. 1 of Leuret & Gratiolet (see below, note 21).

15. *Ibid.,* Plate XV.

16. "Die sylvische Grube", *Arch. Physiol.,* Halle, 1809, 9:195–208, see pp. 196–197.

17. L. Rolando, "Della struttura degli emisferi cerebrali", *Mem. r. Accad. Sci. Torino,* 1830, 35:103–146. Figure 129 is "Fig. 1". (This had appeared in book form with same title, Turin, 1829.)

18. L. Grandeau, *Pierre Gratiolet,* Paris, Hetzel, 1865; P. Broca, "Éloge funèbre de Pierre Gratiolet", *Mém. Soc. Anthrop. Paris,* 1865, 2:cxii–cxviii.

19. L. P. Gratiolet, *Mémoire sur les plis cérébraux de l'homme et des primates,* Paris, A. Bertrand, 1854. See, Clarke & O'Malley *(op. cit.,* Chapt. 2, note 15), pp. 403–407.

20. Planche I, Fig. 2, of *Atlas* which is bound separately. Brain of white Frenchman, "forme restituée".

21. F. Leuret & L. P. Gratiolet, *Anatomie comparée du système nerveux . . .,* 2 vols., Paris, J. B. Baillière, 1839–1857. Vol. 1 by Leuret (see note 14 above) and Vol. 2 by Gratiolet.

22. Planche XXVII, Fig. 1, see footnote 1. In separate *Atlas,* dated, 1857.

23. "Emil Huschke", *Allgemeine Deutsche Biographie,* Leipzig, Duncker & Humblot, 1881, Vol. 13, pp. 449–451.

24. *Schädel, Hirn und Seele des Menschen und der Thiere nach Alter, Geschlecht und Raçe,* Jena, F. Mauke, 1854, Tafel V, Fig. 1. It is from a 29-year old male German, seen from above. See, Clarke & O'Malley *(op. cit.,* Chapt. 2, note 15), pp. 407–409.

25. A. L. Turner, *Sir William Turner, K.C.B., F.R.S.,* Edinburgh, Blackwood, 1919.

26. *The convolutions of the human cerebrum topographically considered,* Edinburgh, Machlachlan & Stewart, 1866. See, Clarke & O'Malley *(op. cit.,* Chapt. 2, note 15), pp. 409–412.

27. *Ibid.,* p. 9.

28. "There does not appear to be any correlation between the gyral pattern and the localization of function including intellectual capacity" (H. C. Elliott, *Textbook of neuro-anatomy,* 2nd edition, Philadelphia, Lippincott, 1969, p. 331).

29. J. Ranke, "Alexander Ecker", *Arch. Anthrop.,* 1887, 17:i-iv.

30. *Die Hirnwindung des Menschen nach eigenen Untersuchungen insbesondere über die Entwicklung derselben beim Föetus,* Braunschweig, F. Vieweg, 1869.

31. *On the convolutions of the human brain,* translated by J. C. Galton, London, Smith, Elder & Co., 1873.

32. Figures 134 A, B are on pp. 7 and 9 of original book (note 30 above) and on pp. 19 and 28 of the English version (note 31).

33. J. Luys, *Iconographie photographique des centres nerveux,* Paris, J. B. Baillière, 1873 (text with an atlas of 70 plates).

34. H. H. Donaldson, "A study of the brains of three scholars. Granville Stanley Hall. Sir William Osler. Edward Sylvester Morse", *J. Comp. Neurol.,* 1928, 46:1–95. Figure 129 is Plate 7.

35. H. C. Elliott, *(op. cit.* above, note 28), Plate III on p. 457. (With permission.)

This phase in the history of cerebral localization is well-known, owing partly to the widespread effect that the discovery of cortical function has had on the neurological sciences both clinical and basic, and partly to the fact that the study of modern concepts begins here; the present situation is but an extension of the pioneer endeavours now to be illustrated. It is not our intention to give a detailed survey of this fascinating development in the history of functional brain localization; instead we have selected appropriate illustrations of the major advances from the great mass of existing pictorial material in the form of cortical "maps". The text accompanying the figures will, of necessity, be lengthier than in earlier chapters because so much was happening in this period which extends from 1870 to 1936.

Pierre Flourens (1794–1867) of Paris[1] more than anyone was responsible for the abnegation of phrenology (see Chapter 10). By stimulation experiments and focal extirpation of the brain in animals he proved, in 1824, to his own and the satisfaction of many others, that although function was located in various parts of the brain the cerebrum was inexcitable, with intellectual and perceptual functions represented diffusely throughout the hemispheres.[2] Thus Flourens was the first to advance a field theory of cerebral equipotentiality[3] (see p. 128). In retrospect his techniques, observations, and deductions were faulty, but such was his authority that his conclusions remained orthodox doctrine for nearly fifty years. Whereas phrenology, as a science, was effectively unseated, the notion of functional localization in the cerebral cortex was not. Phrenology, however, had served its purpose as a useful catalyst, for it had brought together

our two main themes: the morphology of the cerebral gyri and the precise localization of function in the brain.

During the 1860's the description of the cerebral convolutions had reached the ultimate in pictorial representation (Chapter 11). Contemporaneously, histologists were rapidly increasing our knowledge of the neurone,[4] and the layers of cells and fibres in the cortex were being studied, particularly by T. Meynert between 1867 and 1868 who was enlarging on the earlier contributions of J. G. F. Baillarger (1840), R. Remak (1841), and R. A. von Koelliker (1852).[5] Individual cortical constituents were later to be identified, notably by V. A. Betz (1874), W. B. Lewis (1878), and Ramón y Cajal (1891).[6] At the same time attention was now being turned to the vital question of function within the cerebral cortex, and in 1866, Turner (see Figure 133) wrote: "The precise morphological investigations of the last few years into the cerebral convolutions have led to the revival in Paris of discussions, in which the doctrine of Gall and his disciples—that the brain is not one but consists of many organs—has been supported by new arguments and the opinion has been expressed that the primary convolutions, at least, are both morphologically and physiologically distinct organs . . ."[7]

The revolution in concepts of cortical function which was to usher in our present era began in 1870, when two Germans, Gustav Theodor Fritsch (1838–1927) and Eduard Hitzig (1838–1907) of Berlin, in opposition to Flourens, demonstrated the excitability of the cortex and its localized motor functions. They were responsible for only a part of the upheaval, however, for they were preceded by a group of investigators in Paris,[8] including

J. B. Bouillaud (1796–1875),[9] Pierre Broca (1824–1880),[10] and S. A. E. Aubertin (1825–?1893),[11] while in London an important contribution was made by J. Hughlings Jackson (1835–1911).[12] On the basis of clinical and pathological data and, in the case of Jackson, on additional evolutionary and philosophical premises originating with Herbert Spencer (1820–1903),[13] it was concluded that function is precisely represented in the cortex although not as the phrenologists had suggested. These early investigators were primarily concerned with speech and motor activity.

Such views, confirmed first by Fritsch and Hitzig, and then by David Ferrier (1843–1928) of London, opened up a sequence of investigations into this new field of neurophysiology with important clinical undertones. If there were specific cerebral areas representing neurological functions then lesions could be localized in corresponding regions of cortex by means of clinical manifestations. This basic research was an essential prelude to opening up the new field of brain surgery.[14]

Advances were made by physiologists (Figures 137, 138, 139), clinicians (Figure 141), neurosurgeons (Figures 140, 146), and by anatomists (Figures 142, 143, 144, 145) but a combination of disciplines also took place, when, for example, attempts were made to correlate structural and functional data (Figures 144, 145). There were also those who did not subscribe to the concept of localization and, like Flourens, preferred the theory of equipotentiality (see p. 128).

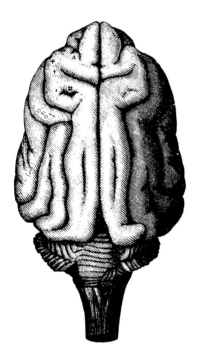

FIGURE 137

FIGURE 137 (LEFT)
In the 1860's clinical evidence for the focal representation of function in the cerebral cortex was accumulating but the basic experimental support for this notion came from the investigations of Fritsch and Hitzig, the results of which were published in 1870.[15] After exposing the brain of a dog they elicited movements of the contralateral limbs by galvanic stimulation of the cortex. Figure 137 is their drawing in which "centres" for movement are indicated: circles for the face, # for the hindlimb; plus-signs for the forelimb and a triangle for the neck. Moreover, in support of their findings, they discovered that removal of the areas they had delineated produced a disturbance of motor function in the opposite limbs. Although at first these findings and interpretations were not universally accepted, nevertheless they began an era of progress which still continues to stimulate new methods of investigation and which has revolutionized ideas of brain function.

FIGURES 138A–B (OPPOSITE)
Shortly after the pioneers Fritsch and Hitzig (Figure 137) had reported their results in 1870, a British school of cortical localizers came into being. The first representative was David Ferrier who, in 1873, carried out animal experiments at the West Riding Lunatic Asylum in order to test the views of Hughlings Jackson concerning the aetiology of unilateral epilepsy, based on the concepts of cortical localization.[16] Having fully confirmed Jackson's views by means of faradic electrical stimulation of the cortex, Ferrier repeated the work of Fritsch and Hitzig, and went on to pursue with

great precision and industry the general problem of the precise localization of cortical function in dogs, monkeys, and other vertebrates. He was particularly concerned in charting the focal "motor points".

Figure 138A shows the left hemisphere of a monkey on which the centres or areas of specific function have been marked with numbers or letters.[17] These relate mainly to motor function (numbers 1–12 and letters a b c d). Circles 13 & 13' localize the centre for vision, an error due probably to damage of neighbouring structures;[18] the centre for hearing is more correctly placed. Ferrier's results concerning the motor cortex in animals are still valid but unfortunately he transposed his findings in the monkey on to Ecker's outline of the human brain (see Figure 134) despite the fact that at that time there was virtually no experimental evidence of human cortical function.[19] Thus in Figure 138B the areas and numbers are located just as in Figure 138A, although he did mention that there were some differences. The two drawings first appeared side by side in 1876.[20] This was an understandable development as clinicians, like Ferrier himself, were keen to apply this new experimental knowledge to urgent problems of cerebral disease in man.

The cortical localizers were soon opposed by a growing faction of researchers who considered that massive inter-neural connections made it impossible precisely to localize function. This "global" concept was based on the theory of cerebral equipotentiality (see Chapter 13) which refers to the ability of any intact cortical area to execute the functions of other parts of the cortex. The main exponent of cerebral equipotentiality and leader of the anti-localizers was F. L. Goltz (1834–1902)[21] of Strassburg. His public encounter with Ferrier in 1881 at the International Medical Congress held in London is an historic event,[22] but provided only the opening exchanges in an argument that still continues unabated. In a pictorial history of brain localization, the anti-localizers are at an obvious disadvantage as they were implicitly opposed to the popular pursuit of cerebral cartography. Nevertheless their importance must not be underrated as they provided a useful and timely counterbalance to the over-exuberance of the more extreme and precise localizers. (See also, Chapter 13.)

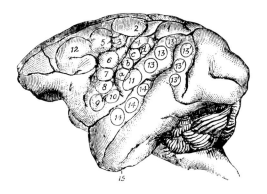

FIGURE 138A

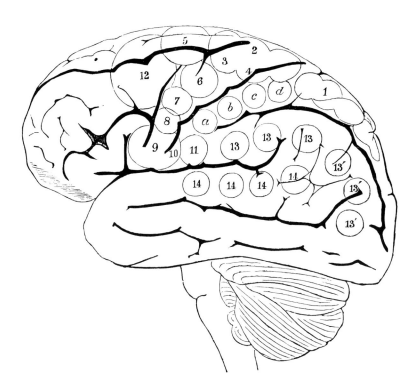

FIGURE 138B

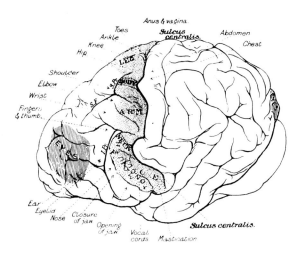 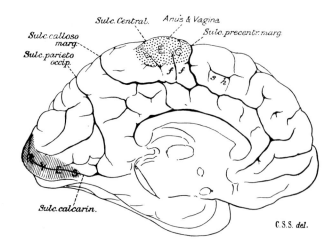

FIGURE 139A–B

FIGURES 139 A–B

Electrical stimulation of the cerebral cortex was now undertaken in several European and American centres. The second member of the British school was Victor Horsley (1857–1916) of University College Hospital, London,[23] who, with his colleagues, first extended Ferrier's investigations on the motor areas of the rhesus monkey, and also carried out similar experiments on the orang-utan and man.[24]

The third British series of experiments on cortical localization, in particular of motor activity, were those conducted during 1901 to 1906 by Charles Sherrington (1857–1952)[25] in collaboration with A. S. F. Grünbaum (1869–1921) and continued in greater detail in 1917 when the latter had changed his name to Leyton.[26] They were carrying Horsley's studies further as they plotted the motor cortex in the higher anthropoid apes. Figure 139A shows the findings of Grünbaum and Sherrington (1902);[27] it reveals the lateral surface of the cerebral hemisphere while Figure 139B illustrates the medial aspect.[28]

As in the case of Ferrier's work (Figures 138 A–B) Grünbaum and Sherrington's results were also transposed on to the human brain, mainly because of the evolutionary proximity of man's brain to that of the higher primates. But as Scarff has pointed out,[29] although there were 74 reports of electrical stimulation of the human motor cortex between 1874 and 1914 none of them gave any accurate information concerning the motor area. As in the case of Flourens (see p. 115) mistakes and deficiencies were due mainly to faulty techniques such as the use of unphysiological stimulation and the failure to achieve a standard threshold current. At the same time there was scanty information concerning the human cerebral cortex which led to faulty or incorrect observations and deductions.

FIGURE 140 (OPPOSITE TOP)

The widespread influence of Grünbaum and Sherrington's work stimulated several neurosurgeons to map the motor cortex in man, as the physiologists had done in animals. Thus Charles K. Mills and Charles H. Frazier of Philadelphia reported on the motor area, 1905–1906;[30] Harvey Cushing did likewise, 1907–1908,[31] followed by Fedor Krause (1857–1937)[32] of Berlin, 1908–1911. Although they all produced a schematic drawing of the motor area, Krause, who is usually claimed as the founder of German neurosurgery, may be taken as a representative of the group. Figure 140 shows his detailed pinpointing of the primary motor area in the left cerebral hemisphere of man.[33]

However, these cortical maps reveal more than was warranted by the experimental findings, and there is no doubt that some of the simian data of Grünbaum and Sherrington among others, had been incorporated. Thus Krause's drawing closely resembles that of Sherrington's (Figure 139A), reproduced on an earlier page of his book. He must have used it to supplement his general lack of data for there was at that time no reliable information on the human cortex in the literature to help him.

FIGURE 141 (OPPOSITE BOTTOM)

The clinical study of the human cortex also led to erroneous conclusions; thus Siegmund Exner's (1846–1926) book of 1881 on cortical localization contained maps based on the clinical manifestations of cerebral lesions.[34] An example of one of them is Figure 141, which is reminiscent of the obsessional physiognomy of Redfield (Figure 120). Exner was among those postulating the existence of precise functional "centres" with a minute parcellation of the cortex, based on the belief that

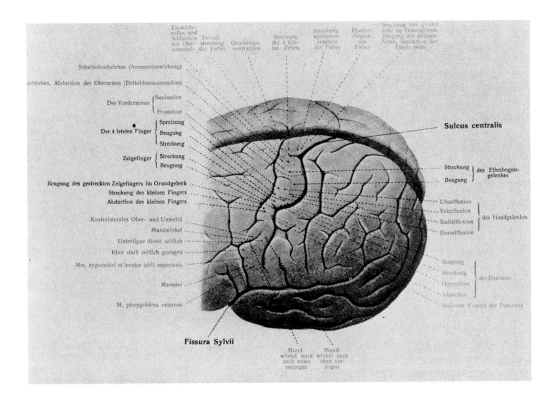

FIGURE 140

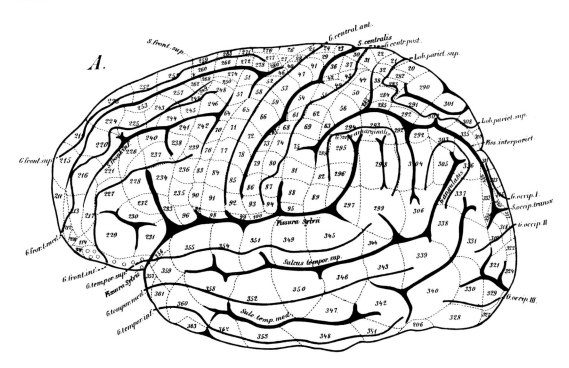

FIGURE 141

the site of a lesion producing a specific functional
disturbance indicated the location of that function.
He is best known for siting his "writing centre" in
the posterior part of the second frontal convolution.[35] Few of his conclusions are now acceptable.

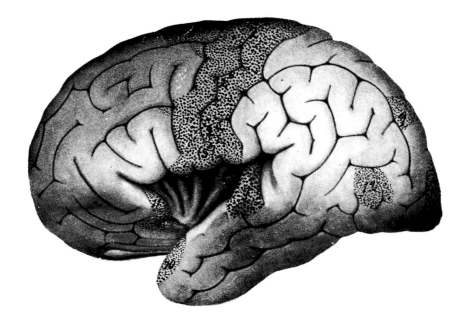

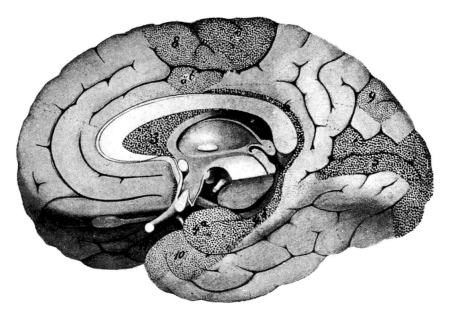

FIGURE 142A

FIGURES 142A–B
Another group of pioneers who studied the
cerebral cortex were the anatomists. Theodore
Meynert (1833–1892) was the first to relate
regional structural differences in the cerebral cortex
to their functions (1867–1868).[36] Paul Flechsig
(1847–1929)[37] was another outstanding representative. As well as pathological data he used his
technique of myelogenesis, based upon observations on the appearance of myelinization in the
sub-cortical white matter of the developing human
foetus and infant. This varies in time, and Flechsig
was able to identify the chronological appearance

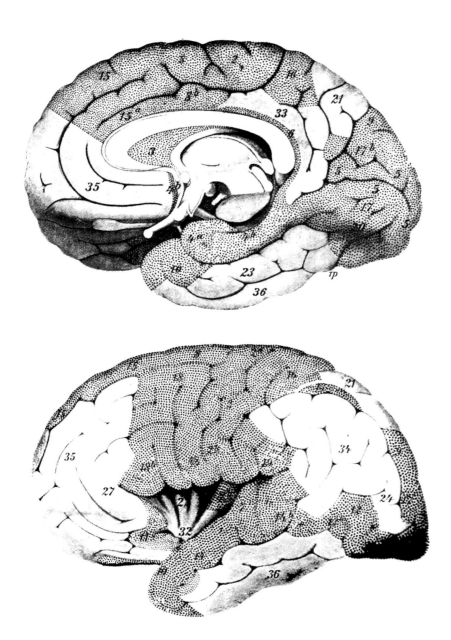

FIGURE 142B

of fibre groups, and thus outlined 36 specific and constant regions of cortex with which they are connected. Function is possible only when myelinization is complete. Figures 142A and B are from his report published in 1904.[38] Figure 142A shows with stippling numbered primary and secondary "projection" motor and sensory areas (1, 2, 4–8, 15) which mature before birth, together with unidentified areas (3, 9–13). Figure 142B illustrates the stippled "association" fields which mature after birth and control intellectual function, reading, etc. In each diagram, the numerals

indicate the sequence of myelinization, the lowest being the earliest. He regarded the parieto-temporo-occipital association areas as being the most important for intellectual activity, as lesions in this zone led to dementia. In this respect, however, it is likely that Flechsig was equating intellectual defects with speech disorders.

These studies generated much useful research and discussion, but a precise assessment of myelogenetic zones is still awaited.

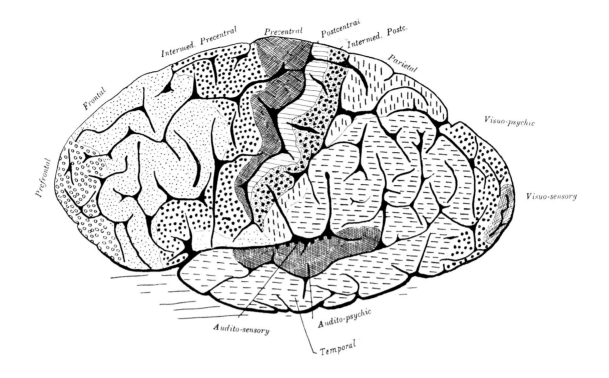

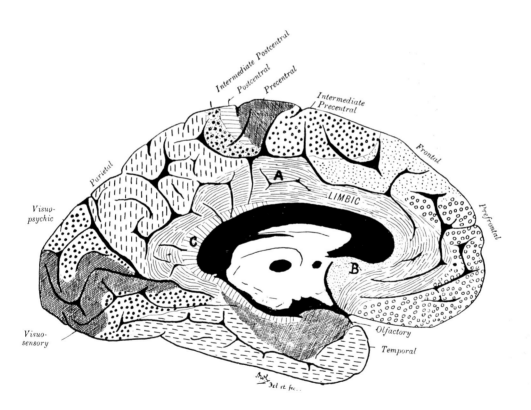

FIGURE 143

FIGURE 143 (OPPOSITE)

Another anatomical approach to the problem of cortical functional representation is architectonics, the microscopical study of the appearances of cells and fibres.[39] Morphologically distinct areas can be identified and hence it seemed reasonable to argue that a direct correlation with function may be found. An Australian, Walter Campbell (1868–1937), together with Brodmann (see Figure 144) and the Vogts (see Figure 145), helped to pioneer work in this exacting field of research.[40] Campbell's studies were based on functional concepts as he believed that the histologist must follow the physiologist and clinician in the investigation of cortical function in order to provide more accurate information on the extent and limits of differentiated areas. He carried out detailed examinations of human and animal brains and, in 1905, published his classic book from which Figure 143 is taken.[41] It depicts the human brain, "with a representation of the extent of the various areas defined . . . from an examination of cortical nerve fibres and nerve cells." Campbell pointed out the important deficiency of all such "maps" occasioned by the artist's inability (in this case the author himself) to show parts of the cortex concealed in the depths of the sulci. Unlike some of his German contemporaries, Campbell was more conservative in identifying distinct architectonic zones and hence his findings have been more widely accepted. This drawing has often been reproduced in textbooks of anatomy.

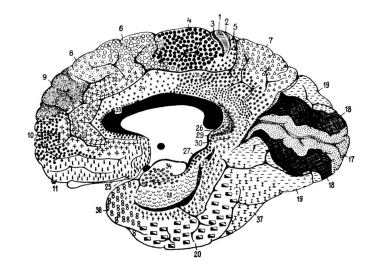

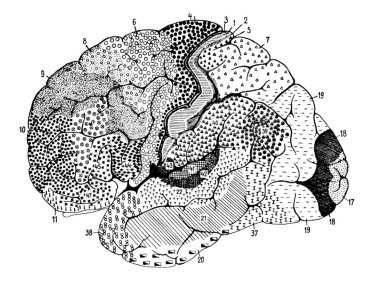

FIGURE 144

FIGURE 144 (RIGHT)

In the field of cyto-architectonics Korbinian Brodmann (1868–1918) was one of Campbell's German counterparts[42] and their investigations, although carried out independently, are essentially in agreement. Brodmann carried the parcellation of the cortex further and was more concerned with comparative studies of the mammalian cortex; his work forms the basis of this modern science. Strongly influenced by Oskar Vogt (see Figure 145) Brodmann with the aid of myelo-architectonics as well as cyto-architectonics helped to bring order into a confused state of knowledge by identifying 52 cortical areas grouped into eleven histological regions. His concept of an increasing differentiation during evolution has been amply confirmed. Brodmann's area numbers are still universally used as depicted in his cortical map (Figure 144) first published in 1908, but here taken from his famous book *Vergleichende Lokalisationslehre der*

Grosshirnrinde which appeared in 1909.[43] As with Krause and others (Figure 140), Brodmann's data on the human cortex does not seem to correlate with the precise areas outlined in his drawing. Nevertheless his studies stimulated much research, and although a good deal of it has been disproved, some of his conclusions are still acceptable. Like Campbell he was primarily concerned with "the advancement of knowledge of function and of pathological manifestations" (p. 285).

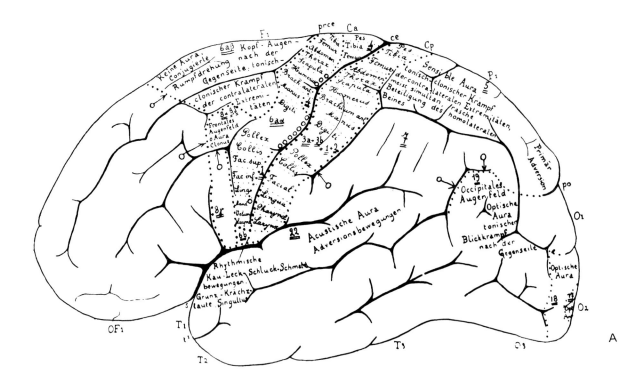

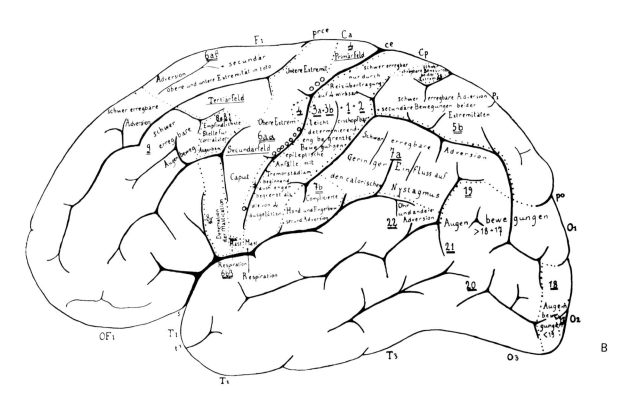

FIGURE 145

FIGURE 145

Oskar (1875–1962) and Cécile Vogt (1870–1959),[44] who had stimulated Brodmann in his cyto-architectonic investigations, dominated the field of cortical localization in the first few decades of the 20th century. In attempting to correlate more closely morphology with physiology they took the parcellation of the cortex to extremes by identifying more than one hundred zones. Their findings have not been generally accepted and, in fact, few have been able to repeat exactly the results of their investigations. Their contributions, nevertheless, were considerable, both anatomical and physiological, inasmuch as they carried out elaborate cyto-architectural studies of the brains of primates and man together with electrical excitation experiments especially in the monkey. It was once more a natural conjunction of the two ideas we have traced, the morphology and function of the cerebral cortex, although differing greatly from the phrenologists' approach (see Chapter 10). By applying the results of their comparative studies the Vogts were able to suggest where a certain cortical function might be localized in man without making a detailed study of the human brain. Thus animal physiology was again being transferred to man, just as Aristotle had done more than two millenia earlier.

The Vogts published their classic monograph on the long-tailed monkey in 1919.[45] In 1926 another historic article appeared,[46] from which Figure 145A is taken, illustrating their improved pattern of physiological fields based on animal histological data derived from their paper of 1919, but delineated on an outline of the human brain. This is their "human homologue". Figure 145B is their "synthetic" map constructed on the basis of their comparative anatomical studies wherein the various physiological fields, reported by Foerster (see Figure 146) in man, were named.

The influence of this work was as widespread as that of the British school of cortical stimulation and ablation (see Figures 138 A–B, 139 A–B) a few decades earlier, but its significance has still not been evaluated fully. However, it is clear that neurochemical and hormonal factors as well as morphological and electrophysiological findings should be taken into account in the study of the human cerebral cortex. The most vigorous and cogent criticism of architectonics was made by Lashley and Clark[47] who represent the non-localizers to be considered in the next chapter .

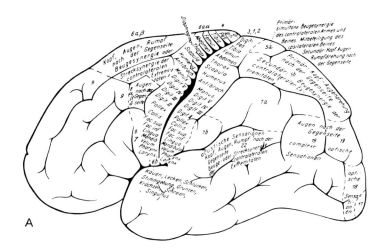

A

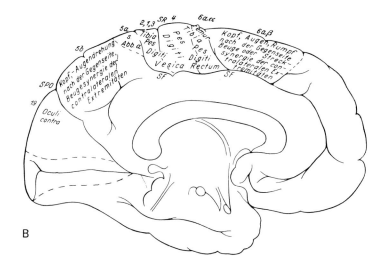

B

FIGURE 146

FIGURE 146

The massive treatise of C. von Economo (1876–1931) on cortical cyto-architectonics based on Brodmann's work, and published in 1925[48] helped to dissipate some of the confusion resulting from the Vogts' plethora of cortical areas, but of greater significance for the advancement of human cortical physiology was the work of O. Foerster (1873–1941) of Berlin.[49] In 1924 Foerster began his stimulation experiments on cortical function as an attempt to repeat in man what the Vogts had done in the monkey. His locations of cortical areas were similar, and as already seen (Figure 146B), the Vogts produced a "synthetic" diagram by superimposing their data on his observations in man. Hereafter, Foerster used his drawing in all subsequent publications with only minor changes.

Figures 146 A–B of 1936 depict his results.[50] The similarities with Figures 145 A–B are obvious, and the numbers follow closely those of Brodmann (Figure 144).

Foerster was a neurosurgeon, and his main interest in this field of research was the localization and excision of epileptogenic foci in the cerebral cortex. A young American, Wilder Penfield (1891–1976), later a naturalized Canadian citizen, worked with him in 1928, and for most of his professional life devoted his considerable energies and talents to a sustained study of the pathology and treatment of epilepsy. Using improved techniques he deviated from the precise areas of the Vogts and Foerster, except in parts of the pre- and post-central gyri and the calcarine but from this work derived some of the must important advances in our knowledge of cortical physiology. They will be discussed in the next chapter.

NOTES

1. J. M. D. Olmsted, "Pierre Flourens", in E. A. Underwood (editor), *Science, medicine ond history. Essays . . . in honour of Charles Singer,* Vol.2, London, Oxford University Press, 1953, pp. 290–302.

2. *Recherches expérimentales sur les propriétés et les fonctions du système nerveux dans les animaux vertèbres,* Paris, Crevot, 1824. Translations of parts of this influential work are in: G. von Bonin, *The cerebral cortex,* Springfield, Ill., C. C Thomas, 1960, pp. 1–21; J. F. Fulton & L.G. Wilson, *Selected readings in the history of physiology,* second edition Springfield, Ill. C. C Thomas, 1966, pp. 286–288. See also, Clarke & O'Malley (*op. cit.,* Chapt. 2, note 15), pp. 483–488 and J. P. Swazey, "Action propre and action commune. The localization of cerebral function", *J. Hist. Biol.,* 1970, 3:213–234.

3. B. Tizard, "Theories of brain localization from Flourens to Lashley", *Med. Hist.,* 1959, 3:132–145.

4. Clarke & O'Malley (*op. cit.,* Chapt. 2, note 15), pp. 67ff.

5. *Ibid.,* pp. 423–437. For Baillarger's paper in translation, see von Bonin (*op. cit.* above, note 2), pp. 22–48. See also, J. L. Conel "Contribution of S. Ramón y Cajal to the knowledge of the cortex", *New Engl. J. Med.,* 1953, 248:541–543.

6. Clarke & O'Malley (*op. cit,* Chapt. 2, note 15), pp. 437–447. For Ramón y Cajal on the cerebral cortex, see von Bonin (*op. cit.* above, note 2), pp. 251–282, who has translated his Chapter from *Histologie du système nerveux de l'homme et des vertébrés,* Paris, A. Maloine, 1909–1911; see also, *Studies on the cerebral cortex [limbic structures] by Santiago Ramón y Cajal,* London, Lloyd-Luke, 1955.

7. *Op. cit.,* Chapt. 11, note 26, p. 27.

8. The events at this famous series of debates in 1861 attended by Bouillaud, Aubertin, Broca, Gratiolet (Figures 130–131) amongst others have often been related. It centred on the problem of the location of language function in the cerebral hemisphere. It was, in fact, a "test case", because if the existence of one functional "centre" could be established then in time others would be identified. See, J. Soury, *Le système nerveux central,* Vol. 1, Paris, G. Carré & C. Naud, 1899, pp. 575–606; F Moutier, *L'aphasie de Broca,* Paris, G. Steinheil, 1908, pp. 17–32; H. Head, *Aphasia and kindred disorders of speech,* Vol.1, Cambridge, University Press, 1926, pp. 12–29; B. Stookey, "A note on the early history of cerebral localization", *Bull. N.Y. Acad. Med.,* 1954, 30:559–578; Clarke & O'Malley (*op. cit.,* Chapt. 2, note 15), pp. 488–497; R. M. Young, *Mind, brain and adaptation in the nineteenth century,* Oxford, Clarendon Press, 1970, pp. 134–149.

9. Extracts from his writings and from those of the other participants in Paris are in Clarke & O'Malley, (*op. cit.,* Chapt. 2, note 15). See also, B. Stookey, "Jean-Baptiste Bouillaud and Ernest Aubertin. Early studies on cerebral localization and the speech center", *J. Amer. med. Assoc.,* 1963, 184:1024–1029.

10. Seo also, von Bonin (*op. cit.* above, note 2), pp. 48–72; R. H. Wilkins, *Neurosurgical classics,* New York & London, Johnson Reprint Corporation, 1965, pp. 61–68.

11. See also, Stookey (*op. cit.* above, note 9) who, however, over-emphasizes the role of Aubertin in the proceedings.

12. W. Broadbent, "Hughlings Jackson as pioneer in nervous physiology and pathology", *Brain,* 1903, 26:305–366; Clarke & O'Malley (*op. cit.,* Chapt. 2, note 15), pp. 499–505; Young (*op. cit.* above, note 8), pp. 197–223; S.H. Greenblatt, "Hughlings Jackson's first encounter with the work of Paul Broca; the physiological and philosophical background", *Bull. Hist. Med.,* 1970, 44:555–570; F. M. R. Walshe, "Some reflections upon the opening phase of the physiology of the cerebral cortex, 1850–1900", in, Poynter (*op. cit.,* Chapt. 2, note 18), pp. 223–224.

13. Clarke & O'Malley, (*op. cit.,* Chapt. 2, note 15), pp. 497–499; Young, (*op. cit.,* note 8 above), pp. 150–203.

14. J. E. Scarff, "Primary cortical centers for movements of upper and lower limbs in man", *Arch. Neurol. Psychiat.,* 1940, 44:243–299.

15. G. Fritsch & L. Hitzig, "Über die elektrische Erregbarkeit des Grosshirns", *Arch. Anat. Physiol.,* 1870, pp. 300–332. Translations into English in: von Bonin (*op. cit.* above, note 2), pp. 73–96; Wilkins (*op. cit.* above, note 10), pp. 15–27; extracts in Clarke & O'Malley (*op. cit.,* Chapt. 2, note 15), pp. 507–511. See also Young (*op. cit.* above, note 8), pp. 224–233.

16. "Experimental researches in cerebral physiology and pathology", *West Riding Lun. Asyl. Med. Rep.,* 1873, 3:30–96. Further results in *The functions of the brain,* London, Smith, Elder & Co., 1876. See, Clarke & O'Malley (*op. cit,* Chapt. 2, note 15), pp. 513–518; Young (*op. cit.* above, note 8), pp. 234–248. See also, H. R. Viets, "West Riding, 1871–1876", *Bull. Hist. Med.,* 1938, 6:477–487.

17. Ferrier, *ibid.,* (1876), Fig.64 on p. 305.

18. A. E. Walker, "Stimulation and ablation. Their role in the history of cerebral physiology", *J. Neurophysiol.,* 1957, 20:435–449.

19. Roberts Bartholow (1831–1904) of Cincinatti alone had reported data from the human brain: "Experimental investigations into the functions of the human brain", *Am. J. med. Sci.,* 1874, 67:305–313. See A. E Walker, "The development of the concept of cerebral localization in the nineteenth century", *Bull. Hist. Med.,* 1937, 31:99–121; Clarke & O'Malley (*op. cit.,* Chapt. 2, note 15), pp. 511–513.

20. Ferrier (1876, *op.cit.* above, note 16). Our Figure 138A is Fig. 64 on p. 305 and Figure 138B is Fig. 63 on p. 304.

21. von Bonin (*op. cit.* above, note 2), pp. 118–158, gives a translation of one of Goltz's important papers published in 1888. Clarke & O'Malley (*op. cit.,* Chapt. 2. note 15), pp. 558–575.

22. See Wilkins (*op. cit.* above, note 10), pp. 119–129.

23. S. Paget, *Sir Victor Horsley. A study of his life and work,* London, Constable, 1919.

24. See, Scarff (*op. cit.* above, note 14), for references to his work .

25. Lord Cohen of Birkenhead, *Sherrington. Physiologist, philosopher and poet,* Liverpool, University Press, 1958; R. Granit, *Charles Sherrington. An appraisal,* London, Nelson, 1966.

26. This paper ("Observations on the excitable cortex of the chimpanzee, orang-utan and gorilla", *Quart. J. exper. Physiol.,* 1917, *11*:135–222) is reprinted by von Bonin (*op. cit.* above, note 2), pp.283–396.

27. "Observations on the physiology of the cerebral cortex of some of the higher apes. (Preliminary communication)", *Proc. Roy. Soc. London,* 1902, *69*:206–209, Plate 4.

28. "Observations on the physiology of the cerebral cortex of the anthropoid apes", *ibid.,* 1903, *72*:152–155.

29. *Op. cit.* above, note 14.

30. "The motor area of the human cerebrum. Its position and its subdivisions, with some discussions of the surgery of this area", *Univ. Pennsylvannia M. Bull.,* 1905–1906, *18*:135–147.

31. "Surgery of the head", in, W.W. Keen (editor), *Surgery, its principles and practice,* Vol. 3, Philadelphia, W. B. Saunders, 1908, pp. 17–276. For an earlier article on motor and sensory responses, see, Fulton & Wilson (*op.cit.* above, note 2), pp. 313–314.

32. "Fedor Krause 1956[*sic*]–1937", in, A. E. Walker, A *history of neurological surgery,* Baltimore, Williams & Wilkins, 1951, pp. 248–249; C. M. Behrend, "Fedor Krause (1857–1937)", in K. Kolle (editor), *Grosse Nervenärzte,* Vol. 3, Stuttgart, G. Thieme, 1963, pp. 199–206.

33. *Chirurgie des Gehirns und Rückenmarkes nach eigenen Erfahrungen,* Vol. 2, Berlin, Urban & Schwarzenberg, 1911, Fig.66 on p.185; see, Clarke & O'Malley (*op. cit.,* Chapt. 2, note 15), pp. 523–526.

34. *Untersuchungen über Localisation der Functionen in der Grosshirnrinde des Menschen,* Vienna, W. Braümuller, 1881, Taf. 1A.

35. For an excellent and brief account of "The history of thought about aphasia", see, R. Brain, *Speech disorders. Aphasia, apraxia and agnosia,* London, Butterworth, 1961, pp. 30–53.

36. Clarke & O'Malley (*op. cit.,* Chapt. 2, note 15), pp. 432–437; von Bonin (*op. cit.* above, note 2) has a translation of a later paper of 1891, "Über das Zusammenwirken der Gehirntheile" on pp. 159–180.

37. *Meine myelogenetische Hirnlehre mit biographischer Einleitung,* Berlin, J. Springer, 1927.

38. "Einige Bemerkungen über die Untersuchungsmethoden der Grosshirnrinde, insbesondere des Menschen", *Ber. Verh. k. sächs Ges. Wiss. Leipz.,* Math.-Phys. Klasse, 1904, *56*:50–104, 177–248, Taf. 1, figs.1–2. See also, von Bonin (*op. cit.* above, note 2), pp. 181–200 for his paper on brain physiology and theories of volition; Clarke & O'Malley (*op. cit.,* Chapt. 2, note 15), pp. 548–554.

39. R. Lorente de Nó gives a brief history in, J. F. Fulton, *Physiology of the nervous system,* third edition, New York, Oxford University Press, 1949, pp. 288–293.

40. W. Haymaker & F. Schiller, *The founders of neurology,* second edition, Springfield, Ill., C. C Thomas, 1970, pp. 102–104.

41. *Histological studies on* the *localisation of cerebral function,* Cambridge, University Press, 1905, Plate 1.

42. *Op. cit.* above, note 40, pp. 99–101.

43. *Vergleichende Lokalisationslehre der Grosshirnrinde in ihren Prinzipien dargestellt auf Grund des Zellenbaues,* Leipzig, J. A. Barth, 1909. See, von Bonin (*op. cit.* above, note 2), pp. 201–230 for translation of Chapter IX. See also, Clarke & O'Malley (*op. cit.,* Chapt. 2, note 15), pp. 450–453 and 554–558.

44. W. Haymaker, "Cécile and Oskar Vogt. On the occasion of her 75th and his 80th birthday", *Neurology,* 1951, *1*:179–218.

45. C. Vogt & O. Vogt, "Allgemeinere Ergebnisse unserer Hirnforschung", *J. Psychol. Neurol.,* 1919, *25*(Suppl.):279–461.

46. "Die vergleichend-architektonische und die vergleichend-reiz-physiologische Felderung der Grosshirnrinde unter besonderer Berücksichtigung der menschlichen", *Die Naturwissenschaften,* 1926, *14*:1190–1194. Our Figures 145 A–B are Fig. 3–4 respectively.

47. K. S. Lashley & G. Clark, "The cytoarchitecture of the cerebral cortex of Ateles: a critical examination of architectonic studies", *J. Comp. Neurol.,* 1946, *85* :223–305.

48. C. von Economo & G. N. Koskinas, *Die Cytoarchitektonik der Hirnrinde des erwachsenen Menschen,* Vienna, J. Springer, 1925. A briefer account in, C. von Economo, *L'architecture cellulaire normale de l'écorce cérébrale,* Paris, Masson, 1927, with its English version, *The cytoarchitectonics of the human cerebral cortex,* London, Oxford University Press, 1929, by S. Parker.

49. K. J. Zülch, *Otfrid Foerster. Physician and naturalist,* Berlin, Springer-Verlag, 1969.

50. O. Foerster, "Motorische Felder und Bahnen", in, O. Bumke & O. Foerster (editors), *Handbuch der Neurologie,* Vol.6, Berlin, J. Springer, 1936, Abb. 69a and b, on p. 50.

CORTICAL LOCALIZATION
IN 1972

13

1. INTRODUCTION

The extensive literature on the localization of cortical function is still lacking in coherence and abounds with inconsistencies. It covers a wide range of disciplines and without mastery of all of them a balanced and critical appraisal is well nigh impossible. Another problem is that of validating and interpreting an accumulation of clinical and experimental evidence from animals and man. How relevant to man is information gleaned from animal studies? What reliance can be placed on subjective evidence? Is the illogical procedure of studying the effects of cortical lesions of any real value in the investigation of normal behaviour in man? What are the effects of a concomitant cortical lesion on deductions about localization? To these general problems there are certain additional difficulties associated with a presentation which is essentially pictorial rather than textual.

There are obvious hazards in attempting a graphic summary of cortical localization, and those indulging in this pursuit have been disparagingly dismissed by Head as "diagram makers". But the theoretical undertones concerning the localization of higher nervous functions are, in fact, quite beyond the reach of even the most diligent cartographer. Hence this text is lengthier, and the illustrations less numerous, than those of preceding chapters. Cortical map-makers run the risk of over-simplifying a complicated subject while ignoring the integrative aspects of brain function. Nevertheless, we intend to adhere unrepentant to our pictorial theme And there may be some, like us, who, having travelled laboriously through the jungle of verbiage with which the subject of cortical localization is overgrown, will be greatly relieved to reach the open country of cortical cartography. We are aware, too, that in presenting a graphic summary of some modern trends in cortical localization we may well have transgressed an important historical and tactical maxim by presenting a lengthy front with but light defence in depth. But in such a full field of enquiry some degree of selectivity is inevitable. In general we have tended to concentrate more on clinical studies rather than on animal experimental work undertaken by physiologists and psychologists. The aftermath of the last war with its heavy toll of penetrating missile injuries of the brain has proved to be a fruitful field of combined enquiry by neurologists, psychiatrists and psychologists. Such surgical advances as commissurectomy and the ablation of various lobes together with psychosurgical procedures for the relief of psychoses or epilepsy; studies of congenitally abnormal brains and direct cortical stimulation have all contributed to the increasing knowledge of cortical function.

This chapter is not intended to be a critical review of recent trends suitable for research workers in the localizing field but simply an illustrated sequel to our survey of the changing concepts of cortical localization in man. In attempting to impose order by means of illustrations on a confused and disorganized field of enquiry we are aware that we are helping to bring the historical wheel full circle as our cortical maps are not unlike those of the phrenologists. Indeed, McFie[1] points out that there is little virtue in unnecessarily changing names, and he regards phrenology to be just as adequate as the newly-coined term neuropsychology: the older term does, at least, recognize the intuitive genius of these pioneers in the localization of intellectual functions.

2. THEORIES OF CORTICAL LOCALIZATION

In the last chapter we have traced the gradual emergence of two opposing theories of cortical localization: those who believed that brain functions, including intellectual processes, can be precisely localized, and others, the anti-localizers who considered that massive inter-neural connections render attempts at precise localization meaningless. During the earlier part of this century the anti-localizers gained considerable impetus from the work of Karl Lashley[2] (1890–1958) who showed that the degree of impairment of maze learning ability in the rat depended not on the site of ablation but on the amount of cortical tissue removed. Lashley followed the global concept of cerebral function based on the theory of cerebral equipotentiality which refers to the ability of any intact cortical area to execute the functions of other parts of the cortex although some loss of efficiency will usually result. This theory of functional equivalence first propounded by Goltz[3] depends, in turn, on the principle of mass action developed by Lashley. The efficiency of cerebral functions, as reflected in complex patterns of behaviour, may be reduced in proportion to the loss of cortical tissue from the whole mass of relatively unspecified parts. Early studies of intelligence supported Lashley's global view, although he was aware that to equate learning capacity with intelligence might be unjustified. With the accumulation of evidence from clinical studies adherents of the global theory began to lose ground, and Lashley[4] himself modified his theory in respect of the human brain to allow for regional subdivisions of verbal and non-verbal cognitive abilities. Thus, as McFie[5] points out, Lashley's original theory of "total equipotentiality" was modified to one of "areal equipotentiality".

Russian views on cerebral localization have been summarized by Luria[6] who adopts the concept of functional pleuripotentialism introduced by Filimonov.[7] This implies that no part of the cortex is solely responsible for a single nervous function as, under certain conditions, each part of the brain may perform other functions. This theory depends, to some extent, on Filimonov's study of the olfactory structures of the dolphin, and other anosmatic animals. He considers that the dolphin's olfactory structures have some function other than smell and the fact that isolated areas of sensory function are found

in the motor cortex and similarly occasional motor zones exist in sensory areas, lends support to these views. In a review of cortical somatic sensory areas Nakahama[9] lends further support to this theory of multiple cortical function by identifying four somato-topically organized regions, each of them concerned with sensory and motor functions. These somatic zones appear to be linked ipsilaterally and contralaterally to each other with feedback circuits between them. According to Luria,[10] this concept of graded localization of function and pleuripotentialism is the basis of "the principle of dynamic localization" formulated by Pavlov.

It would seem that extreme theoretical attitudes on cerebral localization can now be discounted. In particular, the "unitary" or "global" theory of brain function is no longer accepted uncritically.[11–12] Nevertheless, some psychologists, including Vernon[13] and Bruner,[14] still support Lashley's view of mass action as applied to human intelligence. They believe that intelligence is largely determined by environmental factors and explicitly reject the possibility of a correlation with specific areas of the brain.

It may well be that a cautious and qualified interpretation of cortical function may be acceptable in terms of all three theories. Regional specialization of relatively simple multiple functions may well co-exist with global aspects of complex behaviour in man: indeed Chapman and Wolff[15] have tried to reconcile these theories which they regard as "not antagonistic, but indeed, complementary".

3. DIRECT CORTICAL STIMULATION STUDIES

Wilder Penfield[16] and his associates at Montreal have made one of the most important contributions to our knowledge of cerebral localization by direct electrical stimulation of the cortex in fully conscious patients. When a threshold current is applied to the cortex various excitable areas yield responses which may be broadly classified as motor, sensory and psychical (see Figure 147).

Stimulation of the sensory area causes crude sensations of seeing, hearing or feeling, depending on the site. Somatic sensations include such subjective feelings as tingling or a sense of movement, visual responses consisting of moving lights, colours, or stars, and auditory phenomena including buzzing, whispering, singing or thumping sounds. Thus the patient is conscious of only the elementary sensations. Similarly the motor sequence presents with a succession of parts, beginning with the toes

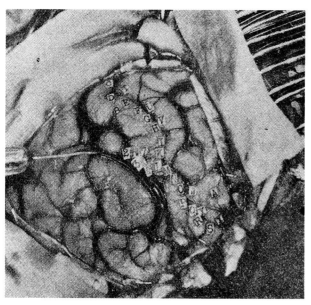

FIGURE 147

FIGURE 147
A photograph at operation showing the electrode poised for cortical stimulation (Penfield and Boldrey, 1937, p. 400, Figure 4).

FIGURE 148
Sensory and motor homunculus. The general order of representation and relative extent occupied in the sensorimotor strip are indicated (Penfield and Boldrey, 1937, p. 432, Figure 28).

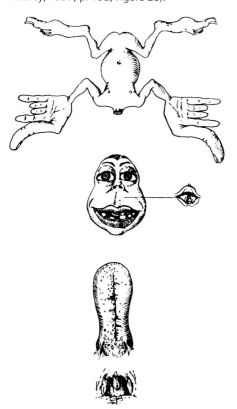

FIGURE 148

and reaches the Sylvian bank with salivation, mastication and swallowing. In general the sensations of each part of the postcentral gyrus and movements of the corresponding zone on the precentral gyrus are related to each other, indicating the presence of interconnecting fibres across the Rolandic fissure. In order to illustrate the order and comparative extent of cortical representation of elements in the sensory and motor sequence, Penfield and Boldrey[17] summarized their results in a combined sensory and motor homunculus (see Figure 148). Later Penfield and Rasmussen[18] separated the sensory homunculus from the motor homunculus, both of which were superimposed around the profile of one hemisphere in order to give a more realistic indication of the extent of representation (see Figures 149 and 150).

The most interesting and controversial information was obtained when the lateral aspects of the temporal lobes were stimulated. When the upper and lateral surfaces of the temporal or "perceptual" cortex were stimulated what Penfield terms "experiental illusions" recalling past memories were evoked. It was as though the subject was watching a play yet conscious of all around him. But the difference was (to use Penfield's picturesque analogy) that the subject "discovers himself on the stage of the past as well as in the audience of the present".[19] Stimulation of parts of the first temporal convolution of either hemisphere causes illusions of distance and the tempo of sounds whereas illusions of familiarity, or the *déjà vu* phenomenon, were confined to the minor hemisphere for speech and handedness.

Somatic aspects of the secondary sensory system were investigated by stimulation of the banks of the upper operculum with taste above and smell below the insula. Motor and sensory responses referrable to the alimentary system were evoked by stimulation of the insula itself; and stiffening of the whole body, various ill-defined sensations of the body and head together with feelings of heat and cold result from a discharge of the anterior mesial temporal lobe. Penfield[20] concludes that "a permanent record of the stream of consciousness" is stored away in the temporal lobe and that "these memories of past events are more complete and detailed than memories that can be voluntarily recalled". This aspect of Penfield's research has most often been misunderstood. He does not suggest that the engram and its thread of facilitation is localized in the temporal cortex immediately beneath the surgeon's electrode, but simply that there may be some scanning mechanism in the temporal cortex capable of activating, at a distance, the thread of facilitation.

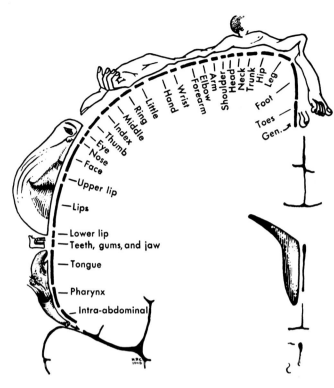

FIGURE 149
Sensory homunculus (Penfield and Rasmussen
1957, p. 44, Figure 17).

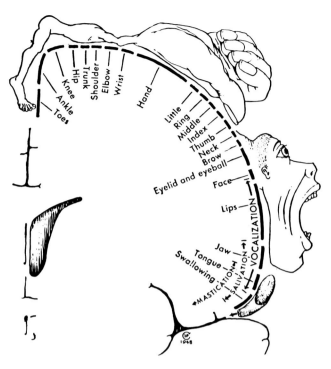

FIGURE 150
Motor homunculus (Penfield and Rasmussen,
1957, p. 57, Figure 22).

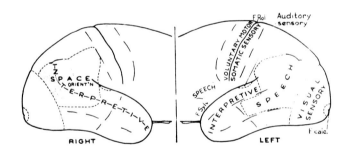

FIGURE 151

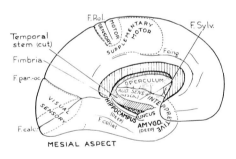

FIGURE 152

FIGURE 151
Lateral surfaces of the human brain showing areas
of language, learning and recall. (Penfield, 1968,
Fig.1.)

FIGURE 152
Mesial aspect of the left hemisphere (after removal
of insula and brain stem) showing the auditory
sensory cortex on the inner surface of the temporal
operculum together with some of the "introspec-
tive" cortex (Penfield, 1968, Fig. 3).

Penfield's extensive research on the human cortex readily lends itself to graphic summarization as in Figures 151 and 152.

One curious omission in Penfield's studies (in contrast to animal experiments) was the absence of erotic sexual arousal after cortical stimulation. A recent study[21] using implanted electroencephalographic electrodes inserted into the septal area caused pronounced sexual arousal in male and female patients. In the female, sexual arousal was stimulated by passing small quantities of acetylcholine or noradrenaline through a cannula into the septal region. The male patient, fitted with a self-

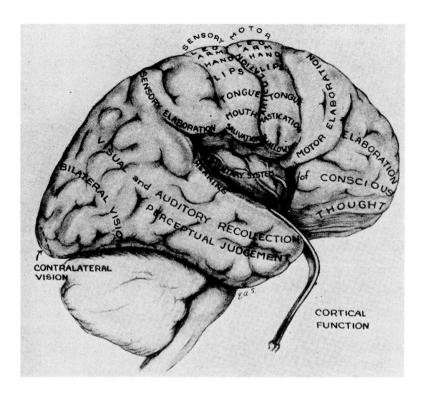

FIGURE 153

A summary of Penfield's conclusions on cortical localization including hypothetical ones such as the "elaboration zones" (from Penfield and Rasmussen, 1957, p. 210, Figure 206).

FIGURE 153

stimulating transistorized device, chose to stimulate the septal region repeatedly causing feelings of pleasure, alertness, goodwill and sexual arousal.

Although Penfield and Rasmussen[22] describe "illusions of introspection" concerning vaguely described reactions to the patient's environment or to his own body by stimulation of the posterior temporal area they never evoked gross disturbances of the body schema. Bollea[23] has reported a full autoscopic illusion after stimulating the area of the parieto-tempero-occipital confluence. Research of such revolutionary and extensive dimensions as that undertaken by Penfield and his associates cannot possibly be expected to escape unscathed from the net of critical commentary. And among psychologists, Piercy,[24] rejects Penfield's theory of the "stream of consciousness" owing to the fact that it is based on the subjective evidence of patients. Even more unacceptable does he find Penfield's[25] statement that "the hippocampus of the two sides is the repository of ganglionic patterns that preserve the record of the stream of consciousness". Piercy mentions that bilateral temporal lobectomy removes only recent memories, leaving remote memory intact.

Among clinicians, Whitty and Lishman[26] point out that the evoked memories described by Penfield have been found only in epileptic patients liable to spontaneous discharges. They suggest that the epileptogenic influence ought to be taken into account as the phenomenon described by Penfield appears to differ from normal recall in its vividness, wealth of detail and sense of immediacy, vesting the whole experience with the cloak of a true hallucination.

Nevertheless, by keeping within the limits imposed by ethical considerations, Penfield and his associates have amassed an immense amount of original information on cortical localization summarized in Figure 153. Their refreshing contributions to a field of enquiry abounding with conflicting theories is indisputably factual, although there may be occasional differences concerning the interpretation of some of their findings.

4. THE PSYCHOLOGIST AND CORTICAL LOCALIZATION

In a survey of brain functions Reitan[27] broadly divides research by psychologists into two groups. Clinical psychologists try to establish valid psychological measurements in patients with localized brain lesions which are then assessed and correlated with independent neurological data. Experimental psychologists tend to be more concerned with the investigation of brain behaviour relationship by undertaking a series of animal experiments. One obvious difficulty is that of assessing the relevance to man of information from animal studies, particularly in the sphere of higher nervous functions. Here we are more concerned with discussing problems facing the clinical psychologists in relation to their contributions to cortical localization.

It is often assumed that the psychological effects of brain lesions in man will be manifested similarly in every subject despite obvious variables. According to McFie[28] the nature of the lesion is one variable with little semeiological significance. Tumours, penetrating injuries, focal EEG abnormalities, atrophic processes and vascular accidents may result in syndromes involving disturbances of higher nervous functions which are indistinguishable. Busch[29] surveyed 662 cases of cerebral tumours and found that glioblastomas are twice as likely to result in mental symptoms as are astrocytomas or meningiomas. Reitan has suggested that a distinction can be made in patterns of intellectual impairment between static and rapidly advancing lesions although psychological signs are, in general, of little value in elucidating the nature of the pathological process. Attempts have been made to investigate other variables such as laterality (Anderson,[30] Reitan,[31] Hécaen et al.;[32] Semmes et al.[33]); localization (Semmes et al.;[34] Reitan[35]); chronicity (Fitzhugh et al.[36]); and age at occurrence of brain damage (Hebb,[37] Fitzhugh and Fitzhugh[38]). Thus one main research problem in clinical psychology is the need for a more rigorous methodological approach together with the assessment of independent and dependent variables.

As an example of a methodological shortcoming, Reitan cites an investigation designed to elucidate frontal lobe function. It is meaningless, he argues, to compare psychological deficits in patients with lesions in this area with a matched group of normal subjects. In order to put forward some hypothesis concerning frontal lobe function it is necessary to compare patients with frontal lobe deficits to another group with similar lesions in another part of the cortex.

Another possible hazard is to disregard the functional efficiency of the whole brain when investigating some localized cortical lesion. Results of psychological testing would obviously vary between one group of patients with localized lesions in otherwise healthy brains compared to a similar group with generalized arteriosclerotic changes.

Finally, the psychologists' tools should be scrutinized. The Wechsler scales, with verbal and non-verbal subtests, is of the utmost importance in psychological assessment. These scales, together with all other commonly used intelligence tests, are American and have never been standardized on a British population. In a strong plea for British standardized tests so that intellectual functions may be more precisely identified, McFie[39] states that a lack of standardization "greatly reduces the value of these tests as cultural differences are likely to affect some subtest scores more than others".

Having mentioned some problems facing the clinical psychologist we should now enquire as to his contributions in cortical localization. The combined efforts of clinicians and psychologists have, in fact, shown that large, and hitherto uncharted areas of the brain, formerly termed "silent areas", are concerned with higher intellectual functions. In particular such neurological disturbances as aphasia, apraxia, agnosia, acalculia, alexia and the like have been related to lesions in specific areas of the brain. The psychologists' contribution to functional localization in the right hemisphere, as McFie[40] points out, seems still to have been ignored (apart from motor and sensory functions) by most authors of current textbooks of psychology and physiology. Hemispheric localization is discussed in detail in the next section but the impairment of some abilities most commonly investigated by the psychologist has been summarized in Figure 154.

One of the most controversial problems concerns the localization of intellectual function. Intelligence is generally considered to be a constellation of mental abilities which enter into our overall performance. In a study of unilateral penetrating missile injuries of the brain Newcombe[41] found a dichotomy between verbal abilities as compared with performance in visual-spatial tasks. She found selective impairment of language, visual perception and spatial orientation "whereas intellectual capacities had been remarkably preserved". But is not some degree of impairment of intelligence implicit in lesions with localizing neurological signs? Can intellectual function be localized? Spearman,[42] and later factor analysts, tried to answer these questions. The "unitary" nature of intelligence has been inferred from the fact that there is a high degree of intercorrelation between different tests designed to measure mental ability.

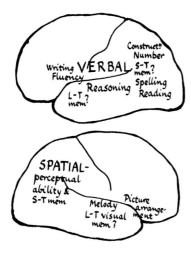

FIGURE 154

Abilities impaired by localized cerebral lesions. L-T, S-T mem. = long term and short term memory (McFie, 1972).

Spearman's simple two-factor theory accounted for these intercorrelations in terms of a general factor corresponding to overall performance, and a specific factor relating to each test. Since then a number of other group factors corresponding to high test correlations have been delineated. In spite of slight differences due to varying statistical techniques, the following five major group factors have been recognized: verbal, spatial, numerical, memory and constructional. McFie[43] suggests that these factorial groups may be correlated with areas of the cortex showing psychological deficits associated with localized lesions causing aphasia, apraxia, alexia, agnosia, acalculia and agraphia. That these intellectual "factors" of the brain are organized in specific regions is supported by the work of Weisenberg and McBride.[44] They studied a series of aphasics with standardized tests and compared them with a group with comparable right hemisphere lesions. Their results were then compared with a group of normal subjects. "Evidence for a distinction between different groups of mental abilities (in normals)", they wrote, "gains additional support from the findings for the pathological groups studied by the same tests. Cases of right-sided cerebral lesions without aphasia . . . were found to be significantly inferior to the normal only on

the arithmetic and some of the non-language tests", while "only a few aphasic patients have anything like as great a difficulty in non-language as in language work". They concluded that there are more or less independent groups of mental abilities which do not show much difference from one another in the normal adult but in localized brain disease "they may be affected unequally".

If it is true that intellectual "factors" of the brain are organized in specific cortical areas then it would seem that, in one sense, modern research on localization is returning to similar concepts to those held by phrenologists with their maps depicting the localization of various "faculties of the mind".

5. CONCEPTS OF THE BODY SCHEME

Interest in the body scheme (or somatognosia) developed historically as a theoretical explanation of clinical observations in brain damaged patients. Unfortunately the term has been corrupted to include psychotic and neurotic disorders. The concept of the body scheme is based on the generally accepted hypothesis that there is a distinct psychological function concerned with body orientation, although opinions vary as to its precise nature and possible localization. Furthermore, the whole body scheme controversy is riddled with semantic difficulties. It has, for example, been regarded by Gerstmann,[45] and Klein[46] as a "conscious awareness" of the body; by Lhermitte[47] as "an image of the body"; by Hauptmann,[48] and Lange[49] as a "cortical representation of the body", whereas Head and Holmes[50] wrote in terms of "a preconscious physiological function". Recently aspects of the body scheme have been critically reviewed by Poeck and Orgass,[51] whose work forms the basis of this account.

First introduced by Bonnier,[52] the term "body scheme" referred to spatial quality in the awareness of various sensory impressions of the body: it was based on the study of patients with neurological disturbances. Munk[53] also expounded a similar theme, and argued that spatial orientation depends on the reactivation of sensorimotor images developed during early childhood. He postulated that there are various sensory zones in the parietal lobes concerned with specific parts of the body: hence the size or site of a lesion would cause a corresponding body image disturbance. This theory was developed by Wernicke[54] who postulated a point to point association between cells in the sensorimotor cortex and their corresponding organ receptors. He believed that nervous impulses had a specific quality, depending on the site of stimulation, whereby the cortex receives various localized sensory modalities enabling the individual to acquire, by experience, spatial images corresponding to the distribution of the receptor sensory organs. Thus, images corresponding to body orientation and to the localization of somatosensory perception together constitute body consciousness as distinct from consciousness of the external world. Pick[55-57] followed the same theoretical route as Munk and Wernicke by adopting a theory of somatognostic orientation due to mental images built up during early life as a consequence of tactile and proprioceptive engrams. He believed that full body orientation in the adult was mainly due to visual images. Pick explained various clinical symptoms in terms of a disturbance of the visual body image: he conceived the possibility of several body schemata subserving various sensory modalities.

A totally different view was taken by Head and Holmes. They suggested that postures or passive movements are recounted preconsciously in relation to preceding postures or movements. Thus the body scheme is the psychological function for comparing the position of a movement with the one immediately preceding it; hence each individual has a constantly changing postural model. Head and Holmes also suggested a second superficial body scheme subserving the ability to localize a point of stimulation on the surface of the body: they were able to demonstrate postural and localizing aspects of the body scheme on a patient who could correctly localize the position of his hand but failed to recognise the site of stimulation. Head and Holmes conceived that past impressions, stored in the sensory cortex, formed preconsciously organized models of the individual's body scheme. They also differentiated between an image and a schema: the latter was regarded as being a preconscious phenomenon whereas an 'image' was consciously appreciated. This subtle difference has tended to be overlooked, or distorted, by subsequent authors, many of whom claim to be disciples of Head and Holmes. Such terms as body scheme, body image, postural schema, somatognosis, *l'image de soi, l'image de notre corps* and spatial image of the body have, at various times, been used in the sense that Head and Holmes used the term body scheme.

The best known current theory of the body scheme is that of Schilder,[58-59] who suggested that various neuropsychological symptoms concerning body orientation should be classified under this general term. Essentially Schilder believed that each individual develops a sensori-motor spatial image of various parts of the body and, like Pick, regarded the body scheme as being built up of predominantly visual-spatial images of various parts of the body. There is an obvious dichotomy between the theories of Head and Holmes and those of Pick and Schilder. The latter received the support of Gerstmann,[60-64] who described a syndrome of right-left disorientation, together with disturbances of calculating and writing associated with finger agnosia. He localized this symptom complex to a circumscribed lesion in the angular gyrus. Gerstmann's syndrome has provoked controversy regarding the concept of the body scheme: there are those, including Benton,[65] Critchley,[66] and Poeck and Orgass,[67] who do not regard the condition as a coherent clinical entity, while Heimburger, Demyer and Reitan[68] do not accept its site of localization.

In a critical survey, Poeck and Orgass[69] have drawn attention to the shortcomings of basing concepts of the body scheme on clinical evidence. The theory that the body scheme undergoes a process of maturation and develops centrally as a result of afferent impulses (Pick;[70-71] Benton[72]) has now been found to be based on the false assumption that children with congenital absence of limbs or after amputation during the first year of life do not experience phantoms. The alleged absence of such phantoms was explained by the assumption that the missing limbs had never been represented in the child's body scheme (Pick;[73] Riese and Bruck[74]). This assumption has been totally invalidated by evidence that children who have been born with congenitally absent limbs do, in fact, develop phantoms comparable with those of adults (Weinstein and Sersen;[75] Weinstein;[76] and Poeck[77]). It must therefore be assumed that somatosensory impulses are not essential to the development of awareness of parts of the body. Furthermore, the importance of visual experience in the orientation of the body scheme has now been found to be inessential. Poeck and Orgass[78-79] have demonstrated that blind children are not handicapped in somatognostic orientation when compared with others with normal visual acuity.

In their critical review Poeck and Orgass[80] have traced the misconceptions and semantic inaccuracies concerning theories of the body scheme which cannot be explained by a unitary theory developed from clinical data and misapplied to describe such unrelated phenomena as phantom limbs, anosognosia, paroxysmal disturbances of body experience, autoscopia and even psychotic and neurotic symptoms. By stressing that cerebral function must subserve the control of body posture and movements, Poeck and Orgass have revived the concept of the "postural schema" first proposed by Head and Holmes.[81]

6. ASYMMETRICAL FUNCTION OF THE HEMISPHERES

The notion of hemispheric dominance developed from Broca's[82] rule that right handedness is associated with cortical representation of language in the left hemisphere. In left handed subjects this assumption does not explain cases of crossed aphasia, *i.e.* aphasia associated with a right hemispheric lesion. Language defects have been examined in a large number of left handed subjects with missile injuries by Conrad,[83] Luria[84] and Russell and Espir:[85] another series including observations by Humphrey and Zangwill,[86] Hécaen and Ajuriaguerra,[87] Goodglass and Quadfasel,[88] Brown and Simmonson,[89] and Hoff,[90] were based on studies of patients with various neurological disorders; and Penfield and Roberts[91] studied speech disorders in relation to cerebral dominance during ablation of epileptogenic zones. They showed that two-thirds of left handed individuals have speech localized in the left hemisphere. Permanent aphasia does not usually occur if the lesion is limited to the right hemisphere as language function tends to be more "ambilateral" in sinistrals—a conclusion supported by Hécaen *et al* and Bingley.[92] Hence, Goodglass and Quadfasel[93] believe that it is unnecessary and incorrect to establish a direct relationship between manual preference and cerebral localization of language function, as left cerebral dominance is more general than right handedness, and right cerebral dominance is much less frequent than the incidence of left handedness.

These studies all emphasize that aphasia is less severe in sinistrals regardless of the hemisphere affected and recovery is more rapid and complete than in right handers. Hécaen and Piercy[94] have shown that patients with paroxysmal dysphasia have handedness differences. In a study of 126 cases of paroxysmal dysphasia of the expressive type they found a significantly higher frequency of left handers than right handers regardless of the hemisphere damaged—a conclusion confirmed by Russell and Espir. In a large series of patients with unilateral lesions Hécaen and Sauguet,[95] compared the frequency of language disturbance in left and right handed subjects. They found that the left hemisphere syndrome in left-handed subjects causes a similar speech disturbance to that of right handers except that there is a lower frequency of defects of verbal comprehension and writing associated with a higher frequency of reading distur-

bances. In the right hemisphere syndrome, left handers were found to have a high incidence of disturbances of oral and written language. The comparison between right and left hemisphere syndromes in left handers shows much less difference in the frequencies of symptoms as compared with those of right handers. Their findings indicate some degree of ambilaterality in left handed subjects who cannot be regarded as a distinct group but should be subdivided into a 'familial' group with a family history of left handedness and a non-familial group. In the latter, disturbance of language and reading is similar in lesions of either hemisphere, whereas in non-familial left handers these disturbances are similar to those found with right handed lesions. They, therefore, conclude that cerebral ambilaterality is not a characteristic of all left handers but only those belonging to the so-called 'familial' groups.

Ettlinger, Jackson and Zangwill[96] were able to trace only fifteen cases of dysphasia resulting from right hemisphere lesions in right-handed patients. More recent reports include those by Espir and Russell. Penfield and Roberts suggest that the incidence of dysphasia in right handed patients is about 1% and approximately 67% with left-sided lesions. Thus it would seem that the traditional theory of right hemisphere dominance for language in sinistrals can no longer be sustained. Zangwill[97] found that 24 out of 54 sinistrals had left hemisphere damage and 13 out of 39 with right hemisphere damage suffered a severe and persistent dysphasia. This survey was extended by Piercy[98] to cover the years 1935–1962. He found 80 left-handed aphasics with left hemisphere lesions and 33 left-handed aphasics with right hemisphere lesions. Piercy suggests that bilaterality for language is probably more common among sinistrals than dextrals although exceptional in both. In summarizing his conclusions Piercy agrees with Goodglass and Quadfasel that left handedness is distinctly more common than right hemisphere specialization for language, but disagrees with the statement of Penfield and Roberts that there is no relationship between handedness and language laterality. Hemispheric differences in language comprehension has been surveyed by Gazzaniga[99] in patients with split brains. In the left hemisphere, speech is unusually disturbed. In the right hemisphere it is greatly limited, and nouns, but not verbs, are understood.

Some functional characteristics of the so-called minor hemisphere were first delineated by Zangwill and his associates. Paterson and Zangwill[100] reported two cases of visual-spatial agnosia due to traumatic lesions of the right cerebral hemisphere. The most pronounced defects were observed in the analysis of spatial relationships and in the execution of constructional tasks under visual control. In a later paper[101] they described a patient with disorders of topographical orientation associated with disturbances of memory and of the body scheme due to a right sided traumatic lesion. More information on the effects of unilateral right sided occipito-parietal lesions was provided by McFie, Piercy and Zangwill.[102] They found apraxia for dressing and the "greater part of the constructional disability can be explained in terms of neglect of the left sided visual space (unilateral spatial agnosia) and a disorganization of discriminative spatial judgement (planotopkinesia)." When they compared unilateral left sided with right sided lesions McFie and Zangwill[103] concluded that left hemisphere damage causes spatial apraxia whereas right sided lesions led to spatial agnosia. Recently Whitty and Newcombe[104] have reported similar disturbances due to unilateral right sided lesions for which they suggest the term 'visual spatial constructional disability'; and studies by Warrington and James[105] confirm that right hemispheric deficits are essentially perceptual. An association between lesions of the right temporal lobe and impairment of the appreciation of tonal patterns has been found by Milner.[106] Studies on visual memory by Warrington and James[107] indicate that memory for new visual material, such as photographs of unfamiliar faces, is impaired in right parietal lesions, whereas recognition of well known faces tends to be disturbed in patients with right temporal lesions. Milner[108] also found that the general deficit of interpretation of pictorial material is associated with lesions in the right hemisphere. Lishman[109] studied the effects of emotional responses after commissurotomy and postulates that the hemisphere functions unequally in the intact brain with the minor hemisphere "sometimes playing the greater part".

Ideomotor apraxia and bilateral somatognosis are, according to Piercy,[110] "almost pathognomonic of left hemisphere lesions". Alexia occurs exclusively with left sided lesions although some disorders such as dressing apraxia and constructional apraxia may occur with lesions of either hemisphere. Warrington, Logue and Pratt [111] studied the localization of auditory-verbal short term memory and reported several cases resulting from lesions in the area of the supramarginal and angular gyri of the left hemisphere. Benton[112] found interhemispheric differences in performance in a comparative study of patients with left, right, and bilateral frontal

lesions and others with post-Rolandic lesions. Shallice and Warrington[113] found an association between profound impairment of short term auditory-visual memory and left parietal lesions; long term memory seems to depend on the integrity of the connexions of the hippocampus and mammilliary bodies. Milner[114] has shown that excision of the left frontal lobe causes a reduction in verbal fluency. In a study of over 200 patients McFie[115] found an association between sensory aphasia and left temporo-parietal lesions. In a review of hemispheric localization, Benton[116] suggests a left hemispheric locus for aphasia, impaired learning, impaired verbal fluency, Gerstmann's syndrome, ideomotor apraxia and impairment of recognition and memory. To this list Brewer[117] adds recognition memory for tests using designs and colours. There appear to be differences of opinion regarding the laterality of lesions causing impairment of calculation (usually associated with left parietal lesions) although some studies have reported acalculia in patients with right sided lesions; arithmetical ability is probably bilaterally represented. Although individual variations are not uncommon, McFie and Zangwill[118] consider that, in general, disorders of the left hemisphere tend to involve manipulative skills whereas those of the right side cause perceptual disorders. After reviewing studies on long term memory impairment Milner concludes that left sided structures are concerned with the retention of verbal material whereas the right hemisphere is more involved in non-verbal memory.

Assumptions concerning asymmetrical hemispheric function based on the assessment of various deficits due to cerebral lesions, have been criticized on the grounds that normal function cannot be implied from a study of disordered function. But a series of psychological studies on normal subjects also reveals asymmetrical hemispheric differences. Kimura[119–120] compared the relative efficiency of the two half fields of vision and also of auditory acuity and demonstrated definite hemispheric differences in both modalities. The laterality effects of voice recognition were studied by Doehring and Bartholomeus[121] by means of ear naming and visual choice response tests. They found a right sided superiority due to left hemisphere dominance for voice recognition. And Hemmelin and O'Connor[122] found differences between the left and right handed reading of Braille due to cortical asymmetry. Hand preference, speed of movement of each hand and the growth of vocabulary were examined by Annett[123–124] in a random sample of normal children between the ages of 3½ and 15 years. She found sex differences in preference and skill indicating that females tend to be more asymmetrical to the right than males. A linear relation was demonstrated between degrees of preference and of relative manual skill. Consistent left handers tended to be superior to right handers in the growth of vocabulary. There was a slight (but unprovable) suggestion that mixed handers had lower vocabulary scores than consistent handers. Thus, there is an ever-growing volume of information from current research refuting the long held concept of hemispheric dominance which has, however, become ingrained in neurological and psychological literature.

Various theories have been suggested to explain functional asymmetry. Orton,[125] for instance, favours a development theory of increasing brain functional asymmetry with incomplete development of cerebral dominance, a view held by Critchley[126] in some cases of developmental dyslexia. Ettlinger *et al.*,[127] Hécaen and Ajuriaguerra[128] and Zangwill[129] believe that cerebral ambilaterality is determined by constitutional factors modified by environmental influences. On the other hand Subirana *et al.*[130] explained unpredictable aphasia in left handers on the basis that different language functions may be represented in different hemispheres. These varying opinions indicate that the neurophysiological concomitants of behavioural laterality are not fully understood. A study by Bryden[131] suggests that cerebral dominance is likely to be determined by several factors. He studied 20 left handers and 20 right handers, all of whom were given a dichotic listening test and a tachistoscopic recognition test. On both tests right handers were significantly more accurate in identifying material presented to the right side while left handers failed to show any consistent left-right differences. But left handers showed a significantly greater variance in laterality scores on the dichotic listening task than did right handers. A group of four familial left handers were more left dominant on both tasks than were the other left handers. There was, however, no significant correlation between laterality scores on the two tasks. Bryden concludes that the performance on both tasks is related to cerebral dominance "which must be viewed as having several components rather than being a unitary process". Critchley,[132] too, points out that laterality may be determined by a multiplicity of influences. Thus handedness, verbal and manipulative skills, hemispheric "dominance" and crossed laterality may all be components in the basic cerebral asymmetry of man.

7. SYNDROMES ASSOCIATED WITH LESIONS IN VARIOUS ANATOMICAL LOBES

It is hoped to illuminate indirectly some aspects of cortical function by summarizing clinical syndromes associated with lesions in various anatomical lobes of the brain. There are, however, several serious objections to this approach. A functional deficit does not necessarily reveal the true function of the part of the cortex concerned. This argument loses some of its force by the researches of Kimura who has shown that there are hemispheric differences in the relative efficiency of perception of the two half fields of vision and the two ears in normal subjects. In a study of a large number of patients with unilateral penetrating missile wounds of the brain twenty years after injury, Newcombe[133] mentioned that the resulting deficits do not always correspond to the anatomical boundaries of the lobes involved. The conventional anatomical subdivisions of the brain into lobes is, of course, purely arbitrary, and does not necessarily correspond to interhemispheric functional differences. Furthermore McFie[134] points out that some syndromes may be due to lesions involving the borders between lobes as, for example, in the parieto-temporo-occipital confluence. This subdivision of the brain can also be criticized on pathological grounds. Marie[135] has observed that a patient's "aphasia is more often determined by the distribution of his arteries than by the topography of his convolutions". Nevertheless, the conventional anatomical subdivisions of the brain have, by long usage, become so ingrained in neurological practice, that this type of summary may be described as a convenient over-simplification.

Frontal Lobes

It was Hughlings Jackson[136] who first regarded the frontal cortex as the repository of the highest and most distinctly human intellectual capacities; it has been variously described as being concerned with "reasoning",[137] "synthesing"[138–139] or "abstracting"[140–141] and as the centre of "biological intelligence".[142] All these suppositions had to be revised when Hebb[143] showed that gross extirpation of the frontal cortex did not affect intelligence; indeed patients with frontal lesions are less impaired intellectually than those with parietal lesions. Thus this association between the frontal lobe and highest intellectual capacity must finally be abandoned

Anterior Part The results of prefrontal damage from psychosurgery have, on the whole, been variable and elusive in their effects on higher cortical function. The only consistent features to emerge are some loss of recent memory, loss of initiative and in particular of foresight, together with personality changes characterized by a variable syndrome including euphoria, indifference, and occasionally, agitated depression. There is a "negative" aspect of pre-frontal lesions in that they may represent an absence of some aspect of the patient's previous behaviour, and also in the sense that characteristic signs of damage to other parts of the hemisphere are not usually found.

Posterior Part Lesions near the precentral motor cortex are liable to impair aspects of voluntary movement. When the second frontal convolution is involved there may be kinetic apraxia, facial apraxia and apraxic anarthria. When the foot of the second and third frontal convolutions in the right hemisphere is damaged there may be motor amusia. Involvement of the same area in the left hemisphere may cause expressive aphasia and, occasionally, motor agraphia.

Temporal Lobes

In general, posterior cortical lesions involve a greater degree of intellectual disability than anterior ones: this generalization is more applicable to the left rather than to the right hemisphere. Posterior temporal lesions are more likely to cause disturbances of language or perception depending on the hemisphere involved. According to Wertheim[144] a lesion of the anterior superior temporal gyrus of either hemisphere may cause sensory amusia.

Scoville and Milner[145] found that bilateral ablation of the infero-medial aspects of the temporal lobes causes a gross amnesic syndrome. After operation patients were able to give a limited, though adequate, account of remote events, but were quite unable to retain new information for more than a few minutes. The syndrome is similar to that seen in Korsakoff's psychosis although confabulation is not quite so pronounced. Severe amnesia has also been reported by Nielsen[146] and Dimsdale *et al.*[147] in extensive lesions of the right temporal lobe; and other memory disturbances such as the *déjà vu* phenomonon have been encountered more frequently with right rather than with left sided lesions.

Whitty and Lishman[148] regard the hippocampus, hy-pothalamus and the periventricular area as the anatomical substrate for memory, although McFie and Piercy[149] take the view that failure on short term memory tests are not associated with lesions of any particular cortical area. They showed that some intellectual abilities were selectively impaired in certain specific sites although, in general, impairment of retention and learning was related to the size rather than the site of the lesion. On the other hand, Whitty and Lishman[150] stress the clinically observed fact that a profound amnesic syndrome may often be associated with a well localized tumour. Milner[151] suggests that the medial temporal structures are concerned with "consolidating" immediate memory which seems to summarize both clinical and experimental observations, although the search for the engram still goes on.

Left Side Temporal lobe functions, though still far from being satisfactorily elucidated, may however, be summarized in terms of functional deficit. Lhermitte and Gautier[152] have stated that receptive aphasia is the major disability associated with left temporal lesions; the more anterior the lesion the more likelihood of disturbances of "motor realisation" of speech whereas posterior lesions disturb the "semantic value of speech and the formulation of sentences". In both areas there may be defective comprehension of speech. Visual aspects of language may be impaired in posterior lesions; those near the temporo-occipital border may cause alexia whereas agraphia is more likely to result from lesions near the temporo-parietal border. In posterior temporal lesions apraxias, somatognosias and acalculia are often found.

Right Side The common disorders for right sided lesions are amusia, amnesia and disturbances of spatial integration. According to Hécaen and Ajuriaguerra[153] the metamorphopsias are also more frequent in right sided lesions. Impairment of tests involving spatial analysis, construction and drawing, together with prosopagnosia are more common in lesions near the occipital lobe whereas hemisomatagnosia occurs in areas near the parietal lobe.

Parietal Lobes

The complexity of parietal lobe functions has been surveyed in Critchley's[154] classic book. Here it is only possible to outline some of the more common syndromes associated with lesions therein. In any event many aspects of parietal lobe function have been discussed in the previous section. McFie and Piercy[155] have drawn attention to the influence on the symptomatology of the size of the lesion. Usually larger lesions are associated with a greater number of symptoms although similar syndromes may occur with lesions of either side. McFie[156] warns against inferring laterality of lesion from a few symptoms such as constructional apraxia as, in the parietal lobes *par excellence,* extensive assessment is necessary before a reliable judgement of laterality can be made.

An association between parietal lobe damage of either side and route finding difficulties when guided by tactile or visual maps has been reported by Weinstein, Semmes, Ghent and Teuber.[157] A similar disturbance of topographical memory was found by Hécaen[158] in association with bilateral post-Rolandic lesions.

Left Side   Receptive language disturbances are associated with lesions along the upper border of the Sylvian fissure and more anterior lesions may cause expressive language disorders. In the angular and supramarginal gyri the symptom complex known as Gerstmann's syndrome is found together with apraxia and asymbolia for pain. Ideomotor and ideational apraxias are associated with left parietal lesions and, as with constructional apraxia, are commonly found in patients with some degree of dementia. In left parietal lesions short term auditory-visual memory is impaired, together with verbal learning and aphasia.

Right Side   A complexity of right sided parietal syndromes has been described as essentially due to a breakdown of spatial perception ranging from disturbance of co-ordination and vestibular disorders, to impairment of constructional ability; these include planotopokinesia (Marie),[159] visual spatialagnosia (Poetzl)[160] apractognosia (Lange)[161] and amorphosynthesis (Denny-Brown and Bamber),[162] and visual-spatial constructional disability (Whitty and Newcombe).[163] Other common features include oculo-motor disturbances, unilateral aso-matognosia, unilateral spatial agnosia, dressing apraxia, prosopagnosia and topographical disorientation. Patients are frequently unaware of these disabilities.

In severe parietal damage there may be acalculia, alexia or agraphia.

Occipital Lobes

Although some occipital lesions may include elements of parietal lobe damage they are most frequently reflected in disturbances of visual perception. The accompanying hemianopia will determine the side of the lesion. McFie[164] points out that it is important to distinguish between disorders due to the use of language and those caused by disturbance of perceptual organization. De Renzi and Spinnler[165] have shown that disorders of colour perception due to language disorders are associated with lesions of the left hemisphere whereas those due to perceptual disorganization are located in the right side.

Left Side   The clinical picture of the left sided syndrome consists of right hemianopia, alexia and colour agnosia. If the lesion is near the occipitoparietal border there may be some degree of receptive dysphasia, dyscalculia, constructional apraxia and simultanagnosia. Although object agnosia usually results from bilateral lesions it may be present in left sided damage. More frequently difficulty in interpreting pictures is found.

Right Side   Disturbance of the primary visual aspects of spatial perception may cause prosopagnosias together with "spatial" dyslexia and dysgraphia.

When elements of the right parietal syndrome are also involved topographical disorientation and dressing apraxia may occur. Large lesions may cause failure of visual recognition and visual hallucinations. Disorders associated with localized lesions of the left and right hemispheres have been summarized graphically in Figure 155 A–B.

8. INTEGRATION OF BRAIN FUNCTION

Inevitably this account of recent trends in cerebral localization is incomplete, as we are primarily concerned with localization within the human cortex. But the recent growth of knowledge concerning brain function would preclude the specialized study of one area to the exclusion of others. Cortical integration with various sub-cortical structures is known to play an important part in regulating higher nervous functions. The pioneer researches of Moruzzi[166] and Magoun[167] have shown that the reticular formation maintains the tone of cerebral neurones, affecting the waking and sleeping state, and thereby directly influencing the integration of cortical function. According to Green[168] the reticular formation has now come to be regarded in much the same way as

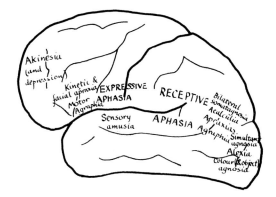

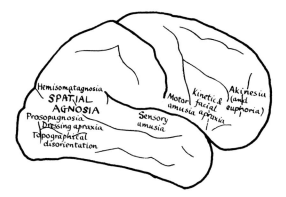

FIGURE 155

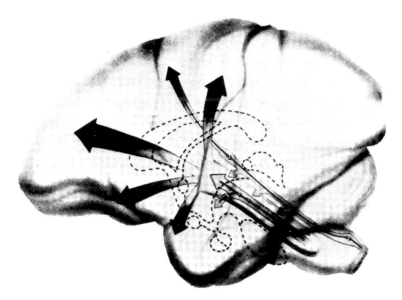

FIGURE 156

FIGURE 155
Disorders associated with localized lesions, (A) left hemisphere; (B) right hemisphere (McFie, 1969).

FIGURE 156
Lateral view of monkey's brain showing the ascending reticular system in the core of the brain stem. It receives collaterals from an afferent pathway and projects widely to cortical areas (Magoun, 1963, Fig. 42).

the cerebral hemispheres were envisaged in the 19th century (see Figure 156). Other sub-cortical structures concerned with the integration of cortical function are the intralaminar thalamic nuclei which are, according to Gastaut,[169] responsible for maintaining the direction of attention. The functional role of the limbic lobe is also of the utmost importance in relation to cortical localization. This complex system has recently been the object of much research, notably by Pribram,[170] and in a recent review of its functional role Smythies[171] seems to accept Papez's hypothesis concerning the higher elaboration of emotion.[172]

What of the future? Anatomists have evolved new techniques for delineating fibre tracts by freezing and

other methods. Histochemical procedures for tracing chemically identifiable neurones, especially by means of specific enzyme activity, are now in use and the elucidation of hormone factors as well as further developments in molecular biology will no doubt contribute to research into cortical morphology and physiology.[173] The electron microscope, fluorescent techniques, and micro-autoradiography will also be used increasingly to tackle the problems of cerebral localization. There are also new electro-physiological techniques including methods of evoked potentials, evoked EEG rhythms, and the insertion in the brain of indwelling electrodes stimulated by radio and even controlled by computer, thus eliminating the effects of anaesthesia and restraint. Vast areas of

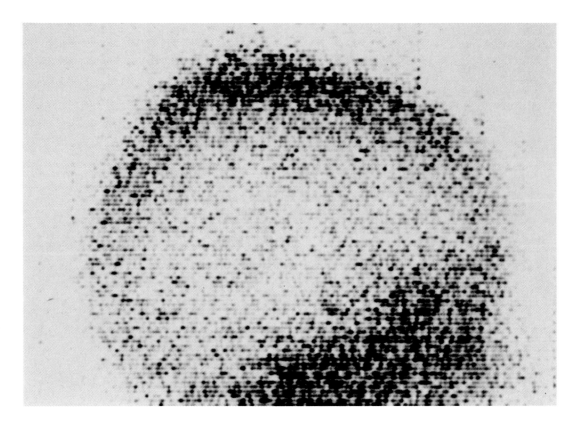

FIGURE 157A

FIGURES 157 A–B
This normal radioactive isotope brain scan was carried out with Indium[113m.], which has a half-life of 1–7 hours. The isotope is injected intravenously and can reveal intracranial space-occupying lesions, owing either to their abnormal vascularity or to their increased uptake of the material. The central area of decreased density is produced by the ventricular system. This then is the most recent method of outlining the tissue of the brain and an increasingly useful method of localizing brain lesions.

research are also being opened up by employing various models of the brain, animate,[174] mathematical and mechanical;[175] and by the application of the principles of cybernetics.

All these and more, together with the psychological approaches already discussed, will be of the greatest significance in future research on the structure and function of the cerebral cortex as it concerns cerebral localization and in attempts to make correlations with bodily function and individual variations in behaviour.

In the clinical sphere improved anaesthesia and surgical techniques have allowed more extensive ablations to be performed without undue risk; and in the realm of diagnosis, brain scanning techniques now probe the substance of the cerebral cortex (see Figure 157 A–B).

NOTES

1. J. McFie, "Recent advances in phrenology", *Lancet,* 1961, 2:360-363.

2. K. S. Lashley, *Brain mechanisms and intelligence,* Chicago, University of Chicago Press, 1929.

3. F. L. Goltz, "Der Hund ohne Grosshirn. Siebente Abhandlung über die Verrichtungen des Grosshirns", *Pflügers Arch.,* 1892, 51:570–614.

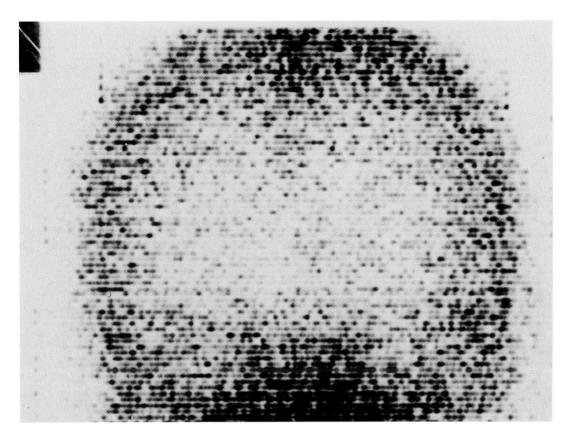

FIGURE 157B

4. K. S. Lashley, "Factors limiting recovery after central nervous lesions", *J. nerv. ment. Dis.*, 1938, *88*:733–755.

5. J. McFie, *(op.cit.* above, note 1), p. 361.

6. A. R. Luria, *Higher cortical functions in man*, London, Tavistock Publications, 1966, pp.23–38.

7. I. N. Filimonov, "Localization of functions in the cerebral cortex and Pavlov's theory of higher nervous activity" *Klinicheskaya Meditsina*, [Russian], 1961, *29*(6).

8. *Idem*, "Architectonics of localization of functions in the cerebral cortex", in, *Textbook of neurology* [Russian], Vol. 1, Moscow, Medgiz, 1957.

9. H. Nakahama, "Somatic areas of the cerebral cortex" *Int. Rev. Neurobiol.*, 1961, *3*:187–250.

10. A. R. Luria *(op. cit.* above, note 6), p.27.

11. J. McFie, "Factors of the brain", *Bull. Br.psychol. Soc.*, 1972, *25*:11–14.

12. F. Newcombe, *Missile wounds of the brain*, London, Oxford University Press, 1969.

13. P. E. Vernon, *The structure of human abilities*, London, Methuen, 1950.

14. J. S. Bruner, "The course of cognitive growth", *Am. Psychol.*, 1964, *19*:1–15.

15. L. F. Chapman & H. G. Wolf, "The human brain—one organ or many?", *Arch. Neurol.*, 1961, *5*:463–471.

16. Of Penfield's voluminous writings we have used the following:

W. Penfield & E. Boldrey, "Somatic motor and sensory representation in the cerebral cortex of man as studied by electrical stimulation", *Brain*, 1937, *60*:389–443.

W. Penfield & T. Rasmussen, *The cerebral cortex of man. A clinical study of localization of function,* New York, Macmillan, 1957.

W. Penfield, "Engrams in the human brain", *Proc. Roy. Soc. Med.,* 1968, *61*:831–840.

W. Penfield, *The excitable cortex in conscious man,* Liverpool, Liverpool University Press, 1958.

17. W. Penfield & E. Boldrey, *ibid.,* p. 432

18. W. Penfield & T. Rasmussen *(op. cit.* above, note 16), pp. 44–57.

19. *Ibid.,* pp. 214–215.

20. *Ibid.*

21. R. G. Heath, "Pleasure and brain activity. Deep and surface encephalograms during orgasm", *J. nerv. ment. Dis.*, 1972, *154*:3–18.

22. W. Penfield & T. Rasmussen *(op. cit.* above, note 16), p. 179.

23. G. Bollea, "Contributo sperimentale alla fisiopatologia del casidetto schema corporeo", *Riv. neurol.*, 1948, *18*:310–352, see p. 337

24. M. Piercy, "The effects of cerebral lesions on intellectual function. A review of current research trends", *Br. J. Psychiat.*, 1964, *110*:310–352.

25. W. Penfield & L. Roberts, *Speech and brain mechanisms.* Princeton, N.J., Princeton University Press, 1959.

26. C. W. M. Whitty & W. A. Lishman, "Amnesia and cerebral disease", in, C. W. M. Whitty & O. L. Zangwill (editors), *Amnesia,* London, Butterworth, 1966, p. 55.

27. R. M. Reitan, "Problems end prospects in studying the psychological correlates of brain lesions", *Cortex, 1966, 2*:127–154.

28. J. McFie, "The diagnostic significance of disorders of higher nervous activity", P. J. Vinken & G. W. Bruyn (editors), *Handbook of clinical neurology,* Vol. 4, Amsterdam, North Holland Publishing Co., 1969, pp.1–12.

29. E. Busch, "Psychical symptoms in neurosurgical disease", *Acta psychiat. neurol. scand., 1940, 15*:257–290.

30. A. L. Andersen, "The effect of laterality localisation of focal brain lesions on the Wechsler-Bellevue subjects", *J. Clin. Psychol., 1951, 7*:149–153

31. R. M. Reitan, "Certain differential effects of left and right cerebral lesions in human adults", *J. comp. physiol. Psychol., 1955, 48*:474–477.

32. H. Hécaen, W. Penfield, C. Bertrand, & R. Malmo, "The syndrome of apractognosia due to lesions of the minor cerebral hemisphere", *Arch.Neurol. Psychiat., 1956, 75*:400–434.

33. J. Semmes, S. Weinstein, L. Ghent, & H. L. Teuber, *Somatosonsory changes after penetrating brain wounds in man,* Cambridge, Mass., Harvard University Press, 1960.

34. *Ibid.*

35. R. M. Reitan, "Psychological defects resulting from cerebral lesions in man", in, J. M. Warren & K. A. Akert (editors), *The frontal granular cortex and behavior,* New York, McGraw-Hill, 1964.

36. K. B. Fitzhugh & R. M. Reitan, "Psychological deficits in relation to acuteness of brain dysfunction", *J. consult. Psychol., 1961, 25*:61–66.

37. D. O. Hebb, "The effect of early and late brain injury upon test scores and the nature of normal adult intelligence", *Proc. Am. phil. Soc., 1942, 85*:275–292.

38. K. B. Fitzhugh & L. C. Fitzhugh, "Effects of early and late onset of cerebral dysfunction upon psychological test performance", *Percept. Mot. skills., 1965, 20*:1099–1100.

39. J. McFie (*op. cit.* above, note 1), p. 363.

40. J. McFie (*op. cit.* above, note 11), p. 12.

41. F. Newcombe (*op. cit.* above, note 12).

42. C. Spearman, *The abilities of man,* London, Macmillan, 1932.

43. J. McFie (*op. cit.* above, note 1).

44. T. Weisenburg & K. E. McBride, *Aphasia,* New York, Hafner, 1964.

45. J. Gerstmann, "Fingeragnosie und isolierte Agraphie. Ein neues Syndrom", *Z. ges. Neurol. Psychiat., 1927, 108*:152–177.

46. R. Klein, "Über die Empfindung der Körperlichkeit", *ibid.,* 1930, *126*:453–472.

47. J. Lhermitte, *L'image de notre corps,* Paris, *Nouvelle revue critique,* 1939.

48. A. Hauptmann, "Die Bedeutung der linken Hemisphäre für das Bewusstsein vom eignenen Körper", *Zentbl. ges. Neurol. Psychiat., 1928, 48*:282–297.

49. J. Lange, "Agnosien und Apraxien", in, O. Bumke & O. Foerster (editors), *Handbuch der Neurologie,* Vol. 6, Berlin, J. Springer, 1936, pp.807–960.

50. H. Head & G. Holmes, "Sensory disturbances from central lesions", *Brain,* 1911–1912, *34*:102–254.

51. K. Poeck & B. Orgass, "The concept of the body schema. A critical review with some experimental results", *Cortex, 1971, 7*:254–277.

52. P. Bonnier, "L'aschématie", *Rev. neurol., 1905, 13*:604–609.

53. H. Munk, *Über die Functionen der Grosshirnrinde,* 2. Aufl., Berlin, A. Hirschwald, 1890.

54. C. Wernicke, *Grundriss der Psychiatrie in klinischen Vorlesungen,* Leipzig, G. Thieme, 1900.

55. A. Pick, "Über Störungen der Orientierung am eigenen Körper," in, *Arbeiten aus der deutschen psychiatrischen Universitäts-Klinik in Prag,* Berlin, S. Karger, 1908, pp. 1–19.

56. A. Pick, "Zur Pathologie des Bewusstseins vom eigenen Körper", *Neurol. Zentbl., 1915, 34*:257–265.

57. A. Pick, "Störung der Orientierung am eigenen Körper. Beitrag zur Lehre vom Bewusstsein des eigenen Körpers", *Psychol. Forsch., 1922, 1*:303–318.

58. P. Schilder, *Das Körperschema Ein Beitrag zur Lehre vom Bewusstsein des eigenen Körpers,* Berlin, J. Springer, 1923.

59. P. Schilder, *The image and appearance of the human body,* London, K. Paul & Trübner, 1935, Psychological Monographs, No.4.

60. J. Gerstmann, "Fingeragnosie. Eine umschriebene Störung der Orientierung am eigenen Körper", *Wien klin. Wschr., 1924, 37*:1010–1012.

61. J. Gerstmann (*op. cit.* above, note 45).

62. J. Gerstmann, "Zur Symptomatologie der Hirnläsionen im Übergangsgebiet der unteren Parietal- und mittleren Occipitalwindung", *Nervenarzt, 1930, 3*:691–695.

63. J. Gerstmann, "Problems of imperception of disease and of impaired body territories with organic lesions. Relations to body scheme and its disorders" *Arch. Neurol. Psychiat., 1942, 48*:890–913.

64. J. Gerstmann, "Some notes on the Gerstmann syndrome" *Neurology, 1957, 7*:866–869.

65. A. L. Benton, "The fiction of the 'Gerstmann syndrome'", *J. Neurol. Neurosurg. Psychiat., 1961, 24*:176–181.

66. M. Critchley, "The enigma of Gerstmann's syndrome", *Brain, 1966, 89*:183–198.

67. K. Poeck & B. Orgass, "Gerstmann's syndrome and aphasia", *Cortex, 1966, 2*:421–437.

68. R. F. Heimburger, W. D. Demter, & R. M. Reitan, "Implications of Gerstmann's syndrome", *J. Neurol. Neurosurg. Psychiat., 1964, 27*:52–57.

69. K. Poeck & B. Orgass (*op. cit.* above, note 51), pp. 273–275.

70. A. Pick (*op. cit.* above, note 55).

71. A. Pick (*op. cit.* above, note 56).

72. A. L. Benton, *Right-left discrimination and finger localization, development and pathology,* New York, Hoeber-Harper, 1959.

73. A. Pick (*op. cit.* above, note 56).

74. W. Riese & G. Bruck, "Le membre fantôme chez l'enfant", *Rev. neurol., 1950, 83*:221–222.

75. S. Weinstein & E. A. Sersen, "Phantoms in cases of congenital absence of limbs", *Neurology, 1961, 11*:905–911.

76. S. Weinstein, "Neuropsychological studies of the phantom", in, A. L. Benton (editor), *Contributions to clinical neuro-psychology,* Chicago, Aldine Press, 1969, pp. 73–106.

77. K. Poeck, "Phantoms following amputation in early childhood and in congenital absence of limbs", *Cortex*, 1964, *1*:269–275.

78. K. Poeck & B. Orgass, "Die Entwicklung des Körperschemas bei Kindern im Alter vom 4–10 Jahre", *Neuropsychologia*, 1964(a), *2*:109–130.

79. K. Poeck & B. Orgass, "Untersuchungen über das Körperschema bei blinden Kindern", *Neuropsychologia*, 1964(b), *2*:131-143.

80. K. Poeck & B. Orgass, (*op. cit.* above, note 51).

81. H. Head & G. Holmes (*op. cit.* above, note 50).

82. P. P. Broca, "Localisation des fonctions cérébrales siège du language articulé", *Bull. Soc. Anthrop. Paris*, 1863, *4*:200–202.

83. K. Conrad, "Über aphasische Sprachstörungen bei hirnverletzten, Linkshänder", *Nervenarzt*, 1949, *20*:148–154.

84. A. L. Luria, *Traumatic aphasia,* The Hague, Mouton, 1969.

85. W. R. Russell & M. L. E. Espir, *Traumatic aphasia,* London, Oxford University Press, 1961.

86. M. E. Humphrey & O. L. Zangwill, "Dysphasia in left-handed patients with unilateral brain lesions", *J. Neurol. Neursrg. Psychiat.,* 1952, *15*:184–193.

87. H. Hécaen & J. Ajuriaguerra, *Les gauchers. Préférence manuelle et dominance cérébrale,* Paris, Presses Universitaires Françaises, 1963.

88. H. Goodglass & F. A. Quadfasel, "Language laterality in left-handed aphasics", *Brain*, 1954, *77*:521–548.

89. J. R. Brown & J. Simmonson. "A clinical study of 120 aphasic patients. I. Observations in lateralization and localization of lesions", *Neurology*, 1957, *7*:777–784.

90. H. Hoff, "Die Lokalisation der Aphasie", *Proc. VIIth Int. Congr. Neurol., 1961*, pp. 23–39.

91. W. Penfield & L. Roberts (*op. cit.* above, note 25).

92. T. Bingley, "Mental symptoms in temporal lobe epilepsy and temporal lobe gliomas", *Acta Psychiat. neurol.*, 1958, *33*:Suppl., p. 120.

93. H. Goodglass & F. A. Quadfasel (*op. cit.* above, note 88).

94. H. Hécaen & M. Piercy, "Paroxysmal dysphasia and the problem of cerebral dominance", *J. Neurol. Neurosurg. Psychiat.,* 1956, *19*:194–201.

95. H. Hécaen & J. Sauguet, "Cerebral dominance in left-handed subjects", *Cortex*, 1971, *7*:19–47.

96. G. Ettlinger, G. V. Jackson, & O. L. Zangwill, "Cerebral dominance in sinistrals", *Brain*, 1956, *79*:569–588.

97. O. L. Zangwill, *Cerebral dominance and its relation to psychological function,* Edinburgh & London, Oliver & Boyd, 1960.

98. M. Piercy, "Testing for intellectual impairment—some comments on the tests and the testers", *J. Ment. Sci.,* 1959 *105*:489–495.

99. M. S. Gazzaniga, *The bisected brain,* New York, Appleton, Century & Crofts, 1970.

100. A. Patterson & O. L. Zangwill, "Disorders of visual space perception associated with lesions of the right cerebral hemisphere", *Brain,* 1944, *67*:331–358.

101. A. Patterson & O. L. Zangwill, "A case of topographical disorientation associated with a unilateral lesion", *ibid.,* 1945, *68*:188–212.

102. J. McFie, M. F. Piercy, & O. L. Zangwill, "Visual spatial agnosia with lesions of the right cerebral hemisphere", *ibid.,* 1960, *78*:167–190.

103. J. McFie & O. L. Zangwill, "Visual constructive disabilities associated with lesions of the left cerebral hemisphere", *ibid.,* 1960, *83*:243–260.

104. C. W. M. Whitty & F. Newcombe, "Disabilities associated with lesions in the posterior parietal region of the non-dominant hemisphere", *Neuropsychologia,* 1965, *3*:175–185.

105. E. R. Warrington & M. James, "Disorders of visual perception in patients with localized cerebral lesions", *ibid.,* 1967, *5*:253–266.

106. B. Milner, "Laterality effects of audition in interhemispheric relations and cerebral dominance", in, V. B. Mountcastle (editor), *Inter-hemispheric relations and cerebral dominance,* Baltimore, Johns Hopkins Press, 1962, pp. 215–243.

107. E. K. Warrington & M. James, "An experimental investigation of facial recognition in patients with unilateral cerebral lesions", *Cortex,* 1987, *3*:317–326.

108. B. Milner, "Memory and the medial temporal regions of the brain", in, K. H. Pribram & D. E. Broadbent (editors), *Biology of memory,* New York, Academic Press, 1970, pp. 29–50.

109. W. A. Lishman, "Emotion, consciousness and will after brain bisection", *Cortex,* 1971, *7*:181–192.

110. M. F. Piercy (*op. cit.* above, note 24).

111. E. K. Warrington, V. Logue, & R. T. C. Pratt, "The anatomical localization of selective impairment of auditory-verbal short term memory", *Neuropsychologia,* 1971, *9*:377–387.

112. A. L. Benton, "Differential behavioral effects in frontal lobe disease", *Neouropsychologia,* 1968, *6*:53–60.

113. T. Shallice & E. K. Warrington, "Independent functioning of verbal memory stores", *Q. J. exp. psychol.,* 1970, *22*:261–273.

114. B. Milner (*op. cit.* above, note 108).

115. J. McFie, "Psychological testing in clinical neurology", *J. nerv. ment. Dis., 1960, 131*:383–393.

116. A. L. Benton, "The problem of cerebral dominance", *Canad. Psychol.,* 1965, *6*:332–348.

117. W. F. Brewer, "Visual memory, verbal encoding and hemispheric localisation", *Cortex,* 1969, *5*:145–151.

118. J. McFie, M. F. Piercy & O. L. Zangwill (*op. cit.* above, note 102).

119. D. Kimura, "Dual functional asymmetry of the brain in visual perception", *Neuropsychologia,* 1966, *4*:275–285.

120. D. Kimura, "Functional asymmetry of the brain in dichotic listening", *Cortex,* 1967, *3*:163–178.

121. D. G. Doehring & R. N. Bartholomeus, "Laterality effects of voice recognition", *Neuropsychologia,* 1971, *9*:425–430.

122. B. Hermelin & N. O'Connor, "Functional asymmetry in the reading of Braille", *Neuropsychologia,* 1971,*9*:431–435.

123. M. Annett, "The growth of manual preference and speech", *Br. J. Psychol.,* 1970, *61*:545–558.

124. M. Annett, "A classification of hand preference by association analysis", *ibid.,* 1970, *61*:303–321.

125. S. T. Orton, *Reading, writing and speech problems in children,* London, Chapman & Hall, 1937.

126. M. Critchley, *Developmental dyslexia,* London, Heinemann, 1964.

127. G. Ettlinger, G. W. Jackson, & O. L. Zangwill (*op. cit.* above, note 96).

128. H. Hécaen & J. Ajuriaguerra, "Le problème de la dominance hemisphèrique: les gauchers lors des lesions hemisphèriques droites et gauches", *J. Psychol. norm. et path.*, 1956, *53*:473–486.

129. O. L. Zangwill (*op.cit.* above, note 97).

130. A. Subirana, J. Corominas, R. Puncernau, L. Oller-Daurella, J. Monteys, & E. Maso-Subirana, "Nueva contribución al estudio de la dominancia cerebral", *Medicamenta,* 1952, pp. 38–82.

131. M. P. Bryden, "Tachistoscopic recognition, handedness and cerebral dominance", *Neuropsychologia,* 1965, *3*:1–8.

132. M. Critchley, *The parietal lobes,* London, Arnold & Co., 1953.

133. F. Newcombe (*op. cit.* above, note 12).

134. J. McFie (*op.cit.* above, note 28), p. 1.

135. P. Marie, "L'Aphasie", in, *Travaux et mémoires,* Vol. 1, Paris, Masson & Cie., 1926, pp.3–181.

136. J. Taylor (editor), *Selected writings of John Hughlings Jackson,* London, Hodder & Stoughton, 1931, 2 vols.

137. G. Rylander, "Personality changes after operations on the frontal lobes", *Acta psychiat. neurol. scand.,* 1939, Suppl. 20.

138. S. Ackerly, "Instinctive, emotional and mental changes following prefrontal lobe extirpation", *Am. J. Psychiat.,* 1935, *92*:717–729.

139. R. M. Brickner, *The intellectual functions of the frontal lobes,* New York, Macmillan, 1936.

140. K. Goldstein, "The significance of the frontal lobes for mental performance", *J. Neurol. Psychopathol.,* 1936, *17*:27–40.

141. I. C. Nichols & J. McV. Hunt, "A case of parietal bilateral frontal lobectomy: a psychopathological study", *Am. J. Psychiat.,* 1940, *96*:1063–1087.

142. W. C. Halstead, *Brain and intelligence. A quantitative study of the frontal lobes,* Chicago, University of Chicago Press, 1947.

143. D. O. Hebb, "Man's frontal lobes. A critical review", *Arch Neurol. Psychiat.,* 1945, *54*:10–24.

144. N. Wertheim, "The amusias" (*op. cit.* above, note 28). The temporal lobes have been extensively reviewed by W. R. Adey "Recent studies of the rhinencephalon in relation to temporal lobe epilepsy and behaviour disorders" *Inter. rev. Neurobiol.,* 1959, *1*:1–46.

145. W. B. Scoville & B. Milner, "Loss of recent memory after bilateral hippocampal lesions", *J. Neurol. Neurosurg. Psychiat.,* 1957, *20*:11–21.

146. J. M. Nielsen, *Memory and amnesia,* Los Angeles, San Lucas Press, 1958.

147. H. Dimsdale, V. Logue, & M. F. Piercy, "A case of persisting impairment of recent memory following right temporal lobectomy", *Neuropsychologia,* 1964 *1*:287–298.

148. C. W. M. Whitty & W. A. Lishman (*op. cit.* above, note 26).

149. J. McFie & M. F. Piercy, "Intellectual impairment with localised cerebral lesions", *Brain,* 1952, *75*:291–311.

150. C. W. M. Whitty & W. A. Lishman (*op. cit.* above, note 26).

151. B. Milner, "The memory defect in bilateral hippocampal lesions", *Psychiat. Res. Rep.,* 1959, *11*:43–57.

152. F. Lhermitte & J. C. Gautier, "Aphasia" (*op. cit.* above, note 28), pp. 84–104.

153. H. Hécaen & J. Ajuriaguerra (*op. cit.* above, note 87).

154. M. Critchley (*op. cit.* above, note 132).

155. J. McFie & M. F. Piercy (*op. cit.* above, note 149).

156. J. McFie (*op. cit.* above, note 28).

157. S. Weinstein, J. Semmes, L. Ghent, & H. L. Teuber, "Spatial orientation in man after cerebral injury", *J. Psychol.,* 1956, *42*:249–263.

158. H. Hécaen, "Clinical symptomatology in right and left hemisphere lesions", in, V. B. Mouncastle (*op. cit.* above, note 106), pp. 215–243.

159. P. Marie (*op. cit.* above, note 135).

160. O. Pöetzl, *Die Aphasielehre vom Standpunkte der klinischen Psychiatrie. Die optisch-agnostischen Störungen,* in, G. Aschaffenburg, *Handbuch der Psychiatrie speziell,* Vol.3 Abt.2(1), Vienna, F. Deuticke, 1928.

161. J. Lange (*op. cit.* above, note 49).

162. D. Denny-Brown & B. Q. Banker, "Amorphosynthesis from left parietal lesions", *Arch. Neurol. Psychiat.,* 1954, *71*:302–313.

163. C. W. M. Whitty & F. Newcombe (*op. cit.* above, note 104).

164. J. McFie (*op. cit.* above, note 28).

165. E. De Renzi & H. Spinnler. "Impaired performance on color tests in patients with hemispheric damage", *Cortex,* 1967, *3*:194–217.

166. G. Moruzzi, "The physiological properties of the brain stem reticular system", in, J. F. Delafresnaye (editor), *Brain mechanisms and consciousness,* Springfield, Ill., C.C Thomas, 1954, pp. 21–53.

167. H. W. Magoun, *The waking brain, ibid.,* 1958.

168. J. D. Green, "The hippocampus", *Physiol. Rev.,* 1964, *44*:561–608.

169. H. Gastaut, "The brain stem and cerebral electrogenesis in relation to consciousness" (*op. cit.* above, note 166), pp. 249–283.

170. K. H. Pribram, "The limbic system", in, D. E. Sheer (editor), *Electrical stimulation of the brain,* Austin, Texas, University of Texas Press, 1961, pp. 311–320.

171. J. R. Smythies, *Brain mechanisms and behavior. An outline of the mechanisms of emotion, memory, learning and the organization of behaviour with particular regard to the limbic system,* 2nd edition, Oxford, Blackwells, 1970.

172. J. W. Papez "A proposed mechanism of emotion", *Arch. Neurol. Psychiat.,* 1937, *38*:725–743.

173. See, for example, S. S. Kety, "Regional neurochemistry and its application to brain function", in, J. D. French (editor), *Frontiers in brain research,* New York & London, Columbia University Press, 1962, pp. 97–120; E. de Robertis, "Molecular organization of synapses for chemical transmission in the central nervous system", in, A. G. Karczmar & J. C. Eccles (editors), *Brain and human behavior,* Berlin, Springer-Verlag, 1972, pp. 22–37.

A book by L. A. Stevens (*Explorers of the brain,* New York, A. A. Knopf, 1971) although pitched at a popular level, gives a good survey of the most recent techniques and advances. Recent studies with implanted electrodes are surveyed in J. M. R. Delgado's *Physical control of the mind,* New York, Harper & Row, 1969.

174. J. Z. Young, A *model of the brain,* Oxford, Clarendon Press, 1964.

175. S. Deutsch, *Model of the nervous system,* New York, J. Wiley, 1967; G. Werner, B. L. Whitsbel, & L. M. Putrucelli. "Data structure and alogorhythms in the primate somatosensory cortex", in Karczmar & Eccles (*op. cit.* above, note 173), pp.164–186.

MODERN CONCEPTS OF CORTICAL LOCALIZATION

14

1. INTRODUCTION

Since the publication of the first edition of this book, there have been remarkable advances in the understanding of the cerebral cortex. Modern concepts of cerebral localization have been influenced by technological advances and refinements in the investigative techniques that can be applied to the study of cortical function. There is now widespread acceptance that certain broad functions are related to specific brain structures. The evidence linking functions to specific structures depends, however, on the nature of the function under consideration. For many years it was argued by physiologists, based upon studies in animals, that there was no strict localization of function in the brain, but that different functions were all interrelated in the intact organism. As mentioned in Chapter 13, Karl Lashley held that the nature of the deficit resulting from removal of portions of the brain was dependent on the amount of brain that was removed.[1] Lashley's original theory of "total equipotentiality" implied that different cortical regions were functionally equivalent. A corollary of this, emphasized by the Russian School and summarized by Alexander Luria (1902–1977), implied that no part of the cortex was responsible solely for a specific function because under certain circumstances it was able to perform other functions.[2]

However, over the last 130 years, an increasing number of neuroscientists have attempted to ascribe functions to specific regions of the brain, and, more specifically, to different areas of the cerebral cortex (see Chapter 12). Much of the early evidence was derived from lesion experiments or clinical studies, and is therefore of ques-

tionable validity. The neurological or behavioral disturbance that follows brain damage does not simply reflect the loss of normal brain function but instead reflects the function in surviving brain tissue, and is best not considered in terms of normal function. As long ago as 1874, John Hughlings Jackson (1835–1911) warned that lesions, not functions, are localized in such circumstances.[3] Moreover, in complex regulatory systems, an apparently similar neurological or behavioral disturbance may result from disrupted function at any point along an extended network or pathway, and the recruitment of other regions of the brain may come to compensate for the original disturbance. Such factors confound clinical attempts to localize functions to discrete regions of the cerebral cortex or hemispheres. Nevertheless, clinical studies first suggested the localization of language function to the left cerebral hemisphere.

The experimental studies in Berlin of Gustav Fritsch and Eduard Hitzig, reported in 1870, showed that electrical stimulation of discrete regions of the cerebral cortex led to distinctive motor responses.[4] Those performed subsequently by David Ferrier in England, also involving electrical stimulation of discrete regions of the brain, provided further evidence to support the concept of cortical localization of certain functions, and in particular of centers responsible for the motor activity of different parts of the body.[5] (See also Chapter 12, p. 116).

In 1881, at the 7th International Medical Congress held in London, there was a dramatic confrontation between Friedrich Leopold Goltz, professor of physiology at the University of Strassburg (Strasbourg), and the cerebral localizers. Goltz reported that ablation of cortical areas in dogs did not lead to the expected deficits. For example, bilateral ablation of the anterior quadrant, including excitable regions, did not produce the permanent paralysis that was predicted from the work involving electrical stimulation. Similarly, after bilateral lesions that destroyed a large area of cortex posteriorly, there were behavioral changes but vision (which had been localized to this region) was preserved.[6] Based on such experiments, Goltz believed that the cortex was responsible for cognitive or psychic functions but that there was no localization of motor or sensory functions. (See also Chapters 12 and 13, pp. 117, 129.) David Ferrier and Gerald Yeo presented the opposing view, pointing out the problem of comparing experimental studies in different animal species and emphasizing their belief that cortical localization is greater in humans and monkeys than in animals such as dogs. They reported on experiments in monkeys in which focal lesions involving the precentral and postcentral gyrus led to contralateral weakness without other deficits, and bilateral lesions of the occipital lobes caused blindness. Then in 1887, Victor Horsley (1857–1916) published maps that also showed areas of motor representation on both sides of the rolandic fissure in humans.[7] The subsequent controversy about the extent of motor representation in relation to the rolandic fissure is discussed in a later section (Section 3).

More recently, careful clinical studies have shown that *cognitive* function can be subdivided into discrete and specific activities that are affected, sometimes in isolation, by localized brain pathology. There may, however, be considerable individual variation in the disturbances that follow isolated cerebral lesions relating in part to anatomical variation (for example, in gyral pattern), to the stability of the lesion, to secondary effects of the lesion on other regions of the brain, and to the interval between lesion onset and clinical evaluation.

Nevertheless, the punctate cortical localization of complex functions in discrete centers, at least as originally envisioned and depicted in maps of the cerebral cortex, seems increasingly unrealistic. Indeed, the concept of localized centers subserving distinct functions to the exclusion of other centers was criticized[8] at the very time of its development by that eccentric scientific genius, Charles Edouard Brown-Séquard (1817–1894). At the present time, it seems likely that several different cerebral regions are interconnected in networks mediating discrete functions. The complexity of any cerebral localization of

functions is exemplified by the subspecialization that exists even in such primary sensory systems as the visual system, where different attributes of a visual stimulus are processed separately by different populations of cortical cells. It is likely that cells in different cortical regions respond to the same object, reflecting different aspects of that object; information from these different cells then has to be integrated, requiring a certain temporal synchrony and the interconnection of different cortical regions. In monkeys, for example, neurons in Brodmann's area 7A of posterior parietal cortex respond both to the retinal location of a visual stimulus and to eye position, so that the spatial location of viewed objects can be determined by combining these signals. The interaction between eye position and visual response is usually nonlinear, and the visual receptive field remains retinotopic whereas the size of the response is modulated by eye position.[9] A neural network model has now been developed that reproduces the nonlinear interactions of eye position and shows how the location of a visual target, independent of eye position, can be extracted from a population of 7A neurons[9] (see Section 3).

Traditional concepts of cerebral localization involved a hierarchical system, in which centers of increasing importance performed integrative and analytical functions of increasing complexity. Primary sensory regions were generally regarded to be interconnected so that the various attributes of a stimulus could be integrated. Connections with limbic areas resulted in memory storage and emotional characterization of the stimulus, and activation of frontal association areas led to further integration so that the intact organism could react appropriately.[10] (The term *association cortex* is used to designate cortical regions other than primary motor and sensory areas.) Aspects of such a traditional hierarchical system may be reflected in convergence in the association cortex, but a serial and unidirectional process is incapable of explaining many aspects of cerebral function. Modern researchers therefore stress the existence of parallel pathways, each being concerned with one aspect of a particular function, that are integrated at multiple levels.[11] Goldman-Rakic has marshalled support for the concept that parallel cortical networks or circuits subserve spatial and nonspatial information processing tasks. This implies an integrated but diffuse system organized in several parallel systems bridging "all major subdivisions of the cerebrum."[12]

Today certain functions are widely accepted as being localized to specific cerebral regions such as the primary motor and sensory areas. However, within such broad regions are even more functionally specialized areas (as is discussed in Section 3). In addition, several different cortical regions appear to be implicated in the same broad category of activity, such as visual, somatosensory, or motor function. For example, cats and monkeys are said to have more than ten visual areas, and between five and ten somatosensory areas.[13] Interactions between the constituents of any given cortical area, between different cortical areas involved in the same general function, and between cortical areas involved in quite different functions must be important in permitting any complex behavioral activity. Activation of numerous cortical and subcortical regions must follow even simple stimuli, so that processing involves large regions of the brain. Both segregation and integration are therefore important aspects of modern concepts of cortical localization of function.[11] Moreover, cerebral regions subserving specialized functions must not only be intact but capable of appropriate activation by other neural structures for those functions to be realized.

With regard to motor activity, several different cortical areas have been implicated, various subcortical regions are involved in feedback loops, and sensory functions may occur in these same, predominantly motor cortical areas. The "motor cortex" is therefore best regarded as simply the output region for various complex neural systems.

Neurocognitive Networks

Neuronal systems that involve the serial processing of information through different centers of increasing complexity would probably be too slow and restrictive to account for certain cognitive processes.[14] A parallel distributed processing system permits many factors to be processed simultaneously and thus is more advantageous in this regard.[15] Such multifocal networks may be localized to one cytoarchitectonic field or adjacent areas. Widely disseminated networks rather than local systems, however, are likely to be involved in complex cognitive functions, such as attention and language.[14] The existence of such diffuse cortical networks would imply that an individual region of association cortex forms an integral part of several networks. Involvement of such a region pathologically may then result in multiple deficits or—in the presence of alternative parallel pathways—in little or no clinical abnormality. Moreover, seemingly similar clinical deficits may result from lesions at diverse sites in the brain.

Neural networks are probably involved in such cognitive functions as the maintenance of attention. Loss of directed attention—or neglect—occurs in humans or monkeys with lesions of various subcortical regions or with lesions of the dorsolateral posterior parietal cortex, the dorsolateral premotor-prefrontal cortex, or the cingulate gyrus.[14] There are extensive reciprocal connections between these three cortical areas. It has therefore been suggested that directed attention depends on an integrated network involving these three cortical regions, each of which provides some slightly different reference for mapping the environment.[14] Sensory representation of external space is subserved by the posterior parietal cortex, the distribution of orienting and exploring movements by the frontal component, and motivational aspects by the cingulate region. This is supported by the observation that in monkeys[16] and humans,[17] sensory inattention or neglect is conspicuous after parietal lobe lesions whereas hemispatial neglect for tasks involving motor activity results with frontal lesions. Cingulate lesions cause contralateral hemispatial neglect, and positron emission tomography (PET) studies in humans show involvement of the cingulate gyrus for attentional activity that selects for action.[18] This topic is discussed further on page 162.

At the neuronal level, experimental evidence suggests that attention may involve enhancement of sensory responses in the posterior parietal cortex or selection—probably by frontal cortex—from amongst a series of motor programs or strategies, some of which may be conflicting.[19] In patients with inattention syndromes, the neglect is multimodal, being independent of the modality of sensory input or motor output. In addition, among patients with right (but not left) cerebral lesions there is evidence of mild ipsilateral as well as severe contralateral spatial inattention, suggesting a right hemisphere dominance for directing attention.[20] Left hemisphere pathology causes only mild contralateral attention deficits, because function of the intact right hemisphere is sufficient to maintain attention.

Plasticity

Cortical maps imply a certain fixed representation that fails to account for the plasticity of the central nervous system.[21] Indeed, as Asanuma has succinctly commented, "a view of the cortex as a static array of hardwired, parallel circuits is blatantly in error."[22] Representation in the cerebral cortex is variable, depending on preceding activity and other factors (Figure 158). The plasticity of the nervous system is one mechanism permitting learning (e.g., improvements in motor performance with practice) to occur.

The somatosensory representation in the sensory cortex is not simply a static somatotopic map based on neuroanatomical connections. The primary somatosensory cortex encompasses Brodmann's architectonic fields 3, 1, and 2, and contains detailed representations of the surface of the body. Following alteration of input to the cortex from the periphery, there is an alteration of the cortical representation of somatosensory function. The somatosensory maps acquired so painstakingly by anatomical cartographers are actually dynamic, and in consequence there is considerable variation in such maps between normal adults. For example, in different monkeys of the same species there is a severalfold difference in the proportional area of cortical representation of a given surface of skin in area 3b, and even greater differences in area 1.[23] Indeed, interindividual differences of cortical representation within a given species may exceed that between different primate species, a finding that has been attributed to differences in skin use among different animals.[23]

Following peripheral nerve degeneration, there is a marked reorganization of somatosensory representation in areas 3b and 1.[21, 24] When the median nerve is cut, for example, cortical neurons previously responsive to cutaneous stimulation within the median nerve territory are "taken over" so that they are responsive instead to stimulation within the territory of the radial or ulnar nerve as a result of some functional reorganization within the central nervous system. Following peripheral nerve transection and surgical reconnection, the subsequent representational maps differ from those present originally so that a single cortical neuron may have several, widely separated receptive fields. Eventually, however, small receptive fields for cortical neurons are reestablished, due presumably to mechanisms involving central input selection or filtering, and topographic order is restored to the cortical map.[25–26] Cortical reorganization seems to reflect differences in synaptic effectiveness rather than anatomical changes such as terminal sprouting.[23] This implies that convergent sensory inputs exist in the normal cortex, but corticocortical pathways may also be important.[27]

Studies in adult humans have also demonstrated cortical plasticity. The normal somatosensory homunculus, mapped by magnetoencephalography (MEG) (see Section 2), shows a wide hand area. Subjects in whom one of

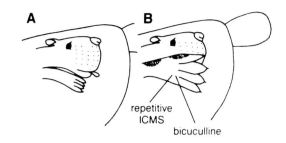

FIGURE 158.
Transient map changes in the rat motor cortex resulting from repetitive intracortical microstimulation (ICMS) or bicuculline application. (A) Control. (B) Repetitive intracortical microstimulation or bicuculline application in the forelimb area results in an enlargement of the forelimb representation, with forelimb movements elicited from sites previously representing the vibrissae or neck. Changes can be identified within hours, and are transient. Shaded zones are dual representation sites. (From Asanuma C., "Mapping movements within a moving motor map", *Trends Neurosci*, 1991, *14*:217–218.)

the upper limbs has been amputated show a conspicuous change in the homunculus (Plate 1), with marked intrusion of the facial representation into the region normally representing the digits and hand.[28] MEG has also been used to investigate the detailed functional organization within the hand area in normal adults and patients with various abnormalities of the hand.[29] In normal adults the somatotopic organization of the cortical hand area has been demonstrated with high spatial precision by recording from the scalp the magnetic fields generated in the region of the parietal somatosensory cortex in response to tactile stimulation of the digits in the contralateral hand. Studies of two adult patients with congenital syndactyly have revealed abnormal cortical topography, with nonsomatotopic spatial representation of the digits; cortical reorganization occurred within weeks of corrective surgery on the hand and correlated with the new functional status of the separated digits.[29]

Cortical reorganization also follows the experimental placement of lesions in the cortex, with neurons adjacent to the lesion gaining new receptive fields. In this way, the body surface originally represented in the lesioned area of cortex comes to be represented in neighboring cortical regions.

Maps of motor function, like those of somatosensory representation, are also dynamic (Figure 158). For example, after the motor nerve to the whiskers is cut in adult rats, electrical stimulation of the whisker area within the primary motor area of cortex leads to forelimb movements.[30–31] Moreover, changes in afferent feedback to the primary motor cortex, such as occurs with changes in static forelimb posture in rats, influence the organization of motor cortex after a brief delay[32] and repeated passive movements of the forelimb increases the size of its cortical representation. It thus appears that the relation between a set of cortical neurons and muscles is dynamic, being influenced by sensory feedback and other mechanisms.[31] Recent work suggests that intracortical connections permit variable interactions between neurons in the primary motor area of cortex, thereby forming the basis of the reorganizational changes that follow central or peripheral injury or that allow for learning to occur. Motor learning encompasses a number of activities such as conditional association and the reorganization of muscle synergies required to develop new motor skills. Accumulating evidence implicates a reorganization of cortical circuits in the primary motor area during learning of motor tasks.[31]

2. DELINEATION OF CORTICAL REGIONS

Anatomical Maps

The best manner of defining cortical regions having specific functional attributes is unclear. It is widely believed that differences in function are reflected by differences in structure. In the past the cerebral cortex was subdivided on the basis of its architecture, and the detailed reports of Korbinian Brodmann[33] in particular, led to complex maps of the brain in which a multiplicity of different regions were delineated on a cytoarchitectonic basis (see Chapter 12). However, there was no unanimity concerning the demarcation of different regions, the number of distinct regions, the criteria for distinguishing regions, or the homologies between species. In many instances, distinctions between regions seemed superficial, trivial, or inapparent to different investigators. Conversely, primary cortical areas that once were deemed to be histologically uniform—and therefore to have a

uniform function—have now been shown to be remarkably heterogeneous. Older histological methods have been extended by new anatomical techniques based upon the distribution of neurotransmitters and other compounds, and recent studies using these techniques have indicated a remarkable diversity among neurons that once were considered to form a homogenous population. Within any individual cortical area, not only do the cells in different layers have different functions but histochemical differences (reflected for example in the modular architecture of the primary visual cortex) and differences in connectivity indicate a separation of different functions.[11] Thus, parallel processing occurs within one cortical region as well as between different regions.

Lesion Experiments and Anatomical Connectivity

For many years, functional-anatomical relationships have been based on studies of humans or animals with relatively large lesions. Histological studies traced the connectivity between the injured region and other areas of the brain, and behavioral studies associated any loss or derangement of behavior with the site of the lesion. However, as has long been recognized, behavioral or functional change after a brain lesion does not necessarily indicate that the site of the lesion is the cerebral region responsible for the normal function that has become deranged.

In recent years, studies of connectivity have been advanced by the development of anterograde or retrograde tracers. These tracer chemicals are injected into a localized region of the brain where they are taken up by portions of the neurons and transported anterogradely or retrogradely along the axons (that is, away from or toward the cell bodies, respectively). This permits fiber connections to be delineated with precision. Further, the strategy of double-labeling two interconnected cortical areas in the same animal provides much additional information.[12] For example, simultaneous injections of two distinct anterograde tracers into the dorsolateral prefrontal cortex and posterior parietal cortex of rhesus monkeys has shown that these two areas are mutually interconnected with each other and that both project to as many as fifteen other cortical areas ipsilaterally, at least three cortical areas contralaterally, and many subcortical areas.[34] The common ipsilateral frontal cortical receiving areas included portions of the supplementary motor area (Brodmann's area 6), dorsal and anterior premotor cortex (area 6), the anterior bank of the arcuate sulcus (area 8), the anterior cingulate cortex (area 24), and orbital prefrontal cortex (area 11); there were also common receiving areas in the parietal and temporal lobes. In most cortical areas, terminals from the frontal injection site alternated with those from the parietal site. However, in projections to the frontoparietal operculum and the superior temporal cortex, terminal labeling from the two cortical areas occurred in the same columns but in different laminae. The extensive common connectivity of the prefrontal and parietal cortices suggested that these areas were part of a larger neural system subserving behavior in a specific cognitive domain,[34] and the different patterns of termination suggested the involvement of different integrative mechanisms.

Electrical Stimulation

As already indicated, electrical stimulation of the cortex has been used in animals to define the function of different cerebral regions and in patients to localize certain functions such as language, especially prior to the surgical treatment of epilepsy and other neurological disorders. More recently, patients have been studied following implantation of arrays of subdural electrodes, or noninvasively by transcranial magnetic stimulation. Electrical stimulation of the brain may activate or block certain functions. Thus, the motor activity initially observed in animals[4, 5] and humans[35] following such stimulation led to the definition of motor centers in the cortex. The early, pioneering studies culminated in the detailed investigations of Wilder G. Penfield (1891–1976) and his colleagues, performed in conscious patients during neurosurgical operations (see Figure 151, Chapter 13), and the mapping of rather grotesque homunculi, representing the localization of motor and sensory functions (see Figures 148–150, Chapter 13) on the cortical surfaces.[36] Similarly, stimulation of the striate cortex in the occipital region led to sensations of light. By contrast, stimulation of certain other cortical areas led to impairment or blocking of speech and language.[37]

With cortical stimulation, it is possible to compare functional performance before, during, and after stimulation. In humans, stimulation with current at intensities that do not produce seizures may interfere with task performance while the current is applied, with recovery occurring once stimulation is discontinued. This has been used to define brain areas that are involved in the performance of a specific task. Functional involvement is assumed when the task cannot be performed satisfactorily while a specific area is stimulated. However, any site defined by this means may be only one of several involved in the function being tested, and task perfor-

mance may be good even after resection of this region. Moreover, regions adjacent to a lesioned area rapidly gain new receptive fields,[23] either because of the development of new connections or a functional reorganization of existing synaptic connections and activity.

The effects of electrical stimulation are, in any event, difficult to interpret because cortical stimulation may have both local (cortical) effects and more distant effects from intracortical spread of current or stimulation of subcortical fiber tracts. Moreover, different motor maps can be obtained from the same brain by varying the stimulus parameters. Studies in anesthetized animals are also difficult to interpret because the response of the cortex may have been modified pharmacologically.

Imaging Techniques

Modern imaging techniques have had a major impact on concepts of cerebral function and have permitted studies of specific functions in humans. New imaging techniques provide an ancillary approach to investigating the functional localization of the brain in normal subjects and patients with neurological diseases. X-ray computed tomography scanning (CT), magnetic resonance imaging (MRI), and magnetic resonance angiography (MRA) are important means of visualizing noninvasively the structural anatomy of the brain, thereby permitting anatomoclinical correlations in patients with focal cerebral lesions. In patients with focal, hemispheric structural pathology, specific functions cannot be ascribed to the involved part of the brain on the basis of the associated neurological deficits, however, because metabolic (and thus functional) changes occur in regions distant to the visualized structural lesions.[38] Electroencephalography (EEG), magnetoencephalography (MEG), positron emission tomography (PET), single photon emission computed tomography (SPECT), and functional MRI (f MRI) are means of studying cerebral function in normal subjects and patients with cerebral pathology.

Computed Tomography (CT) The technique depends on the absorption by different tissues of different amounts of x-rays depending on tissue density. X-rays taken of the head at a number of different angles through a plane will, after computer processing, allow an image of the head to be reconstructed. CT imaging of the head provides good visualization of the cortical gyri and ventricular system of the brain, but only limited differentiation of gray and white matter.

Magnetic Resonance Imaging and Angiography (MRI, MRA) MRI, which does not require exposure to ionizing radiation, provides outstanding anatomical resolution of the brain, and excellent differentiation of gray and white matter. MRIs reflect the spatial distribution and chemical environment of water protons. Using a combination of selective radiofrequency pulses and precise magnetic gradient coils, the magnetic relaxation properties and location of protons can be calculated. Mathematical manipulation allows presentation as an image (MRI) or as a chemical spectrum (MR spectroscopy).

MRA permits the visualization of blood vessels by techniques that depend on motion-related phase and frequency shifts of the blood to generate contrast. Spatial resolution is such that vessels of about 2 to 3 mm in diameter can be routinely visualized.

Magnetic Resonance Spectroscopy (MRS) Certain nuclei resonate at different frequencies in the same static magnetic field when located in different chemical microenvironments, thereby permitting different resonances to be assigned to specific sites in different molecules.[39] Initial studies in humans were based on especially strong hydrogen proton resonances such as from N-acetylaspartate, but technological improvements now permit the study of weaker resonances such as lactate, glutamate, and creatine.[39] Phosphorous spectroscopy permits identification of high energy phosphates (such as adenosine triphosphate [ATP]) and calculation of tissue pH. These techniques, which can record focal changes in, for example, cerebral pH over short periods of time, will eventually permit the analysis of a range of chemicals in the brain. Recent advances have extended previous limitations such that large-area spectroscopic imaging has become feasible. Efforts are underway to develop libraries of metabolic changes in various disease states.

Positron Emission Tomography (PET) This technique utilizes positron emitting isotopes (such as oxygen[15] or fluorine[18]) which are integrated into tracer chemicals having known biological properties. A labeled chemical is administered to subjects either intravenously or by inhalation, and the distribution of the radioisotope is then determined in three-dimensional space by an array of external detectors, and is held to reflect cerebral blood flow. The technique has been used to measure regional cerebral metabolism or oxygen utilization, a variety of regional biochemical processes, and local cerebral blood flow. There are focal increases in glucose metabolism and blood flow in regions of the cerebral cortex during performance of motor or cognitive tasks or with sensory stimulation in normal subjects, as shown in Plate 2.[40–46] It is assumed that such changes primarily reflect excitatory processes that have a direct functional role in effecting the function under study, whereas increases in neuronal activity (and thus in cerebral blood flow) may lead to inhibition in other cerebral regions, and thus have a less direct functional role.[47] Other concerns about the use of PET in inferring cerebral function also exist and have been reviewed by Sergent.[47] Among the more important objections is the erroneous assumption that any increase in cerebral blood flow mirrors the contribution of the affected region to a particular aspect of the task under investigation and that this cerebral region always has the same role regardless of context or any other cerebral operations involved.

In one recent study, within-arm somatotopy was demonstrated in several cerebral motor areas of normal subjects performing a visuomotor tracking task during sequential imaging.[46] Segmental limb movements were associated with changes in cerebral blood flow in the contralateral motor, supplementary motor, cingulate, and parietal cortex. Analysis of responses showed an overlapping somatotopic distribution in the motor cortex, with thumb responses most ventrolateral and shoulder responses most dorsomedial; there was also somatotopy in the supplementary motor cortex and the cingulate cortex, with finger responses anterior to shoulder responses. Recent studies have also shown that, in patients with structural cerebral lesions, the technique can be used for functional localization of motor cortex.[48]

Analysis of cognitive processes is more complex[47] and there are certain inconsistencies between the results of different investigators. Moreover, with cognitive tasks in particular, PET studies may provide information about changes in blood flow in different cerebral regions during task performance (that is, may provide information about which cerebral areas are involved), but provides only limited information on the temporal relationships involved during the activation of these different areas.

Single Photon Emission Computed Tomography (SPECT) SPECT involves the administration intravenously or by inhalation of chemicals containing isotopes (such as xenon[133] or iodine[123]) that emit single photon radiation, especially as gamma rays. SPECT has been used to evaluate normal and pathological brain function, and especially cerebral perfusion and receptor distributions. It promises to become a valuable tool in extending understanding of cerbral function.

Functional Magnetic Resonance Imaging (*f* MRI)   Functional MRI offers the prospect of discrete anatomical localization of function superimposed on three-dimensional images of the brain, that is, it provides both anatomical and functional information (Plate 3). The technique involves the intravenous administration of gadolinium diethylenetriaminepentaacetic acid which, as it passes through the cerebral vasculature, lowers signal intensity on MRI in relation to blood flow. When studies are performed at rest and then after some activation procedure, the change in signal intensity can provide some indication of the effect of the activation procedure on local cerebral perfusion. An alternative approach does not require a bolus tracer injection. It involves using pulse sequences showing changes in signal intensity that reflect changes in the oxygen concentration of venous blood at sites of altered neuronal activity. Deoxyhemoglobin is paramagnetic relative to oxyhemoglobin and the surrounding brain tissues. With focal cerebral activity there is an increase in oxygen supply to discrete regions of the brain, leading to a higher concentration of oxygenated blood. Oxygen consumption does not necessarily increase in parallel with the increased blood flow, however, and there is a reduction in deoxyhemoglobin concentration within the venous system of the active area. Images are acquired rapidly, so that changes in signal in relation to underlying activity can be recognized.

The gadolinium technique was used first to provide a map of activated cortical areas in humans exposed to a visual stimulus. There was a significant increase in regional blood volume within the anatomically defined primary visual cortex, especially in the medial-posterior regions of the occipital lobes along the calcarine fissures. There were also areas of increased activation in regions beyond the primary visual area.[49]

Electroencephalography (EEG)

The electrical activity of the brain that is recorded from the scalp reflects primarily the activity of cells in the superficial layers of the cerebral cortex. The temporal resolution of EEG is in the order of milliseconds (so that events can be recorded that are too brief to be recognized by PET or MRI), but the spatial resolution is not as good as with certain imaging techniques. Computerized analysis

and signal averaging techniques, however, have provided fresh impetus to the use of this approach. Similarly, recordings from the surface of the brain (electrocorticography or ECoG), from grids of subdural or epidural electrodes, or from within the depth of the brain (depth electrography) utilizing structural imaging approaches have improved the spatial resolution and provided much new information about cerebral localization.

The spatial detail of the scalp-recorded EEG has recently been improved in the research setting by increasing the number of recording electrodes and mathematically modeling the volume conduction of cerebral potentials to the scalp based upon anatomical information derived from the MRI of individual subjects. By such an approach, there is a reduction of the "blurring" that occurs as a result of conduction though the highly resistive bone of the skull. Technical details are provided by Gevins and associates.[50] With this approach, it is possible to monitor the subsecond changes in cerebral activity that accompany perceptual and cognitive processing. The aim of the applied modeling method is to find a hypothetical point dipole to account for the field measured at the scalp, that is, to fit mathematically the site, orientation, and strength of a hypothetical point source of electrical current to the electrical potentials (or magnetic fields) recorded over the scalp. In fact, however, a single dipole is not a physiologically realistic model, if only because extensive areas of brain are activated by almost any stimulus.[51]

Magnetoencephalography (MEG)

MEG measures the magnetic fields generated by electric current flow in the brain, and permits the source of electrical events to be determined. The magnetic field of the brain is very much weaker than that of the earth or of many items found in an urban environment. Therefore, recording the brain's magnetic field requires sophisticated apparatus (a superconducting quantum interference device or SQUID) isolated from the environment. The recent development of multichannel devices has made it possible to map the amplitude of the extracranial magnetic field over the scalp and thereby localize the source of the field within the head. Localization is based on the concept of dipole modeling, the current source being deduced from the magnetic field pattern (Plate 4). However, several current sources can account for the recorded pattern, and any proposed source is therefore designated an "equivalent" source capable of generating a field pattern similar to that recorded.

The probable source of cerebral magnetic fields are electric currents generated in relation to synchronously activated cortical neurons. MEG is complementary to EEG, being especially sensitive to tangential current sources whereas the latter is more sensitive to radial current sources. The MEG thus records fissural activity, which is important because the greater part of the cerebral cortex is fissural. It has a greater spatial resolution than EEG (in the order of 1 to 2 mm under favorable conditions),[52] but is relatively insensitive to deep sources. The technique has been used in recent years to study the cortical activity generated spontaneously or in response to cognitive processes. It has shown, for example, that there are significant differences in the activity elicited in the human brain by sound stimuli, depending on whether the subject is required to pay attention to the stimulus.[52] The spatiotemporal information provided by MEG is also important in studying aspects of signal processing in the brain. This is exemplified by investigations of the ongoing spontaneous activity in the range of 8 to 13 Hz (the so-called alpha rhythm) that is found normally over the cerebral cortex and is suppressed by cognitive tasks over areas of cortex participating in those tasks.[53] When a subject is required to seek a rhyme for a visually displayed word on a screen, suppression of alpha activity begins immediately over the visual area and lasts for more than 500 ms, whereas there is a delay of about 100 ms before suppression begins over the temporal area, indicating the interplay between the two areas.

Evoked Potentials

The cerebral potentials elicited by somatosensory, auditory or visual stimuli have been used in humans and animals in attempts to localize the corresponding primary afferent cortical areas. However, the use of auditory evoked potentials to map the primary auditory cortex in humans is limited by the invasive technique that is required, and mapping of the primary visual cortex by visual evoked potentials has not been successful. Somatosensory evoked potentials can be recorded easily and directly from the cerebral cortex because of their large size. They have been used in localization studies performed for clinical purposes. For example, when direct recordings are made from the cortex, certain components of the response to median nerve stimulation are localized to the immediate rolandic-perirolandic region and show a clear phase reversal across the rolandic fissure. This is useful in defining the rolandic fissure for surgical reasons, but provides only limited information concerning the more subtle aspects of cerebral function.

Recent technological advances, however, have increased the information that can be derived from electrophysiological studies of cerebral function in normal humans. Evoked potential studies utilizing an increased number of electrodes and some means of increasing the spatial resolution of signals, such as the Laplacian derivation or the finite element deblurring method, hold promise of contributing significantly to the analysis of functional specialization in the cerebral cortex. Topographic maps of sensory or cognitive evoked potentials generally display the voltage recorded over different regions of the scalp at a specific time selected to correspond to the latency of the evoked potential component under consideration. The latency of this component, however, may well vary at different electrode sites, because several areas of the brain are likely to be involved in any particular function, especially one involving a behavioral response. Gevins and his associates have been concerned with the development of a practical method for characterizing evoked potential components in terms of their spatial topography and their temporal relations at different sites on the scalp.[54-55] Such relationships can be studied by various quantitative techniques, but they have developed the method of evoked potential covariance analysis, based upon the concept that the neural processes associated with higher cognitive functions must involve the coordination of activity in different regions of the brain and that the coordination of two or more neuronal populations during task performance should be reflected by a consistent relationship between the morphology of the evoked potential waveforms generated by these populations, with a consistent time interval between them. Covariance of this sort does not in itself establish the existence of direct corticocortical connections or interactions, nor does it indicate the anatomical basis of the electrophysiological findings, but the findings can be related to those obtained by other techniques to provide a better appreciation of the functional specialization of the cerebral cortex. The approach developed by Gevins and his collaborators requires data collection and preprocessing for artifact removal, computer averaging of the cerebral responses, and spatial enhancement of the signal. The correlations between electrical activity (multilag cross-covariance functions) are then computed between all pairs of electrodes. The locations and width of these intervals depend on the timing and duration of components of the evoked potential under study.[56]

Studies using this approach are of especial interest with regard to cognitive function. They suggest that individual cognitive functions are associated with a sequence of spatiotemporal patterns of coordinated processing that involves widely distributed areas of sensory, association, and motor cortex. They are exemplified by the findings obtained during a skilled motor response task that involved the production of a precisely graded ballistic pressure response of either the right or left index finger to a visually presented stimulus (Plate 5). The results of this and similar studies suggest the functional association of different cerebral areas during the performance of a cognitive task (Plate 6). The moment-by-moment changes in the evoked potential covariance patterns have been taken to reflect processing by different neural networks as cognitive requirements change during different stages of task performance.

Magnetic Fields

Recordings of magnetic fields have also been used to study and localize cerebral activity generated in discrete cortical regions in response to various sensory stimuli or cognitive tasks. Locating a neuronal source is achieved more satisfactorily magnetically than electrically because a simpler model of the head can be used and the conductivity of intervening tissue can be neglected because it does not influence the field pattern[53] The first study involving this technique to localize a neuronal source involved recording the magnetic field over the scalp following somatosensory stimulation.[57] The cortical cells activated by the somatosensory stimulus produce a rapidly changing magnetic field, and if these cells occupy an area less than a few square centimeters, the current distribution can be approximated by a dipole.[52] Recent studies with this approach have permitted the somatosensory cortex (and other sensory cortical regions) to be mapped in healthy human subjects.

3. CORTICAL LOCALIZATION OF SELECTED FUNCTIONS

Motor and Somatosensory Function

Based on perceptive clinical observations, Hughlings Jackson originally envisioned a hierarchical organization of the motor system.[58] Subsequent experimental studies in animals employing electrical stimulation showed that stimulation at certain sites of the cerebral cortex led to contraction of muscles. Over the years, several discrete cortical motor areas have been recognized, but there is no unanimity concerning their site, function, or even nomenclature. In primates the posterior precentral gyrus includes the primary motor area of cortex (MI, sometimes designated MsI because it also has some sensory

functions), which corresponds closely to Brodmann's area 4. The area immediately anterior to this—Brodmann's area 6—is also a motor region and is generally considered as at least two separate areas: the supplementary motor area medially, and the premotor or lateral premotor area laterally. Other motor areas within area 6 have also been recognized by some, but not other, authors. The border between area 4 and area 6 is not clearly demarcated.

In addition, on the medial surface of the cortex there is a cingulate motor area (in Brodmann's area 24) and a region involved in eye movement, while laterally the frontal eye fields are situated just anterior to area 6, in area 8. The parietal lobe also contains motor areas, and it is misleading to consider the primary somatosensory regions (in areas 3, 1, and 2) as having no motor role. Indeed, for many years there has been controversy concerning the extent to which the prerolandic motor region of the cortex should be distinguished from postrolandic regions to which some authors—including both Sir Charles Sherrington (1857–1952) and Harvey Cushing (1869–1939)—attributed purely sensory function.[59-60] Most textbooks still follow the rigid demarcation proposed by Sherrington and his colleagues although increasing evidence indicates that this view is too narrow. Woolsey and his colleagues[61] found by their stimulation experiments that the "perirolandic" region has both sensory and motor functions and subsequently showed that primary motor responses could be elicited from the postcentral gyrus even after chronic removal of the perirolandic and supplementary motor areas.[62] This and other evidence[63] suggests a broad and overlapping cortical representation of sensorimotor function (despite the perpetuation in many texts of the Sherringtonian distinction between sensory and motor function). Recent experience, involving electrical stimulation in epileptic patients prior to neurosurgical resection of a seizure focus, provides support for this view.[64-65]

Studies involving electrical stimulation, both in humans and animals, led to the publication of topographically organized maps of the motor representation in the primary motor cortex.[36,61] The grotesque figurines (homunculi of Penfield) so depicted reflected the cortical regions (within the confines of the primary motor cortex) from which movements of different parts of the body could be elicited, and which—it was therefore assumed—were responsible for movement of those bodily parts (see Figures 148 and 150, Chapter 13). Although there are certain methodological limitations associated with stimulation techniques, important information has emerged from these studies.[66–67] First, there are clearly multiple cortical outputs to individual muscles and to the individual lower motor neurons innervating these muscles. Second, there is extensive overlap of the cortical output to different muscles or lower motor neurons. Individual lower motor neurons, muscles, or movements can be activated from relatively large, often discontinuous, cortical regions. Individual cortical cells usually project to more than one muscle, typically to a particular set of muscles and often inhibiting antagonistic muscles.[66] Overlapping representations of different muscles permits synergistic, functionally relevant movements to occur.[66–67]

The somatotopic organization of the primary motor cortex for movements of different parts of the body in normal humans has subsequently been confirmed by MEG recordings[68] and by techniques involving the noninvasive (transcranial) electrical or magnetic stimulation of the brain.[69] In addition, evidence has been acquired of somatotopic representation in the other motor areas of cerebral cortex.[61] Recent studies in nonhuman primates have confirmed the somatotopic organization of the supplementary motor area and shown homuncular representation in the cingulate cortex[70–71] and electrical stimulation in humans at the time of corticography provides support for the somatotopic organization of the supplementary motor area.[72] Such an organization must be interpreted with a certain caution. Glees and Cole[73] reported forty-five years ago that there was rapid recovery of skilled motor functions after small lesions of the motor cortex (Brodmann's area 4) in monkeys. Resection of the electrically defined thumb area of the cortex, for example, was followed within two days by functional recovery, and cortical stimulation then elicited thumb movements from regions where stimulation had previously elicited only hand movements. They concluded that neighboring cortical areas have the ability to control the functions of previously removed or undercut cortical regions. Such cerebral plasticity was discussed earlier.

Various studies have indicated an increase in cerebral blood flow in the primary motor cortex (Brodmann's area 4) in response to volitional motor activity (Plates 7 and 8). Roland and associates[74] showed that there was increased blood flow to the contralateral primary motor and sensory hand region in response to simple finger movements, whereas performance of complicated finger-sequencing tasks produced changes in blood flow within the supplementary motor areas bilaterally as well as in the contralateral primary motor and sensory cortex. Such studies suggest that the supplementary motor area is a higher-order center involved in generating and programming complex movements, and this has been supported by studies in humans undergoing corticectomies.[75]

The results of PET and functional MRI studies have sometimes been conflicting. Fox and coworkers found in PET studies that the supplementary motor area was active during all motor tasks regardless of their complexity, and assigned it a role in establishing motor set and in the preparation to move, independent of task complexity.[76] By contrast, a recent preliminary study involving functional MRI showed that a number of sites in the frontal and parietal regions are activated by movements, the precise number depending on the type of movement that is performed.[77] The posterior precentral gyrus is activated in humans only during motor performance, whereas more frontal and parietal motor cortical areas are activated during complex motor performance and mental rehearsal for such performance. The supplementary motor area and premotor cortex participated especially during complex sequential motor activity. During an imagined complex motor activity, signal changes were observed especially in the supplementary motor area and, to a lesser extent, in the premotor cortex; there was no activation in primary motor or sensory cortex.

It seems that the motor cortex receives inputs from—and, in turn, projects to—multiple regions, including the thalamus, other cortical areas including primary somatosensory and association cortex, and the basal ganglia. The various motor areas of cortex are also interconnected. The primary motor cortex appears to be involved especially in the fine control of force and position.[31] The supplementary motor area is implicated in the planning and initiation of complex movements.[74–75,77–78] It is also involved in movement sequences that are dependent on feedback mechanisms. The lateral premotor area may be important in using sensory (for example, visual) cues to prepare or direct movements.[31, 79]

The somatosensory cortex has been mapped in humans and animals by direct electrical stimulation of the brain,[80–81] by recording the cortical potentials evoked by mechanical stimulation of the body surface,[81] or by recording somatosensory evoked potentials from the cortical surface following electric stimulation of peripheral nerves.[82–83] Some of the earliest studies indicated that more than one cortical region could be activated by somatosensory stimuli. The first widely accepted somatic cortical receiving area to be described has come to be designated SI (or SmI), and a subsequently described region is referred to as SII (or SmII), but the functional relationship between these two major areas is unclear. Other somatosensory areas have also been described in certain animal species. In monkeys, at least four areas within the primary somatosensory cortex (SI)—that is, within Brodmann's areas 3, 1, and 2—contain distinct maps of the contralateral body surface.[84] Direct cortical recording of the cerebral responses elicited by somatosensory stimulation of patients undergoing epilepsy surgery has provided more detailed information concerning the organization of somatosensory cortex in humans. Thus, analysis of the spatiotemporal features of the median-derived somatosensory evoked potential reveals two cortical sources (based on dipole modeling) in the postcentral gyrus[85] in accord with experiments in animals, which have suggested multiple cortical somatosensory representations of cutaneous body surface in the postcentral gyrus. In humans, direct cortical stimulation (during epilepsy surgery) has elicited contralateral sensations after stimulation of SI, but bilateral parasthesias with SII stimulation, and this accords with experimental evidence that SII has bilateral input.[86] The SII region is located within the parietal lobe on the superior bank of the sylvian fissure and in the adjacent cortex over the convexity.

PET studies and noninvasive MEG studies have provided further information about the functional organization of the human somatosensory cortex. PET studies, for example, have been used to localize three distinct sites in the human SI following cutaneous stimulation by mechanical vibration of the lips, fingers, and toes. The location of the primary somatosensory response varied systematically with the stimulus site and formed a consistent homunculus in each of eight subjects, confirming earlier descriptions of the human SI based on intraoperating studies.[44] MEG approaches depend on mapping the somatosensory evoked magnetic fields with a large-array biomagnetometer. Yang and coworkers have mapped the somatosensory homunculus (Plates 1 and 4) by plotting the somatosensory cortical locations corresponding to various tactile sites on the fingers, hand, arm, and face in different subjects.[87] They calculated source localizations using a single equivalent dipole model and transposed the localizations onto the subject's cranial MRI to determine the site of the individual dipoles in a given subject. They found separate locations for discrete

regions on the face and head, with the sites of facial representation clustered inferiorly to those representing the hand and digits. Sources of the somatosensory evoked field by these and other authors[57, 85, 88–89] are in general accord with the somatosensory homunculus defined by the intracranial studies of Penfield and Jasper[90] in 1954. Bilateral representations have been found in SI for face area, with MEG recordings.[89] In the SII region, there is bilateral representation; signs of somatotopic organization may be found but are often difficult to detect.[89]

Language

For more than 100 years, language functions have been ascribed to the left hemisphere based on studies involving clinicopathological correlations and relating the loss of linguistic function to the site of cerebral pathology. Clinical case-material suggests that the right hemisphere also has some language function, by affecting prosody.[91–92] It now seems accepted widely that the posterior one-third of the left inferior frontal gyrus (Broca's area, corresponding especially to Brodmann's area 44) is essential for the expression of language, and a region encompassing the posterior portion of the middle and superior temporal gyri (Brodmann's area 22) and the adjacent parietal operculum (Wernicke's area) is required for the comprehension of language. Lesions of Broca's area have been associated with disturbances of speech output, with mutism, expressive difficulties, and speech that is telegrammatic, paraphasic (incorrect word usage) and nonfluent; lesions of Wernicke's area are traditionally associated with fluent, well-formed, paraphasic speech circumlocutions, and profound difficulty in the comprehension of speech. In fact, lesions confined to Broca's area produce a much more restricted and transient speech disturbance than that generally referred to as Broca's aphasia, which typically results from a much larger lesion in the sylvian region, involving the operculum, insula, and subjacent white matter.[93] The importance of connections between these two major areas has also been emphasized, and disturbances of language attributed to lesions interrupting these pathways (conduction or transcortical aphasia). It has thus been envisioned that language involves serial processing, from comprehension to speech production, in an orderly manner.[94–95] Unfortunately, accumulating evidence conflicts with this simple model.

Complex linguistic functions require the involvement of many cerebral regions. The data relating specific disturbances of language to the location of brain lesions is incomplete. For example, Willmes and Poeck[96] studied the location of CT lesions in relation to language function in 221 patients (grouped by performance on the Aachen aphasia test) into global, expressive (Broca), receptive (Wernicke), and amnestic aphasias. No unequivocal association between aphasia type and lesion location was found; discrepancies were too great to permit them to be dismissed simply as exceptions from the general rule. Moreover, to consider certain aphasic syndromes as simply expressive or receptive may be deceptively facile. Thus, expressive (motor) aphasia involves such disturbances as agrammatism (or impaired syntactic processing) that are difficult to account for in purely motor terms.[96] Similarly, patients with expressive aphasia from lesions in Broca's area may have difficulties in comprehension due to word-order errors[97] and problems with assigning syntactic structure during sentence processing;[98] indeed, Broca's area is activated in PET studies when subjects simply listen to commands or a story.[40, 99]

Studies on humans undergoing surgery for epilepsy suggest that models of cortical language organization may require separate systems for different language functions, which are activated in parallel.[100–101] These systems include not only discrete frontal and temporoparietal areas but neurons present more diffusely in the cortex. There is, in fact, evidence even from clinicopathological studies that several different systems subserve different aspects of language function. For example, frontal or temporoparietal lesions may disproportionately impair written as opposed to oral language,[102] and polyglots may lose the ability to communicate in one language but not another after certain cerebral lesions.[103]

The intracarotid amobarbital perfusion test[104] is important in defining lateralization of hemispheric function, whereas intraoperative techniques have been used to localize function, especially language, within the hemisphere. Ojemann[105] reported that in about 15 percent of his patients the right hemisphere had at least some involvement in speech production; among these patients, language was localized exclusively in the right hemisphere in between one-half and one-third of cases, while in the remainder language representation was bilateral.[106] In Ojemann's studies, there was no statistically significant relation between left-handedness and language lateralization (that is, involvement of the right hemisphere in language) as judged from amobarbital studies, provided

that patients were excluded if they were left-handed because of left hemisphere damage.[106]

Intraoperative studies have confirmed that the posterior inferior frontal Broca's area is indeed necessary for speech output, with speech arrest following stimulation in this region. The occurrence of electrocorticographic changes with naming indicates that this area is active throughout the language process, even when speech is not actually produced. Stimulation studies have also identified essential areas for speech production more widely (Figure 159) than previously recognized, however, and especially in the perisylvian cortex, more anteriorly in the inferior frontal gyrus, and in parts of the superior temporal gyrus and anterior parietal operculum.[100, 105] Stimulation in these regions impairs the sequential orofacial movements used in speech production and also the identification of speech sounds.[107]

Intraoperative investigation has also suggested that the relationship between speech production and perception is an overlapping one. Temporal lobe microelectrode studies have indicated that some neurons in the left superior temporal gyrus respond in the same way to both speech production and perception.[101] Commonly, however, in areas of the temporal lobe that are not essential for language, neuronal activity was influenced only by speech production or speech perception (rather than by both), and—if responses did occur to both—the changes were in opposite directions with perception and production.[101] For example, if neurons responded to both, their activity was increased with speech perception and inhibited by speech production. Certain neurons, including some in the nondominant temporal cortex, exhibited specific patterns of activity in response to the perception of specific words.[108] Some cells became active in response to certain phonemes or to a particular syllable during the perception of polysyllabic words.[108] These and other related findings suggest that there are specific subdivisions in the neural mechanisms of speech perception, involving cells in both hemispheres.

It seems, then, that neuronal activity related to linguistic functions can be recorded from much wider regions than the areas previously regarded as essential for language function, and from both the dominant and non-dominant hemisphere. In the dominant hemisphere there are multiple, partially separate systems for different aspects of language, such as for naming in one language, for naming in another language, for reading, and for recent verbal memory. In each there may be several

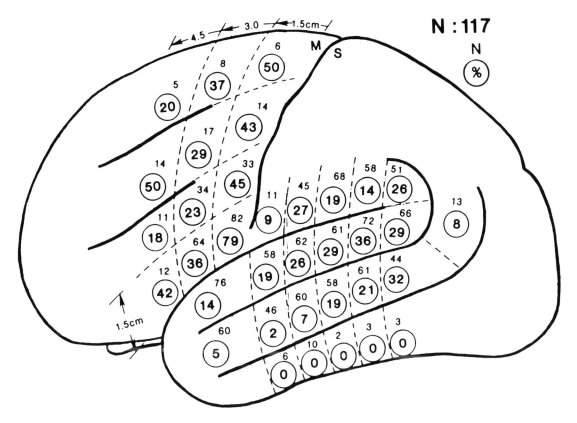

FIGURE 159

FIGURE 159
Variability in localization of sites required for naming in 117 patients. The data were obtained by electrical stimulation of the left, language-dominant hemisphere. The cortex is divided into zones identified by dashed lines. Upper number in each zone is the number of patients in whom a site was tested in that zone; lower circled number is the percentage of those patients in whom significant naming errors were evoked at sites in that zone. M and S indicate motor and sensory cortex, respectively. (From Ojemann G., Ojemann J., Lettich E., Berger M., "Cortical language localization in left, dominant hemisphere", *J. Neurosurg.*, 1989, *71*:316–326.)

essential cortical areas and widely dispersed neurons. Patterns of localization may vary with gender and with verbal ability.

Studies involving evoked potentials (Plate 9) and PET have also provided fresh insights into the relation of different parts of the brain to language. The regional changes that occur in average cerebral blood flow during the processing of auditory or visually presented words provides support for the concept of multiple parallel routes between discrete sensory-specific, phonological, articulatory, and semantic coding areas.[109] In particular, passive auditory or visual presentation of words led to activation of modality-specific primary and nonprimary sensory regions; no region was activated by both auditory and visual presentation. With visual presentation, activation was in the striate cortex and regions of the prestriate occipital cortex. The responses in primary striate cortex were similar to those produced by other visual stimuli, but the extrastriate occipital regions seemed to be activated only by the visual presentation of words. This suggested that these latter regions represent a network coding for visual word-form. With auditory stimuli, activation occurred bilaterally in primary auditory cortex, and in the left temporoparietal, anterior superior temporal, and inferior anterior cingulate cortex. The temporoparietal and anterior superior temporal regions were not activated by auditory stimuli unless these included words. Cortical areas involved in motor output and articulatory coding were activated when words were repeated aloud after their visual or auditory presentation.[109] Such regions have included parts of the primary sensorimotor cortex and supplementary motor area, and perisylvian regions. Activation occurred near Broca's area in the left perisylvian region, but also occurred on the right; this bilateral sylvian activation occurred also when subjects simply moved the mouth and tongue. This finding, then, does not support the concept of specialization of this region specifically for speech or linguistic function, but rather for motor programming of output in general.[109]

Cognitive Functions

The neural substrates of cognitive processes are probably more widespread than those underlying simple motor and sensory functions, and whether they can be localized precisely is unknown. The prefrontal cortex was suggested by Nauta to be unique in its relations with both interoceptive and exteroceptive sensory domains.[110] For many years it has been held that the output of various sensory regions converges on the prefrontal cortex, although in fact there is no individual region within this cortical area in which these sensory projections terminate. Instead, they appear to project in parallel on different small regions of prefrontal cortex.[12]

With PET scanning, for example, the approach to studying cognitive processing is similar to that used for evaluating other cerebral functions. Studies performed in the resting state are subtracted from those made during the performance of a cognitive task to identify the functional changes associated with task performance, but not all variables are easily controlled in such studies, and seemingly minor stimulus variables may influence the findings.[47] Moreover, it may be misleading to equate the degree to which cerebral blood flow increases just with the extent of cerebral involvement in the function under consideration; factors such as task difficulty and familiarity with the task may also influence cerebral blood flow.[47]

As was indicated on page 150, there is evidence to suggest that attention depends on a neural network involving frontal, parietal and cingulate cortex and various subcortical regions. O^{15} PET studies provide support for this view. They have shown increased blood flow in the right prefrontal and superior parietal cortex during activity requiring sustained attention to sensory stimuli.[111] Another area that has been involved by PET studies in attentional processes is the anterior cingulate gyrus.[112] These studies also suggest that the cerebellum is involved in certain cognitive activities. For example, the cerebellum is activated in motor sequence learning,[113] as well as during spontaneous or repetitive speech.[114] The novelty of the stimulus influences the degree to which cerebral blood flow is increased in the anterior cingulate gyrus[115] and the cerebellum.[113]

Alexia

In acquired alexia, a cerebral lesion causes an impaired ability to read or to comprehend what is read. Norman Geschwind, based in part upon the earlier work of Joseph Jules Dejerine (1849–1917) and others, defined a series of cerebral regions that are necessary for the reading and comprehension of written words.[116] He suggested that visual information is transmitted from the left visual association areas to the angular gyrus where it is coded phonologically. Connections are also made with the posterior temporal region for semantic coding, and then the left inferior frontal region (via the arcuate fasciculus) for speech output.

Benson and coworkers have described the features of different types of alexia.[117–118] These and other clinical studies suggest that visual information reaching the left calcarine cortex (Brodmann's area 17) is transmitted to the visual association areas (areas 18 and 19) and then to the left angular gyrus. Corresponding visual information is projected across the splenium from areas 18 and 19 on the right to the left. Another possible connection is from the right visual association areas to the right angular gyrus, with subsequent transmission across the corpus callosum to the left angular gyrus.[116] However, such wiring diagrams are misleading and simplified, for the reasons indicated earlier. Nevertheless, damage to the left occipital region causes pure alexia, without any other language disturbance—patients can write words, but cannot read what they have written. More specifically, lesions in the periventricular white matter region at the temporo-occipito-parietal junction in the left hemisphere will disconnect the input from both right and left visual association cortices to the necessary language areas and cause pure alexia.[119]

Damage to the left perisylvian region may lead to alexia. A lesion of the angular gyrus can cause alexia and agraphia, with preservation of spoken language. Other conjoined clinical abnormalities may include anomia, ideomotor apraxia, and sometimes acalculia, right-left disorientation, and finger agnosia.[118] In other patients with pathology in the perisylvian region, alexia is associated with aphasia. With frontal pathology, agrammatism is often present.

One form of alexia—neglect alexia—is associated with disturbances of attention and occurs with pathology involving the territory of the right middle cerebral artery, especially with parietal damage.[120]

Agraphia

Agraphia may occur as an isolated phenomenon or in association with aphasia or alexia. Isolated or pure agraphia is characterized by a selective disturbance of the ability to write, without any other disturbance of language. This disorder has generally been related to frontal lobe lesions, particularly lesions at the lower end of the second frontal convolution (Exner's area), but it has become increasingly clear that a single center for writing does not exist.[121] Among patients with this form of agraphia, many different sites for the underlying pathology have now been described. Indeed, pure agraphia may occur in patients with an acute confusional state. Among the lesion sites that have been implicated in addition to Exner's area are the posterior perisylvian region, superior parietal lobe, left occipital lobe, posterior insular and posterior putamen, basal ganglia, and other subcortical structures.

Agraphia has been described in association with both expressive (Broca's) aphasia, receptive (Wernicke's) aphasia, and with conduction aphasia or transcortical aphasia. The occurrence of agraphia with alexia, without the concomitant occurrence of aphasia, usually relates to a parietal lobe lesion.

Vision

Individual areas of the primary visual cortex (V1) have parallel and independent outputs to different visual areas of the prestriate visual cortex (Figure 160). In fact, there is functional specialization in the human visual cortex. In V1, cells concerned with different aspects of a visual scene, such as color, motion, or form, are segregated, as are also cells situated in V2, which is the immediately adjoining prestriate cortex. The connectivity of V1 with V2 represents a parallel output, with the connection of functionally similar cells. Both V1 and V2 also connect with other specialized visual areas in prestriate cortex in a manner emphasizing the existence of parallel and independent outputs based on functional specialization within the visual system. Thus, direction-sensitive cells of V1 project to V5 (situated at the junction of Brodmann's areas 19 and 37) and also to selected regions of V2 that project in turn to V5. By contrast, cells in V1 that are orientation-selective project to V3 and to parts of V2 that also project to V3.

In V3, which has been characterized especially in macaque monkeys, most cells are sensitive to orientation rather than to the color or wavelength of the stimulus.

Recent PET studies have shown that cerebral areas that are maximally activated when subjects view color (as opposed to equiluminous grey and white) displays are located in the region of the lingual and fusiform gyri, just beyond the striate cortex, especially in the left hemisphere.[122] This area has been designated V4 in humans. When humans are asked to view a pattern of random black and white squares when it is stationary and then when it is moving in different directions, subtraction and comparison of the scans shows that the V5 region has maximal activity when subjects view moving stimuli.

Clinical case studies provide some confirmation of the distinctive nature of the specialized cortical areas for vision referred to above. Cerebral achromatopsia designates the loss of ability to discriminate colors following certain cerebral lesions. This is in contrast to color

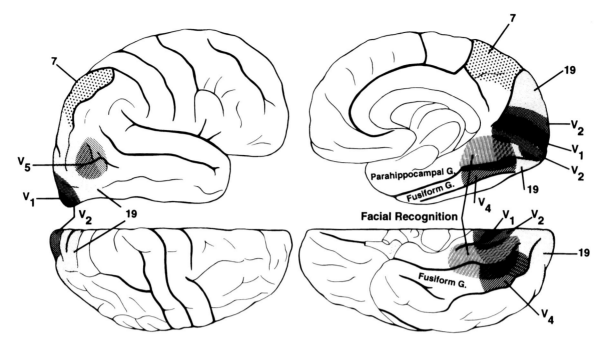

FIGURE 160

The major cortical areas devoted to vision in the human brain. These areas are shown from various perspectives of the right cerebral hemisphere. Numbers signify Brodmann's areas of the cortex, which are now known to receive input from other visual areas. Areas V1 and V2, which are primary and secondary visual processing areas, approximately encompass Brodmann's areas 17 and 18. Areas V4 and V5, which are believed to be areas for processing color and motion, have no direct correlates with any of Brodmann's areas. Brodmann's area 19 probably contains area V3, the boundaries of which have not yet been identified. (From Celesia G. G., De Marco P. J., "Anatomy and physiology of the visual system", *J. Clin. Neurophysiol.*, 1994, *11*:482–492.)

agnosia, in which colors are seen but not recognized, and from color anomia in which colors cannot be named even though they can be seen and recognized. Despite references to cerebral achromatopsia that extend back for more than one hundred years, clinicians have been reluctant to accept the syndrome perhaps because of its rarity. The recent PET studies alluded to above, however, provide support for its existence.

Other patients may have a visual impairment of all modalities except color vision, a disorder that has been termed chromatopsia by Zeki.[122] The explanation for this syndrome is unclear at the present time, but it does provide support for the existence of parallel pathways within the cerebral cortex and should not be dismissed simply because it is difficult to comprehend.

The perception of motion (Plate 10) may also be impaired specifically after certain cortical lesions, leading to the condition of akinetopsia or "motion blindness."[122] Zihl and associates described a patient with a selective disturbance of movement vision after bilateral brain damage in an area encompassing V5 as located from PET studies.[123] Kinetopsia is the syndrome in which patients can see movements in a field in which vision is otherwise lost. Rare cases have been described, but rejected by many clinicians and whether this disorder truly exists remains unclear.

Recent studies on vision, then, indicate a greater complexity of specialization than has previously been conceived, with parallel processing of different submodalities but, at the same time, greater integration between cortical and subcortical regions concerned with vision (Figure 161). V3 and V5 are supplied from cells in a deeper layer of V1, and also receive input from certain regions of V2 which, in turn, are supplied by V1. Area V5, in turn, projects back to V1, but also influences cells in V1 that do not directly project to it but project instead to area V3. As Zeki[122] points out, it thus unites two subdivisions of the visual system, one concerned primarily with motion and the other with form.

The specialized visual cortical areas have direct connections with each other, and also are connected either directly or indirectly with parietal and temporal areas. Most of the projection from V5 is to parietal cortex, but there is also a projection to temporal cortex. Conversely, V4 projects mainly to temporal cortex but also connects consistently with parietal cortex. Area V3 projects both to V4 and V5, and these in turn project to parietal and temporal areas which are interconnected.

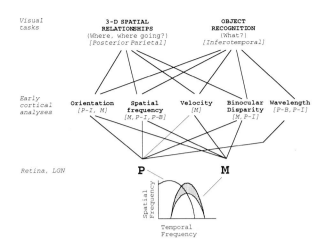

FIGURE 161

Convergence and divergence in visual processing. Lines represent major information-flow from subcortical parvocellular (P) and magnocellular (M) streams that originate within the retina and pass through the lateral geniculate nucleus (LGN) (bottom). In the V1 and V2 cortical regions, these are reorganized into a tripartite system (the P-B, P-I and M streams) for early cortical analysis (middle). Two general tasks of vision requiring more complex processing are also shown (top level). The hatched portion of the M cell curve represents their nonlinear component of processing. The processing streams associated with each property in the middle row are assigned on the basis of a high incidence of selectivity recorded physiologically (Courtesy of Van Essen D. C., Anderson C. H., Felleman D. J.: "Information processing in the primate visual system: an integrated systems perspective," *Science*, 1992, *255*:419–423. Copyright 1992 American Association for the Advancement of Science.)

Activity in any one of these specialized visual areas is thus readily passed on to other areas through these interconnections.

Fox and colleagues mapped the retinotopic organization of human visual cortex using PET.[43] Oxygen[15]-labeled water, delivered intravenously, was used as the blood-flow tracer. They found that changes in stimulus location caused systematic and highly significant change in the location of responses within the visual cortex. Based upon numerous case reports, it was already widely appreciated that the central retina projects to the vicinity of the occipital pole, while peripheral retina projects more rostrally, the superior retina projecting above the calcarine fissure and the inferior retina projecting beneath it. Cortical electrical stimulation produces visual illusions (phosphenes), and the location of these varies with the site of stimulation. The cortical projection zone of the retina has been mapped by this means, but has conformed only in broad outline to the expected arrangement predicted by the study of clinical deficits in patients with defined cerebral lesions.[124] Subsequent studies by Dobelle and Mladejovsky[125] suggested that any discrepancies may relate, at least in part, to technical difficulties and variables rather than simply to physiological factors. The PET studies recently published have yielded findings that accord with the conventional concept of retinotopic organization of the visual cortex.

Zeki[126] has recently discussed the concept of the visual association cortex, pointing out that the meaning of the designation "association" is vague and that many neurologists seem to imagine that it is association cortex which gives visual "impressions" their meaning and thus that it represents "higher" functions. In his analysis, Zeki points out that the so-called visual association cortex consists in fact of multiple visual areas rather than a single area with uniform architecture. Moreover, recent studies have shown that the visual areas of association cortex have different functions, rather than simply undertaking the same task at increasing levels of complexity as was implied by the earlier doctrine of exclusive hierarchies. Thus, area V5 subserves visual motion. Area V4 is specialized for color and form in association with color, and V3 is specialized for dynamic form. Areas of the visual association cortex (or prestriate cortex) receive parallel inputs from area V1, so that the cortex undertakes a number of visual operations in parallel, enabling it to construct a visual image. How these specialized visual areas interact to provide a unified image is less clear. There is no evidence that cells in the prestriate areas or visual association cortex

are influenced to any significant extent by stimuli other than visual ones, so that the concept of association cortex as originally envisioned is not supported by the data available at the present time.

In area V1 or V2, cells concerned with a specific attribute are grouped together, but in the prestriate areas there is more specialization so that in area V5 the cells are primarily directionally selective and unresponsive to wavelength, whereas those in area V4 are wavelength selective. Even in area V1, visual signals are segregated into distinct functional submodalities from which the more specialized areas receive their cortical input. The same is true of area V2.

Is there any real reason to suppose that seeing depends upon the integrity of area V1 and that understanding of visual information depends upon the functional integrity of surrounding areas? The occurrence of agnosia, akinetopsia, and achromatopsia has led Zeki to suppose that each visual area contributes explicitly to visual perception in a way that requires no further processing, and that the patient can see and understand based upon that contribution. This implies that the ability to perceive a particular visual attribute, such as color, is not dependent upon the integrity of the entire visual pathway. An achromatopsic patient can discriminate between different wavelengths, but cannot utilize this information to construct colors, which is similar to the deficit seen in monkeys when a lesion is made in area V4.

Subjects with lesions in area V1 and who therefore are blind are nevertheless sometimes able to discriminate certain visual stimuli correctly or more frequently than would be expected by chance alone. This phenomenon of "blindsight" has been taken to suggest either that processing in area V1 is necessary for a conscious awareness of visual stimuli or that operations performed by the specialized areas in prestriate cortex have to be referred back to area V1, or both. It seems that area V1 is an essential component of the process permitting conscious experience of visual stimuli. However, a recent study involving PET scanning has shown that during visual motion stimulation, signals may reach the cortical area involved in the perception of visual motion without necessarily passing through area V1, and that in such circumstances a patient may be consciously aware that the stimulus in his blind field is moving with correct identification of the direction of motion.[127] Such conscious awareness of visual motion is not as faultless as when there is an intact area V1 in addition to an intact V5. This study shows that, in fact, area V1 does not have a monopoly in mediating conscious vision and that other areas in some manner contribute directly to conscious visual experience.

Hearing

The auditory system has been studied by a variety of different approaches, both in humans and animals. Experimental studies in animals have shown that the tonotopic organization of the cochlea persists throughout the auditory pathway to the primary auditory cortex.[128–129] The primary auditory cortical receiving area in Old World monkeys, apes, and humans is located on the caudal aspect of the superior temporal plane of the superior temporal gyrus. In the macaque monkey, low-frequency auditory stimuli are represented rostrolaterally in the primary auditory cortex and high-frequency stimuli caudomedially.[128] Surrounding the primary auditory cortex are four other fields that can be distinguished histologically and by the distribution of frequencies within them.

In humans, the primary auditory area AI is generally held to be represented by Brodmann's areas 41 and 42, and the second auditory area (AII) by Brodmann's areas 21 and 22, but the auditory cortex is difficult to define either anatomically or physiologically. Anatomical studies have shown interhemispheric asymmetries in the temporal regions, especially in the perisylvian region. Intraoperative studies have revealed that crude auditory sensations can be elicited by electric stimulation of Heschl's gyri, that is, the anterior and posterior transverse temporal gyri[90] and cortical evoked potentials to auditory stimulation can be recorded from the lateral surface of the exposed temporal lobe. Celesia summarized in 1976 his experience in recording these potentials in 19 patients undergoing surgery for partial seizures.[130] Responses could be recorded from a limited area around the lips of the posterior two-thirds of the sylvian fissure and in a small area on the supratemporal plane corresponding to Heschl's gyri. The findings obtained by binaural and by ipsilateral and contralateral monaural stimulation indicated that each ear is represented bilaterally (but with a contralateral predominance) in the primary auditory cortex. The limits of human experimentation precluded the testing of tones of different frequencies to determine whether there was tonotopical representation.

PET has been used to study the metabolic changes in normal human brain to monaurally and binaurally presented verbal and nonverbal auditory stimuli. The metabolic responses to auditory stimuli were determined by the content of the stimulus and the strategy by which the subject analyzed it, rather than the side of stimulation.[40] Many studies have suggested an important role for the perisylvian temporal cortex in the analysis of auditory stimuli. The temporal regions in both hemispheres appear to be involved, at least to some extent. Processing of complex stimuli such as words requires the activation of more widespread areas of the brain than the processing of certain nonspeech sounds.[131–132] Thus, PET studies of human volunteers showed increased activity of the primary auditory cortex in response to noise bursts, whereas acoustically matched speech syllables activated secondary auditory cortex bilaterally.[131] Functional MRI was used by Binder and associates[133] to visualize brain regions involved in auditory speech perception in five normal subjects, who listened to auditory stimuli that included nonspeech noise, meaningless speech sounds, single words, and narrative text. There were signal changes in the superior temporal gyrus and superior temporal sulcus bilaterally in all subjects. Speech stimuli were associated with significantly more widespread changes than were noise stimuli, but there was considerable variability between subjects in the topography of these changes. Other studies have also shown that speech stimuli activate a more widespread region of the temporal lobe than noise and nonspeech stimuli, and different speech stimuli produce similar activation patterns.[131–132, 134] PET studies have further shown that the changes induced by a 4000 Hz tone are located deeper and more posteriorly in the contralateral hemisphere than those induced by a 500 Hz tone.[132]

MEG has also been used to localize cortical sources responding to ipsilateral and contralateral auditory stimulation,[135] and neuromagnetic measurements for localizing projections of different frequencies in the human auditory cortex have indicated similarly that there is tonotopic organization of the auditory cortex,[136–137] as illustrated in Plate 11.

4. CLINICAL FEATURES RELATED TO LOCALIZED PATHOLOGY

As indicated earlier, function cannot be inferred reliably from the neurological deficit resulting from localized cerebral pathology. Nevertheless, a brief summary of the clinical sequelae of lesions of the various lobes of the cerebral hemispheres may be of some interest to clinicians and helps to place in perspective the experimental and more specific findings already discussed, both in this chapter and in Chapter 13.

Frontal Lobe Syndromes

The frontal lobes, which occupy approximately one-third of the cerebral hemispheres in humans, are traditionally divided into the precentral cortex (Brodmann's area 4) immediately anterior to the rolandic fissure, the premotor cortex (areas 6, 8, and 44) in front of this, the heteromodal prefrontal cortex which includes Brodmann's areas 9–12, and 45–47, and the paralimbic cortex of the anterior cingulate, paraolfactory and caudal orbitofrontal regions. As mentioned in Chapter 13, Hughlings Jackson first designated the frontal cortex as the area where the highest human intellectual capacities reside, a designation that had to be revised after Hebb performed the experiments discussed below. Others variously described the frontal cortex as being concerned with "reasoning,"[139] synthesizing[140–141] or "abstracting"[142–143] and as the center of "biological intelligence."[144] Hebb[145] showed that removal of much of the frontal cortex did not affect intelligence; indeed patients with frontal lesions are less impaired intellectually than those with parietal lesions. Thus, the association between the frontal lobes and highest intellectual capacity must be modified.

Recent functional imaging studies have shown that the frontal lobe has a greater diversity than was previously recognized.[99] Depending on the task, different areas within the frontal lobe and its main divisions are activated. In many circumstances, homologous regions are activated bilaterally, although with quantitative differences between the two sides.[99]

Pathology involving the frontal lobe leads to a clinical disturbance characterized by changes in mood, personality, and behavior. Following prefrontal leucotomy (which severs the frontal connections bilaterally), patients become apathetic, may be incontinent, and sometimes develop akinetic mutism. Improvement occurs with time, but diminished initiative and other behavioral changes persist, with altered social habits, emotional liability, inability to organize daily schedules, and poor judgment. Patients seem preoccupied with immediate events (at the expense of past or future activities), and may have deficits in performance on certain psychological tests. Unilateral frontal lobectomy leads to mild clinical changes, with some impairment of initiative and planning ability.

Some patients with frontal lobe lesions seem to have little, if any, clinical deficit on neurological or psychological examination, although the findings obtained in a clinical setting may not be representative of the behavioral state of the patient in other environments.[146–147] The clinical silence of even large lesions of the frontal lobes has led to suggestions that prefrontal cortex is involved in functions that are less "hard-wired" than other functions, and that it has more of an integrative role than other cortical areas, generating behavior programs that are appropriate to a particular context.[146]

Certain symptoms may nevertheless be conspicuous in patients with frontal lobe lesions. Disturbances of memory occur in some patients with extensive, bilateral frontal pathology, but whether this and other cognitive changes relate directly to the frontal lesion, diencephalic involvement, or an associated hydrocephalus is unclear. Inattention may contribute to any memory disturbance. There may be difficulty in recalling the context in which information was obtained.[148] There is a reduction in initiative, a loss of spontaneity, and a certain indifference or unconcern about personal affairs or previous interests. Patients are often inattentive, easily distractable, impulsive, shallow, echopraxic, and have poor concentration and judgement. Demented patients with predominantly frontal pathology behave inappropriately, are often incontinent, and become socially uninhibited and excessively jocular. Anomia may be present. When spatial neglect occurs, it is usually relatively mild. Frontal pathology may reportedly impair certain aspects of musical function, but there is little convincing evidence in this regard. Frontal lesions may lead to difficulty in initiating movement of the contralateral arm or leg, especially when the lesion involves the right hemisphere.

Lesions of the anterior cingulate gyrus bilaterally lead to akinetic mutism. Patients are typically aphonic, and make little or no attempt at vocalization.[149] Stimulation of the anterior cingulate gyrus in humans causes affective changes; hallucinatory manifestations; arousal or alerting reactions; movements of the digits and hand, mouth, legs and eyes; and associated, integrated movements of the hand and mouth.[150]

Unilateral stimulation of the supplementary motor area causes speech arrest or vocalization, or speech abnormalities with distortion and palilalia (repetition of phrases). There may be accompanying limb, facial, and ocular movements.[149] Irritative lesions, especially left-sided ones, may lead to palilalia and vocalizations,[151] and destructive lesions of the left supplementary motor area may cause mutism, followed by transcortical motor aphasia as recovery occurs.[152] Spontaneous speech is limited, agrammatism occurs, and there is akinesia of the upper limbs, especially contralaterally. The effect of bilateral lesions of the supplementary motor area is poorly defined.

Lesions of the left premotor area lead to the syndrome of Broca's aphasia. Agrammatism (telegrammatic speech, with a relative lack of small grammatical words) probably relates to involvement of premotor cortex. Isolated lesions of Broca's area (Brodmann's area 44) cause transient difficulties with the expression of speech without there necessarily being any syntactic errors, and—as mentioned earlier—seem not to produce the classic Broca's aphasia syndrome.

Temporal Lobe Syndromes

Three major functional systems have been localized to the temporal lobes: the visual projections inferolaterally (Brodmann's areas 37, 20, and 21), the auditory areas laterally in the superior temporal gyrus (areas 41, 42, and 22), and the limbic structures involved with emotions and memory mediobasally.[153] Visual and auditory information is directed from the temporal neocortex to the limbic structures. The activation of limbic structures by a spontaneous or electrically induced seizure leads not only to emotional responses but also to complex visual and auditory hallucinations, illusions of familiarity, and memory flashbacks.[154] Recent studies suggest that the occurrence of such psychic phenomena during seizures depends upon activation of both limbic structures and temporal neocortex, reflecting the engagement of a neuronal network involving the medial and lateral aspects of the temporal lobe.[155–156]

Unilateral lesions involving the anterior temporal lobe may lead to a contralateral upper quadrantanopia. Bilateral medial temporal lobe lesions cause global amnesia when the hippocampi are involved. Bilateral ablation of the inferomedial aspects of the temporal lobes causes a gross amnesic syndrome.[157] (See also Chapter 13, p. 139.) Patients have a limited but adequate recall of remote events, but cannot retain new information for more than a few minutes. Severe amnesia has also been reported by others[158–159] in extensive lesions of the right temporal lobe; other memory disturbances, such as the déjà vu phenomenon, have been encountered more frequently with right- than left-sided lesions. (See also Chapter 13, p. 139.) In humans, lesions of the right hippocampus are associated particularly with deficits of spatial memory and learning, and the left hippocampus with impaired memory for verbal material.[14, 160]

Unilateral destruction of the primary auditory projection area is asymptomatic, but bilateral lesions lead to cortical deafness (an inability to recognize sounds). If the auditory areas are intact, lesions inferolaterally of the dominant temporal lobe lead to difficulty in the visual recognition of words; similar lesions in the nondominant hemisphere impair the visual recognition of nonverbal material and the auditory recognition of melodies.

Lesions of the left temporal lobe (in patients with left hemispheric specialization for language) lead to difficulty in the comprehension and recall of verbal material. Visual aspects of language may be impaired by posterior lesions; those near the temporo-occipital border may cause alexia, whereas agraphia is more likely with lesions near the temporo-parietal border. In posterior temporal lesions apraxias, somatognosias (an impaired appreciation of the body schema), and acalculia are often found. Lesions of the right temporal lobe are accompanied by impairment of various visual nonverbal tasks,[153] including disturbances of memory and spatial integration, and, as Hécaen and Ajuriaguerra[161] pointed out (see Chapter 13, p. 136), the metamorphopsias (visual illusions) are also more frequent in right-sided lesions. Impairment of tests involving spatial analysis, construction, and drawing, together with prosopagnosia (a failure to recognize faces despited preserved vision) are more common in lesions near the occipital lobe whereas hemisomatognosia occurs in areas near the parietal lobe.

Parietal Lobe Syndromes

Various deficits follow lesions of the parietal lobe. Somatosensory disturbances are characterized either by loss of sensation or of discriminitive sensibility, sensory inattention, or by the occurrence of abnormal sensations, as occurs in focal sensory seizures. A pseudothalamic syndrome has also been described and is characterized by unpleasant dysesthesias and spontaneous pain in the absence of any disturbance of tactile or position sense or stereognosis. Astereognosis may occur, with an inability to recognize the shape or physical characteristics of an object (such as its texture or weight) by touch or an inability to recognize the identity of objects in the absence of any disturbance of primary sensation. Ataxia may also occur in the absence of postural loss.

Some patients with parietal lesions develop muscle wasting, for uncertain reasons. The wasting is not due simply to disuse.

Lesions of the posterior-inferior part of the parietal lobe may involve the optic radiation, causing a contralateral homonymous hemianopia or quadrantanopia.

In patients with parietal lobe lesions, there may be disturbances in spatial perception of the body, as evidenced by right-left disorientation, finger agnosia, autotopagnosia (the inability to name or indicate different parts of the body), asymbolia for pain (inappropriate response to pain, which is not consciously related to the patient's own body), and anosognosia or loss of awareness of one side of the body, regardless of whether or not it is paralyzed.

Gerstmann's syndrome (which consists of agraphia, acalculia, right-left disorientation, and finger agnosia) has been related to a lesion involving the left angular gyrus, but the localization or lateralization of causal lesions has been questioned and the existence of the entire syndrome has been the subject of controversy.

Posterior parietal lesions, such as those made by gunshot wounds, may lead to disturbances in visual localization, motion recognition, size comparisons, counting, stereoscopic vision, visual attention, and ocular mobility. Unilateral visuospatial neglect is well described and may occur with lesions of either hemisphere. Balint's syndrome is characterized by optic ataxia (eye-hand incoordination), impaired visual attention, impaired estimation of distance, and apraxia (psychic paralysis) of gaze (an inability to displace the gaze voluntarily from the point of fixation in the peripheral field, despite the preservation of automatic or random eye movements). Mild disturbances of visual attention may be manifest as simultanagnosia (the inability to recognize the meaning of a picture even though its constituents can be appreciated correctly).

Various forms of apraxia have been related to parietal lobe lesions. These include ideomotor apraxia (movements cannot be performed on request despite a full understanding of what is required and the ability to perform similar movements spontaneously), ideational apraxia (sequential or complex movements cannot be performed even though each component step can be performed separately), constructional apraxia (objects cannot be constructed from their component parts), dressing apraxia (clothing cannot be put on because of difficulty in correctly orienting items in relation to the body). A variety of language disorders occurs in patients with parietal lobe lesions, but speech is considered separately on pages 159–162.

Biparietal lesions may lead to an impairment of intellectual function. Lesions of the right parietal lobe have been associated particularly with confusional states or even with psychoses.

Occipital Lobe Syndromes

Pathology in both occipital lobes leads to bilateral visual loss (cortical blindness). Some patients deny that they are blind (Anton's syndrome). Patients with a large, unilateral, occipital lesion have a contralateral homonymous hemianopia, with sparing of macular vision because of the dual vascular supply of the cortical region subserving the macula, and perhaps also because of retinal ganglion cell overlap.[162]

Lesions involving the left occipital region may result in color anomia, which is often associated with alexia without agraphia, visual agnosia, and a right homonymous hemianopia.

Disturbance of the primary visual aspects of spatial perception may cause prosopagnosia, "spatial dyslexia" (reading disorders due to unilateral spatial agnosia), and dysgraphia in patients with right occipital lesions.

5. CONCLUDING COMMENT

It is becoming increasingly clear that the operation of the nervous system during the performance of a particular function depends on the patterns of excitation and inhibition in neuronal populations that are often widely dispersed in different regions of the cerebral cortex. The belief that distinct functions are restricted to discrete cortical regions, as envisioned in an earlier part of this century, has become increasingly untenable. Recent work has emphasized the plasticity of the cortex, which is not simply a hard-wired array of neuronal circuits but a dynamic system that is modified or reorganized by preceding activity and feedback, and the importance of parallel distributed cortical networks with mutual reciprocal interconnections between different cortical areas. Further technological refinements and experimental observations will doubtless necessitate the modification of these concepts as greater insight into the operation of the brain is obtained.

NOTES

1. K. S. Lashley, *Brain mechanisms and intelligence*, Chicago, University of Chicago Press, 1929.

2. A. R. Luria, *Higher cortical functions in man*, London, Tavistock Publications, 1966, pp. 23–38.

3. J. Hughlings Jackson, "On the nature of the duality of the brain", *Brain*, 1915, 38:80–86. (Reprinted from *Medical Press & Circular*, 14 January 1874.)

4. G. Fritsch & E. Hitzig, "Über die elektrische Erregbarkeit des Grosshirns", *Arch. Anat. Physiol.*, 1870, 37:300–332.

5. D. Ferrier, *The functions of the brain*, London, Smith, Elder & Co., 1876.

PLATES

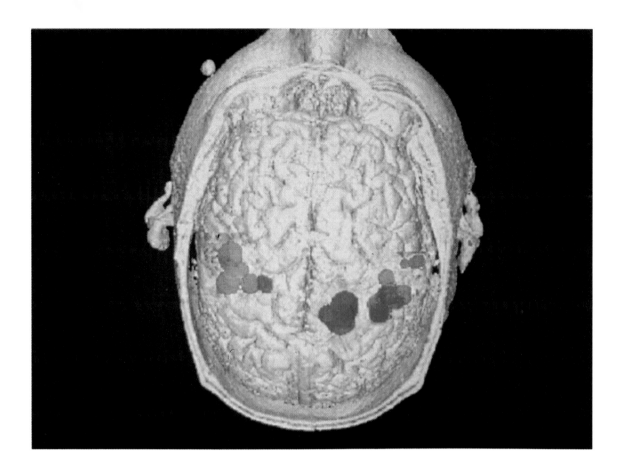

PLATE 1

Top view of a combined MEG and three-dimensional surface-rendered MRI of an adult whose right arm was amputated below the elbow when he was eleven years old. The right hemisphere is normal and shows the primary somatosensory face area (red) lateral, anterior and inferior to the hand localizations (green), which are in turn lateral, anterior and inferior to the upper arm region (blue). The left hemisphere shows the face (red) and upper arm region (blue) extending into the expected hand territory, reflecting reorganization of the sensory map as result of the amputation. (Adapted from Yang T. T., Gallen C., Schwartz B., Bloom F. E., Ramachandran V. S., Cobb S. "Sensory maps in the human brain," *Nature*, 1994, *368*:592–593.)

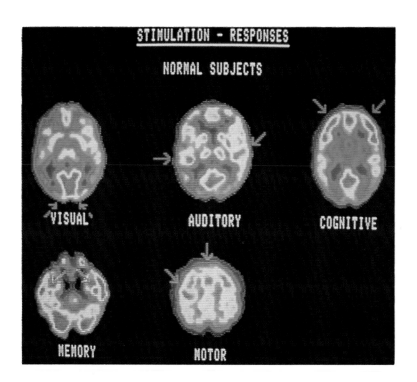

PLATE 2

Glucose metabolism of the active human brain. Each image represents a single slice from a fluorodeoxyglucose PET study depicting glucose metabolism in individual normal subjects as they performed specific tasks. On this color scale, red indicates areas of high metabolic activity; shades of blue and green represent low metabolic activity. In each case regions appropriate to the functional localization of properties in the brain are active when subjects perform visual, auditory, cognitive, memory, or motor tasks. (Reprinted from Phelps M. E., Mazziotta J. C.: "Positron emission tomography: human brain function and biochemistry, *Science*, 1985, 228, 799–809. Copyright 1985 American Association for the Advancement of Science.)

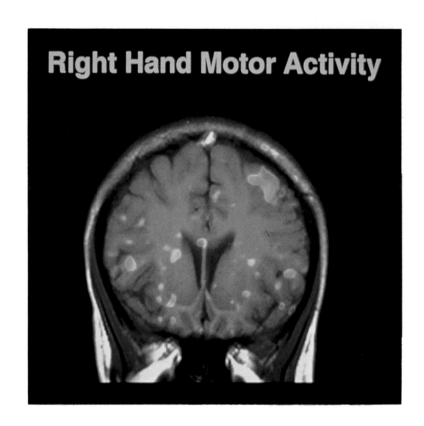

Right Hand Motor Activity

PLATE 3

Functional magnetic resonance image (*f*MRI) of a normal subject performing a motor task. Top: The coronal image of a normal subject is taken through the motor cortex during the performance of a motor task with the right hand. The left hemisphere is on the reader's right. Note the increased signal in the primary motor cortex in the hand area of the left hemisphere, shown in red. Bottom: The *f*MRI signal intensity in the left motor area when the subject alternately rested and moved the right hand is plotted. These measurements of the motor response time course were obtained without administering ionizing radiation or exogenous contrast material but merely by measuring differences in oxygenation of hemoglobin concentrations of the venous blood in the brain tissue. (Courtesy of C. Stern, K. Kwong, B. Rosen, J. Belliveau, M. Cohen, MGH-NMR Center, Charlestown, Massachusetts.)

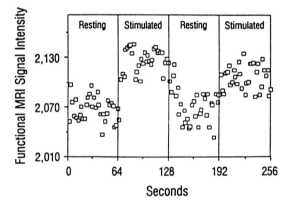

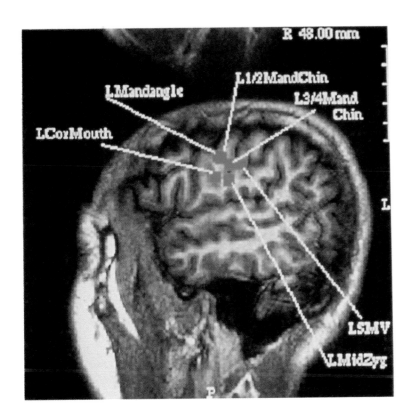

PLATE 4

Sagittal section of the brain in a normal subject showing locations of dipoles corresponding to tactile sites on the left face. A large-array biomagnetometer was used to map the cortical locations corresponding to distinct tactile sites, and source localizations were calculated using a single equivalent current dipole model and transposed on to an MRI of the subject's head to determine the anatomical focus of individual dipoles. L$^{1}/_{2}$MandChin and L$^{3}/_{4}$MandChin, half-way and three-quarters of the distance from the left mandibular angle to the chin, respectively; LMidZyg, left midzygomatic region; LCorMouth, left corner of mouth; LMandAngle, left mandibular angle; LSMV, left submental vertex. (Adapted from Yang T.T., Gallen C. C., Schwartz B. J., Bloom F. E., "Noninvasive somatosensory homunculus mapping in humans by using a large-array biomagnetometer", *Proc. Natl. Acad. Sci. USA*, 1993, *90*:3098–3102.)

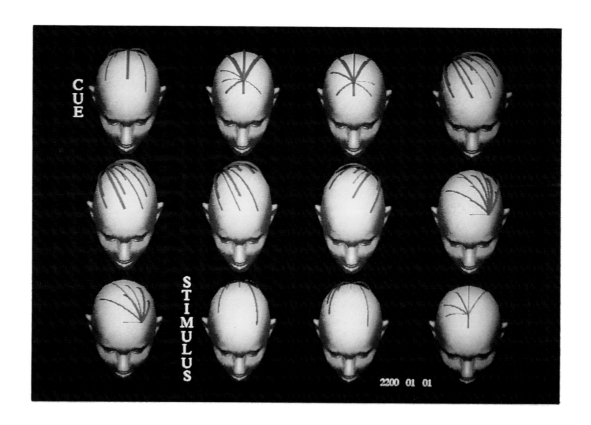

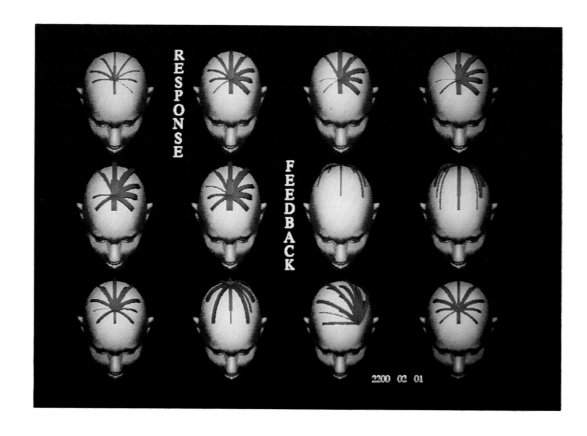

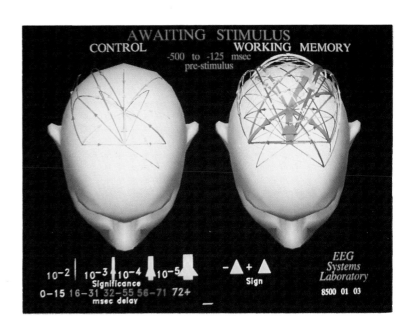

AWAITING STIMULUS
CONTROL   WORKING MEMORY
-500 to -125 msec
pre-stimulus

10^{-2} | 10^{-3} 10^{-4} 10^{-5} − ▲ + ▲   EEG
Significance   Sign   Systems
0-15 16-31 32-55 56-71 72+   Laboratory
msec delay   8500 01 03

PLATE 5 (OPPOSITE)
Series of twenty-four heads showing how the scalp location with the highest total covariance with other areas changes during a simple four-second motor task. Time is increasing from left to right; each successive head is about 100 ms later than the preceding one. A visual CUE prepared the subject for a visual STIMULUS number from 1 to 9 (top); a graded pressure RESPONSE (bottom) was then required with the right index finger according to the size of the number. A visually presented FEEDBACK number showed the subject his response accuracy. In the encoding interval immediately after each visual event, the covariance hot spot occurs posteriorly over visual cortex. By contrast, immediately preceding the appearance of the stimulus the hot spot shifts to the left frontal region as the subject mentally prepares to encode the number and respond to it. Following the response, the covariance hot spot occurs centrally, with the largest covariances over left central sensorimotor cortical areas responsible for controlling the finger movement. Finally, covariances are again focused over left frontal cortex as the subject integrates feedback information and updates strategies in anticipation of the next trial. Data from seven subjects are averaged. The width of a line corresponds to the significance of the covariance, with the thinnest line representing p<.05. The color violet indicates a positive covariance, the color blue negative covariance. (From Gevins A., Cutillo B., DuRousseau D., Le J., Leong H., Martin N., Smith M. E., Bressler S., Brickett P., McLaughlin J., Barbero N., Laxer K.: "Imaging the spatiotemporal dynamics of cognition with high-resolution evoked potential methods," *Human Brain Mapping*, 1994, *1*:101–116. Copyright 1994. Reprinted by permission of John Wiley & Sons, Inc.)

PLATE 6
Mental activity involves moment-by-moment changes in the interactions of different cerebral areas. The particular pattern of interactions involved with a specific thought process—a neurofunctional network—can be measured by evoked potential covariance analysis. Neurofunctional network patterns are shown in a split-second instant when five subjects stared at a blank video screen awaiting a visual stimulus (a single digit number). In the Working Memory condition, subjects had to remember the two previous stimulus numbers, and the patterns are far more complex than in the control condition, in which they did not. Involvement of left posterior cortical areas may reflect verbal coding of the numeric stimuli. (From Gevins A. S., Cutillo B. A., "Spatiotemporal dynamics of component processes in human working memory", *Electroencephalogr. Clin. Neurophysiol.*, 1993, *87*:128–143.)

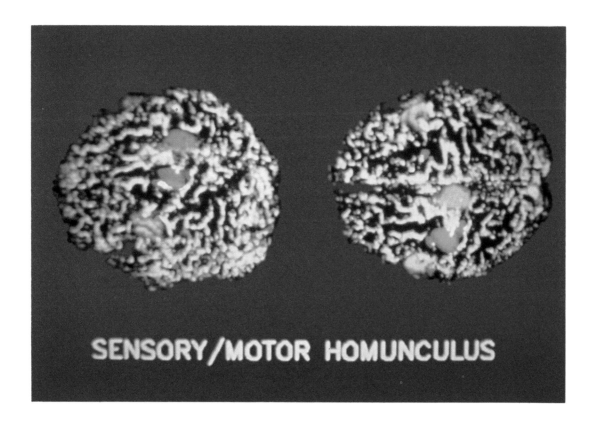

SENSORY/MOTOR HOMUNCULUS

PLATE 7

The sensory-motor homunculus of the human brain. These images are three-dimensional renderings of structural MRI studies depicted in shades of gray as seen from the left lateral view (left image) and from above (right image). Colored areas represent blood flow activations in a single normal subject who performed a visual tracking task with the right foot (green), right index finger (red), and the tongue (pink). Note that the task performed with the extremities is associated with discrete and purely contralateral responses, whereas that performed with the tongue shows discrete but bilateral activation (the tongue was moving across the midline). (From Grafton S. T., Woods R. P., Mazziotta J. C., Phelps M. E., "Somatotopic mapping of the primary motor cortex in humans: activation studies with cerebral blood flow and positron emission tomography", *J. Neurophysiol.*, 1991, *66*:735–743.)

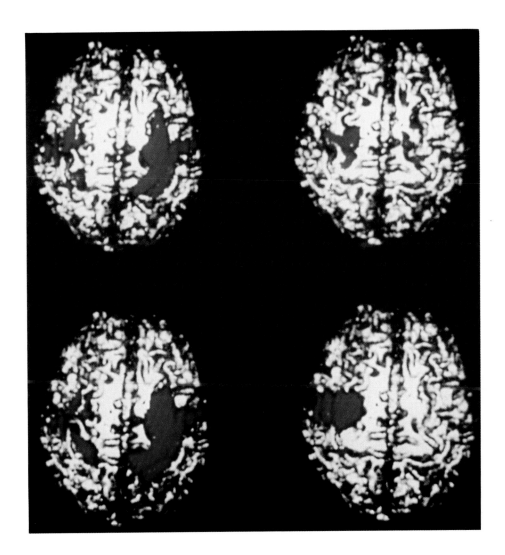

PLATE 8

Four combined MRI and PET studies of the same subjects performing a motor task. The black-and-white images represent three-dimensional reconstructions of a normal right-handed subject's brain seen from above with the right hemisphere on the left and the frontal lobes on top. The red areas show significant increases in blood flow as the subject performed a task using the index finger to follow a moving target on a television screen. The bottom right image shows the subject performing the task for the first time using the dominant right index finger. Controlled by the opposite left hemisphere, this task produced a discrete increase in blood flow over the contralateral motor cortex. The bottom left image shows the same subject performing the same task for the first time using the nondominant left hand. The area of brain activated is larger and is not discretely limited to the contralateral side. Rather, there seems to be functional participation of both halves of the brain in performing this task. In the top row of images the subject is performing the same task (i.e., using the right hand in the right image, and the left hand in the left image), but after fifteen minutes of practice. It can be seen that the areas of response, when the task is performed with either hand, are significantly smaller than they were when first attempted (bottom row). Thus, despite only a few minutes of training, the brain has responded by decreasing the amount of tissue required to perform a previously novel task. More activity still occurs when the task is performed with the less proficient, nondominant (left) hand, a feature seen with many tasks involving the motor system. (Courtesy of J. C. Mazziotta, R. Woods, S. Grafton, University of California, Los Angeles.)

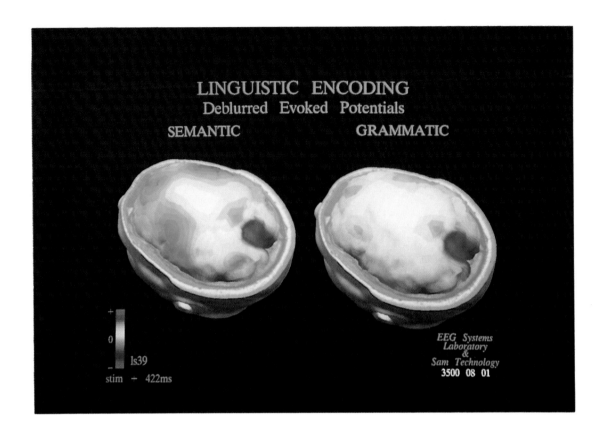

PLATE 9
High resolution EEG images obtained during an experiment on the neural basis of language. Data are from an instant 422 ms after presentation of a word stimulus requiring either a semantic or grammatic judgement. In the semantic condition subjects had to decide whether two words were antonyms, whereas in the grammatic condition they decided whether they formed a grammatically correct sentence. The distinguishing feature of the two conditions is the activation of left frontal cortex (probably Broca's area) in the grammatic condition. (From Gevins A., "High-resolution EEG enters imaging arena", *Diagnostic Imaging*, 1993, *15*:77–84.)

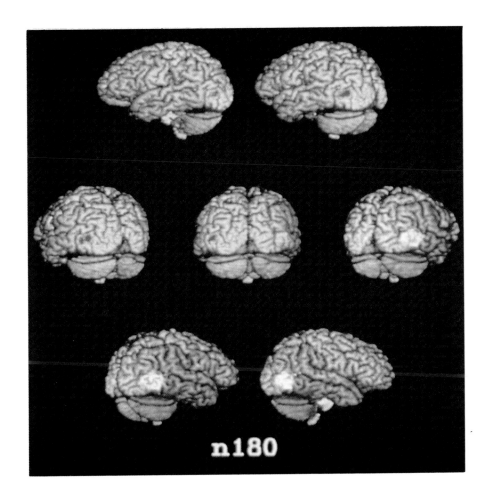

PLATE 10

Brain mapping used in the study of normal vision. Seven views are shown of the three-dimensionally rendered brain of a single normal subject performing a visual task. The structural anatomy image is derived from serial MRI studies that have been three-dimensionally rendered with the skull and meninges removed. The red areas indicate increased cerebral blood flow derived from PET when this subject observed a moving visual stimulus, as compared to a stationary visual stimulus. The result demonstrates two regions at the junction of the temporal and occipital lobes critical to the processing and interpreting visual motion. Damage to these areas leads to a behavioral syndrome where patients misunderstand visual information that is moving. Experiments in monkeys have demonstrated a visual motion center in a homologous portion of the brain. (From Watson J. D. G., Myers R., Frackowiak R. S. J., Hajnal J. V., Woods R. P., Mazziotta J. C., Shipp S., Zeki S., "Area V5 of the human brain: evidence from a combined study using positron emission tomography and magnetic resonance imaging", *Cerebral Cortex*, 1993, *3*:79–94. By permission of Oxford University Press.)

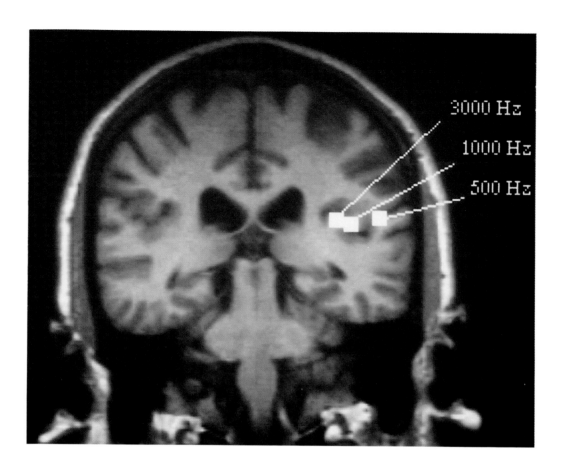

PLATE 11

MEG auditory tonotopic mapping. Evoked magnetic dipole localizations for three separate tones have been plotted on this normal subject's coronal T1-weighted magnetic resonance image. All points fall along the superior temporal gyrus, with high-frequency tones located medial to low-frequency tones. (Courtesy of H. Rowley, University of California, San Francisco.)

6. F. L. Goltz, *Über die Verrichtungen des Grosshirns*, Bonn, Gesammelte Abhandlungen, 1881. See also C. G. Phillips, S. Zeki & H. B. Barlow, "Localization of function in the cerebral cortex: past, present and future", *Brain*, 1984, *107*:327–361.

7. V. Horsley, "Remarks on ten consecutive cases of operations upon the brain and cranial cavity to illustrate the details and safety of method employed", *Br. Med. J.*, 1887, *1*:863.

8. C. E. Brown-Séquard, "Cerebral localization", *Forum*, 1888, *5*:166–177. See also M. J. Aminoff, *Brown-Séquard: A Visionary of Science* New York: Raven Press, 1993, pp. 134–139.

9. D. Zipser & R. A. Andersen, "A back-up propagation programmed network that simulates response properties of a subset of posterior parietal neurons", *Nature*, 1988, *331*:679–684.

10. D. N. Pandya & B. Seltzer, "Association areas of the cerebral cortex", *Trends Neurosci.*, 1982, *5*:386–390.

11. S. Zeki & S. Shipp, "The functional logic of cortical connections", *Nature*, 1988, *335*:311–317.

12. P. S. Goldman-Rakic, "Topography of cognition: parallel distributed networks in primate association cortex", *Annu. Rev. Neurosci.*, 1988, *11*:137–156.

13. J. H. Kaas, "The organization of neocortex in mammals: implications for theories of brain function", *Annu. Rev. Psychol.*, 1987, *38*:129–151.

14. M-M. Mesulam, "Large-scale neurocognitive networks and distributed processing for attention, language, and memory", *Ann. Neurol.*, 1990, *28*:597–613.

15. J. L. McClelland, D. E. Rumelhart & G. E. Hinton, "The appeal of parallel distributed processing", in, D. E. Rumelhart & J. L. McClelland, and the P.D.P. Research Group, *Parallel distributed processing*, Vol. 1, Cambridge, MIT Press, 1986, pp. 3–44.

16. K. M. Heilman, D. N. Pandya & N. Geschwind, "Trimodal inattention following parietal lobe ablations", *Trans. Am. Neurol. Assoc.*, 1970, *95*:259–261.

17. K. R. Daffner, G. L. Ahern, S. Weintraub & M-M. Mesulam, "Dissociated neglect behavior following sequential strokes in the right hemisphere", *Ann. Neurol.*, 1990, *28*:97–101.

18. M. I. Posner, S. E. Petersen, P. T. Fox & M. E. Raichle, "Localization of cognitive operations in the human brain", *Science*, 1988, *240*:1627–1631.

19. M. E. Goldberg & M. A. Segraves, "Visuospatial and motor attention in the monkey", *Neuropsychologia,* 1987, *25*:107–118.

20. S. Weintraub & M-M. Mesulam, "Right cerebral dominance in spatial attention. Further evidence based on ipsilateral neglect", *Arch. Neurol.*, 1987, *44*:621–625.

21. M. M. Merzenich, J. H. Kaas, J. T. Wall, M. Sur, R. J. Nelson, & D. J. Felleman, "Progression of change following median nerve section in the cortical representation of the hand in areas 3b and 1 in adult owl and squirrel monkeys", *Neuroscience*, 1983, *10*:639–665.

22. C. Asanuma, "Mapping movements within a moving motor map", *Trends Neurosci.*, 1991, *14*:217–218.

23. W. M. Jenkins & M. M. Merzenich, "Reorganization of neocortical representations after brain injury: a neurophysiological model of the bases of recovery from stroke", *Progress in Brain Research*, 1987, *71*:249–266.

24. M. M. Merzenich, R. J. Nelson, M. P. Stryker, M. S. Cynader, A. Schoppmann, & J. M. Zook, "Somatosensory cortical map changes following digit amputation in adult monkeys", *J. Comp. Neurol.*, 1984, *224*:591–605.

25. M. M. Merzenich, "Sources of intraspecies and interspecies cortical map variability in mammals: conclusions and hypotheses", in, M. J. Cohen & F. Strumwasser (editors), *Comparative neurobiology: modes of communication in the nervous system*, New York, John Wiley & Sons, 1986, pp. 105–116.

26. J. T. Wall, J. H. Kaas, M. Sur, R.J . Nelson, D. J. Felleman & M. M. Merzenich, "Functional reorganization in somatosensory cortical areas 3b and 1 of adult monkeys after median nerve repair: possible relationships to sensory recovery in humans", *J. Neurosci.*, 1986, *6*: 218–233.

27. E. Smits, D. C. Gordon, S. Witte, D. D. Rasmusson & P. Zarzecki, "Synaptic potentials evoked by convergent somatosensory and corticocortical inputs in raccoon somatosensory cortex: substrates for plasticity", *J. Neurophysiol.,* 1991, *66*:688–695.

28. T. T. Yang, C. C. Gallen, V. S. Ramachandran, S. Cobb, B. J. Schwartz & F. E. Bloom, "Noninvasive detection of cerebral plasticity in adult human somatosensory cortex", *NeuroReport,* 1994, *5*:701–704.

29. A. Mogilner, J. A. I. Grossman, U. Ribary, M. Joliot, J. Volkmann, D. Rapaport, R. W. Beasley & R. R. Llinas, "Somatosensory cortical plasticity in adult humans revealed by magnetoencephalography", *Proc. Natl. Acad. Sci. USA*, 1993, *90*:3593–3597.

30. J. P. Donoghue, S. Suner & J. N. Sanes, "Dynamic organization of primary motor cortex output to target muscles in adult rats. II. Rapid reorganization following motor nerve lesions", *Exp. Brain Res.*, 1990, *79*:492–503.

31. J. P. Donoghue & J. N. Sanes, "Motor areas of the cerebral cortex", *J. Clin. Neurophysiol.*, 1994, *11*:382–396.

32. J. N. Sanes & J. P. Donoghue, "Organization and adaptability of muscle representations in primary motor cortex", in, R. Caminiti, P. B. Johnson, Y. Burnod, (editors), *Control of arm movement in space*, Berlin, Springer-Verlag, 1992:103–127.

33. K. Brodmann, *Vergleichende Lokalisationlehre der Grosshirnrinde*, Leipzig, Barth, 1909.

34. L. D. Selemon & P. S. Goldman-Rakic, "Common cortical and subcortical target areas of the dorsolateral prefrontal and posterior parietal cortices in the rhesus monkey: evidence for a distributed neural network subserving spatially guided behavior", *J. Neurosci.*, 1988, *8*:4049–4068.

35. R. Bartholow, "Experimental investigations into the functions of the human brain", *Am. J. Med. Sci.*, 1874, *67*:305–313.

36. W. Penfield & E. Boldrey, "Somatic motor and sensory representation in the cerebral cortex of man as studied by electrical stimulation", *Brain*, 1937, *60*:389–443.

37. W. Penfield & L. Roberts, *Speech and brain mechanisms*, Princeton, Princeton University Press, 1959.

38. M. E. Phelps, J. C. Mazziotta & S-C. Huang, "Study of cerebral function with positron computed tomography", *J. Cereb. Blood Flow Metab.*, 1982, *2*:113–162.

39. R. G. Shulman, A. M. Blamire, D. L. Rothman & G. McCarthy, "Nuclear magnetic resonance imaging and spectroscopy of human brain function", *Proc. Natl. Acad. Sci. USA*, 1993, *90*:3127–3133.

40. J. C. Mazziotta, M. E. Phelps, R. E. Carson & D. E. Kuhl, "Tomographic mapping of human cerebral metabolism: auditory stimulation", *Neurology*, 1982, *32*:921–937.

41. J. C. Mazziotta & M. E. Phelps, "Positron computed tomographic studies of cerebral metabolic responses to complex motor tasks", *Neurology*, 1984, *34*:116–120.

42. P. T. Fox, M. A. Mintun, M. E. Raichle, F. M. Miezin, J. M. Allman & D. C. Van Essen, "Mapping human visual cortex with positron emission tomography", *Nature*, 1986, *323*:806–809.

43. P. T. Fox, F. M. Miezin, J. M. Allman, D. C. Van Essen & M. E. Raichle, "Retinotopic organization of human visual cortex mapped with positron-emission tomography", *J. Neurosci.*, 1987, *7*:913–922.

44. P. T. Fox, H. Burton & M. E. Raichle, "Mapping human somatosensory cortex with positron emission tomography", *J. Neurosurg.*, 1987, *67*:34–43.

45. M. D. Ginsberg, J. Y. Chang, R. E. Kelley, F. Yoshii, W. W. Barker, G. Ingenito & T. E. Boothe, "Increases in both cerebral glucose utilization and blood flow during execution of a somatosensory task", *Ann. Neurol.*, 1988, *23*:152–160.

46. S. T. Grafton, R. P. Woods & J. C. Mazziotta, "Within-arm somatotopy in human motor areas determined by positron emission tomography imaging of cerebral blood flow", *Exp. Brain Res.*, 1993, *95*:172–176.

47. J. Sergent, "Brain-imaging studies of cognitive functions", *Trends Neurosci.*, 1994, *17*:221–227.

48. S. T. Grafton, N. A. Martin, J. C. Mazziotta, R. P. Woods, F. Vinuela & M. E. Phelps, "Localization of motor areas adjacent to arteriovenous malformations: a positron emission tomographic study", *J. Neuroimag.*, 1994, *4*:97–103.

49. J. W. Belliveau, D. N. Kennedy, R. C. McKinstry, B. R. Buchbinder, R. M. Weisskoff, M. S. Cohen, J. M. Vevea, T. J. Brady & B. R. Rosen, "Functional mapping of the human visual cortex by magnetic resonance imaging", *Science*, 1991, *254*:716–719.

50. A. Gevins, J. Le, N. K. Martin, P. Brickett, J. Desmond & B. Reutter, "High resolution EEG: 124-channel recording, spatial deblurring and MRI integration methods", *Electroencephalogr. Clin. Neurophysiol.*, 1994, *90*:337–358.

51. A. Gevins, "High-resolution EEG enters imaging arena", *Diagn. Imag.*, 1993, *15*:77–84.

52. R. Hari & O. V. Lounasmaa, "Recording and interpretation of cerebral magnetic fields", *Science*, 1989, *244*:432–436.

53. S. J. Williamson, Z-L. Lu, D. Karron & L. Kaufman, "Advantages and limitations of magnetic source imaging", *Brain Topogr.*, 1991, *4*:169–180.

54. A. Gevins, "Dynamic cognitive networks in the human brain", in, G. Buzsaki et al. (editors), *Temporal coding in the brain*, Berlin, Springer-Verlag, 1994, pp. 273–289.

55. A. Gevins, B. Cutillo, D. DuRousseau, J. Le, H. Leong, N. Martin, M. E. Smith, S. Bressler, P. Brickett, J. McLaughlin, N. Barbaro, K. Laxer, "Imaging the spatiotemporal dynamics of cognition with high-resolution evoked potential methods", *Human Brain Mapping*, 1994, *1*:101–116.

56. A. S. Gevins, S. L. Bressler, N. H. Morgan, B. A. Cutillo, R. M. White, D. S. Greer & J. Illes, "Event-related covariances during a bimanual visuomotor task. I. Methods and analysis of stimulus- and response-locked data", *Electroencephalogr. Clin. Neurophysiol.*, 1989, *74*:58–75.

57. D. Brenner, J. Lipton, L. Kaufman & S. J. Williamson, "Somatically evoked magnetic fields of the human brain", *Science*, 1978, *199*:81–83.

58. J. Hughlings Jackson, "Evolution and dissolution of the nervous system", in, J. Taylor (editor), *Selected writings of John Hughlings Jackson*, London, Hodder & Stoughton, 1932, pp. 45–75.

59. H. Cushing, "A note upon the faradic stimulation of the postcentral gyrus in conscious patients", *Brain*, 1909, *32*:44–53.

60. A. S. . Leyton & C. S. Sherrington, "Observation on the excitable cortex of the chimpanzee, orangutan and gorilla", *Q. J. Exp. Physiol.*, 1917, *11*:135–222.

61. C. N. Woolsey, P. H. Settlage, D. R. Meyer, W. Sencer, T. P. Hamuy & A. M. Travis, "Patterns of localization in precentral and "supplementary" motor areas and their relation to the concept of a premotor area", *Res. Publ. Assoc. Res. Nerv. Ment. Dis.*, 1952, *30*:238–264.

62. C. N. Woolsey, "Organization of somatic sensory and motor areas of the cerebral cortex", in, H. F. Harlow & C. N. Woolsey (editors), *Biological and biochemical bases of behavior*, Madison, University of Wisconsin Press, 1958, pp. 63–81.

63. S. Uematsu, R. P. Lesser & B. Gordon, "Localization of sensorimotor cortex: the influence of Sherrington and Cushing on the modern concept", *Neurosurgery*, 1992, *30*:904–913.

64. S. Uematsu, R. Lesser, R. S. Risher, B. Gordon, K. Hara, G. L. Krauss, E. P. Vining & R. W. Webber, "Motor and sensory cortex in humans: topography studied with chronic subdural stimulation", *Neurosurgery*, 1992, *31*:59–72.

65. H. Lüders, R. P. Lesser, D. S. Dinner, H. H. Morris, J. F. Hahn, L. Friedman, G. Skipper, E. Wyllie & D. Friedman, "Commentary: Chronic intracranial recording and stimulation with subdural electrodes", in, J. Engel, Jr. (editor), *Surgical treatment of the epilepsies*, New York, Raven Press, 1987, pp. 297–321.

66. D. R. Humphrey, "Representation of movements and muscles within the primate precentral motor cortex: historical and current perspectives", *Fed. Proc.*, 1986, *45*:2687–2699.

67. R. Lemon, "The output map of the primate motor cortex", *Trends Neurosci.*, 1988, *11*:501–506.

68. D. Cheyne, R. Kristeva & L. Deecke, "Homuncular organization of human motor cortex as indicated by neuromagnetic recordings", *Neurosci. Lett.*, 1991, *122*:17–20.

69. L. G. Cohen & M. Hallett, "Methodology for non-invasive mapping of human motor cortex with electrical stimulation", *Electroencephalogr. Clin. Neurophysiol.*, 1988, *69*:403–411.

70. R. P. Dum & P. L. Strick, "The origin of corticospinal projections from the premotor areas in the frontal lobe", *J. Neurosci.*, 1991, *11*:667–689.

71. G. Luppino, M. Matelli, R. M. Camarda, V. Gallese & G. Rizzolatti, "Multiple representations of body movements in mesial area 6 and the adjacent cingulate cortex: an intracortical microstimulation study in the macaque monkey", *J. Comp. Neurol.*, 1991, *311*:463–482.

72. I. Fried, A. Katz, G. McCarthy, K. J. Sass, P. Willamson, S. S. Spencer & D. D. Spencer, "Functional organization of human supplementary motor cortex studied by electrical stimulation", *J. Neurosci.*, 1991, *11*:3656–3666.

73. P. Glees & J. Cole, "Recovery of skilled motor functions after small repeated lesions of motor cortex in macaque", *J. Neurophysiol.*, 1950, *13*:137–148.

74. P. E. Roland, B. Larsen, N. A. Lassen & E. Skinhoj, "Supplementary motor area and other cortical areas in organization of voluntary movements in man", *J. Neurophysiol.*, 1980, *43*:118–136.

75. D. Laplane, J. Talairach, V. Meininger, J. Bancaud & J. M. Orgogozo, "Clinical consequences of corticectomies involving the supplementary motor area in man", *J. Neurol. Sci.,* 1977, *34*:301–314.

76. P. T. Fox, J. M. Fox, M. E. Raichle & R. M. Burde, "The role of cerebral cortex in the generation of voluntary saccades: a positron emission tomographic study", *J. Neurophysiol.*, 1985, *54*:348–369.

77. S. M. Rao, J. R. Binder, P. A. Bandettini, T. A. Hammeke, F. Z. Yetkin, A. Jesmanowicz, L. M. Lisk, G. L. Morris, W. M. Mueller, L. D. Estkowski, E. C. Wong, V. M. Haughton & J. S. Hyde, "Functional magnetic resonance imaging of complex human movements", *Neurology*, 1993, 43: 2311–2318.

78. H. J. Freund, "Premotor area and preparation of movement", *Rev. Neurol.* (Paris), 1990, *146*:543–547.

79. R. E. Passingham, "Cues for movement in monkeys (Macaca mulatta) with lesions in premotor cortex", *Behav. Neurosci.*, 1986, *100*:695–703.

80. W. Penfield & T. Rasmussen, *The cerebral cortex of man*, New York, Macmillan, 1950.

81. C. N. Woolsey, T. C. Erickson, W. E. Gilson, "Localization in somatic sensory and motor areas of human cerebral cortex as determined by direct recording of evoked potentials and electrical stimulation", *J. Neurosurg.*, 1979, *51*:476–506.

82. C. Baumgartner, D. S. Barth, M. F. Levesque, W. W. Sutherling, "Functional anatomy of human hand sensorimotor cortex from spatiotemporal analysis of electrocorticography", *Electroencephalogr. Clin. Neurophysiol.*, 1991, *78*:56–65.

83. C. C. Wood, D. D. Spencer, T. Allison, G. McCarthy, P. D. Williamson & W. R. Goff, "Localization of human sensorimotor cortex during surgery by cortical surface recording of somatosensory evoked potentials", *J. Neurosurg.*, 1988, *68*:99–111.

84. J. H. Kaas, M. Sur, R. J. Nelson, & M. M. Merzenich, "The postcentral somatosensory cortex: multiple representations of the body in primates", in, C. N. Woolsey (editor), *Cortical sensory organization*, Vol. 1. Multiple somatic areas, New Jersey, Humana Press, 1981, pp. 29–45.

85. C. Baumgartner, A. Doppelbauer, L. Deecke, D. S. Barth, J. Zeitlhofer, G. Lindinger & W. W. Sutherling, "Neuromagnetic investigation of somatotopy of human hand somatosensory cortex", *Exp. Brain Res.*, 1991, *87*:641–648.

86. H. Burton, "Second somatosensory cortex and related areas", in, E. G. Jones & A. Peters (editors), *Cerebral cortex*, New York, Plenum Press, 1986, pp. 31–98.

87. T. T. Yang, C. C. Gallen, B. J. Schwartz & F. E. Bloom, "Noninvasive somatosensory homunculus mapping in humans by using a large-array biomagnetometer", *Proc. Natl. Acad. Sci. USA*, 1993, *90*:3098–3102.

88. J. Suk, U. Ribary, J. Cappell, T. Yamamoto & R. Llinas, "Anatomical localization revealed by MEG recordings of the human somatosensory system", *Electroencephalogr. Clin. Neurophysiol.*, 1991, *78*:185–196.

89. R. Hari, J. Karhu, M. Hamalainen, J. Knuutila, O. Salonen, M. Sams & V. Vilkman, "Functional organization of the human first and second somatosensory cortices: a neuromagnetic study", *Eur. J. Neurosci.,* 1993, *5*:724–734.

90. W. Penfield & H. Jasper, *Epilepsy and the functional anatomy of the human brain*, Boston, Little, Brown & Co., 1954.

91. E. D. Ross & M-M. Mesulam, "Dominant language functions of the right hemisphere? Prosody and emotional gesturing", *Arch. Neurol.*, 1979, *36*:144–148.

92. S. Weintraub, M-M. Mesulam & L. Kramer, "Disturbances in prosody: a right-hemisphere contribution to language", *Arch. Neurol.*, 1981, *38*:742–744.

93. J. P. Mohr, M. S. Pessin, S. Finkelstein, H. H. Funkenstein, G. W. Duncan & K. R. Davis, "Broca aphasia: pathologic and clinical", *Neurology*, 1978, *28*:311–324.

94. N. Geschwind, "The organization of language and the brain", *Science*, 1970, *170*:940–944.

95. A. R. Damasio, "Concluding remarks: neuroscience and cognitive science in the study of language and the brain", in, F. Plum (editor), *Language, communication, and the brain*, New York, Raven Press, 1988.

96. K. Willmes & K. Poeck, "To what extent can aphasic syndromes be localized?", *Brain*, 1993, *116*:1527–1540.

97. A. J. Gallaher & G. J. Canter, "Reading and listening comprehension in Broca's aphasia: lexical versus syntactical errors", *Brain Lang.*, 1982, *17*:183–192.

98. A. D. Friederici, "Production and comprehension of prepositions in aphasia", *Neuropsychologia*, 1981, *19*:191–199.

99. P. E. Roland, "Metabolic measurements of the working frontal cortex in man", *Trends Neurosci.*, 1984, *7*:430–435.

100. G. A. Ojemann, "Cortical organization of language", *J. Neurosci.*, 1991, *11*:2281–2287.

101. G. A. Ojemann, "Cortical organization of language and verbal memory based on intraoperative investigations", *Progress in sensory physiology*, Vol. 12, Berlin, Springer-Verlag, 1991, pp. 193–230.

102. D. Benson, "The third alexia", *Arch. Neurol.*, 1977, *34*:327–331.

103. M. Paradis, "Bilingualism and aphasia", *Stud. Neurolinguistics*, 1977, *3*:65–122.

104. J. Wada & T. Rasmussen, "Intracarotid injection of sodium amytal for the lateralization of cerebral speech dominance", *J. Neurosurg.*, 1960, 17:266–282.

105. G. A. Ojemann, "Cortical stimulation and recording in language", in, A. Kertesz (editor), *Localization and neuroimaging in neuropsychology*, San Diego, Academic Press, 1994, pp. 35–55.

106. R. P. Woods, C. B. Dodrill & G. A. Ojemann, "Brain injury, handedness, and speech lateralization in a series of amobarbital studies", *Ann. Neurol.*, 1988, 23:510–518.

107. G. Ojemann & C. Mateer, "Human Language cortex: localization of memory, syntax, and sequential motor-phoneme identification systems", *Science*, 1979, 205:1401–1403.

108. O. Creutzfeldt, G. Ojemann & E. Lettich, "Neuronal activity in the human lateral temporal lobe. II. Responses to the subjects own voice", *Exp. Brain Res.*, 1989, 77:476–489.

109. S. E. Petersen, P. T. Fox, M. I. Posner, M. Mintun & M. E. Raichle, "Positron emission tomographic studies of the cortical anatomy of single-word processing", *Nature*, 1988, 331:585–589.

110. W. J. H. Nauta, "The problem of the frontal lobe: a reinterpretation", *J. Psychiatr. Res.*, 1971, 8:167–187.

111. J. V. Pardo, P. T. Fox, M. E. Raichle, "Localization of a human system for sustained attention by positron emission tomography", *Nature*, 1991, 349:61–64.

112. J. V. Pardo, P. J. Pardo, K. W. Janer & M. E. Raichle, "The anterior cingulate cortex mediates processing selection in the Stroop attentional conflict paradigm", *Proc. Natl. Acad. Sci. USA*, 1990, 87:256–259.

113. I. H. Jenkins, D. J. Brooks, P. D. Nixon, R. S. J. Frackowiak, R. E. Passingham, "A PET study of the functional anatomy of motor sequence learning", *Neurology*, 1993, 43: Suppl. 2, A188.

114. M. E. Raichle, "Anatomical Explorations of mind", *Semin. Neurosci.*, 1990, 2:307–315.

115. K. F. Berman, C. Randolph, J. Gold, D. Holt, D. W. Jones, T. E. Goldberg, R. E. Carson, P. Herscovitch & D. R. Weinberger, "Physiological Activation of frontal lobe studied with positron emission tomography and oxygen^{15} water during working memory tasks", *J. Cereb. Blood Flow Metab.*, 1991, 11:S851.

116. N. Geschwind, "Disconnexion syndromes in animals and man", *Brain*, 1965, 88: 237–294.

117. D. R. Benson, J. Brown & E. B. Tomlinson, "Varieties of alexia", *Neurology*, 1971, 21: 951–957.

118. D. R. Benson, "Alexia", in, J. A. M. Frederiks, (editor), *Handbook of clinical neurology*, Vol. 45, Amsterdam, Elsevier, 1985, pp. 433–455.

119. A. R. Damasio & H. Damasio, "The anatomic basis of pure alexia", *Neurology*, 1983, 33:1573–1583.

120. M. Behrmann, M. Moscovitch, S. E. Black & M. Mozer, "Perceptual and conceptual factors in neglect dyslexia: two contrasting case studies", *Brain*, 1990, 113:1163–1183.

121. D. P. Roeltgen, "Localization of lesions in agraphia", in, A. Kertesz (editor), *Localization and neuroimaging in neuropsychology*, San Diego, Academic Press, 1994, pp. 377–405.

122. S. Zeki, "Parallelism and functional specialization in human visual cortex", *Cold Spring Harbor Symposia on Quantitative Biology*, 1990, 55:651–661.

123. J. Zihl, D. Von Cramon & N. Mai, "Selective disturbance of movement vision after bilateral brain damage", *Brain*, 1983, 106:313–340.

124. G. S. Brindley, "Sensory effects of electrical stimulation of the visual and paravisual cortex in man", in, R. Jung (editor), *Handbook of sensory physiology*, Berlin, Springer-Verlag, 1973, pp. 583–594.

125. W. H. Dobelle & M. G. Mladejovsky, "Phosphenes produced by electrical stimulation of human occipital cortex, and their application to the development of a prosthesis for the blind", *J. Physiol.*, 1974, 243:553–576.

126. S. Zeki, "The visual association cortex", *Curr. Opin. Neurobiol.*, 1993, 3:155–159.

127. J. L. Barbur, J. D. G. Watson, R. S. J. Frackowiak & S. Zeki, "Conscious visual perception without V1", *Brain*, 1993, 116:1293–1302.

128. M. M. Merzenich & J. F. Brugge, "Representation of the cochlear partition on the superior temporal plane of the macaque monkey", *Brain Res.*, 1973, 50:275–296.

129. M. M. Merzenich, J. H. Kaas & G. L. Roth, "Auditory cortex in the grey squirrel: tonotopic organization and architectonic fields", *J. Comp. Neurol.*, 1976, 166: 387–402.

130. G. G. Celesia, "Organization of auditory cortical areas in man", *Brain*, 1976, 99:403–414.

131. R. J. Zatorre, A. C. Evans, E. Meyer & A. Gjedde, "Lateralization of phonetic and pitch discrimination in speech processing", *Science*, 1992, 256:846–849.

132. J. L. Lauter, P. Herscovitch, G. Formby & M. E. Raichle, "Tonotopic organization in human auditory cortex revealed by positron emission tomography", *Hearing Res.*, 1985, 20:199–205.

133. J. R. Binder, S. M. Rao, T. A. Hammeke, F. Z. Yetkin, A. Jesmanowicz, P. A. Bandettini, E. C. Wong, L. D. Estkowski, M. D. Goldstein, V. M. Haughton & J. S. Hyde, "Functional magnetic resonance imaging of human auditory cortex", *Ann. Neurol.*, 1994, 35:662–672.

134. R. Wise, F. Chollet, U. Hadar, K. Friston, E. Hoffner & R. Frackowiak, "Distribution of cortical neural networks involved in word comprehension and word retrieval", *Brain*, 1991, 114:1803–1817.

135. A. C. Papanicolaou, S. Baumann, R. L. Rogers, C. Saydjari, E. G. Amparo & H. M. Eisenberg, "Localization of auditory response sources using magnetoencephalography and magnetic resonance imaging", *Arch. Neurol.*, 1990, 47:33–37.

136. G. L. Romani, S. J. Williamson, L. Kaufman & D. Brenner, "Characterization of the human auditory cortex by the neuromagnetic method", *Exp. Brain Res.*, 1982, 47:381–393.

132. C. Pantev, M. Hoke, K. Lehnertz, B. Lutkenhoner, G. Anogianakis & W. Wittkowski, "Tonotopic organization of the human auditory cortex revealed by transient auditory evoked magnetic fields", *Electroencephalogr. Clin. Neurophysiol.*, 1988, 69:160–170.

138. J. Taylor (editor), *Selected writings of John Hughlings Jackson*, London, Hodder & Stoughton, 1931, 2 vols.

139. G. Rylander, "Personality changes after operations on the frontal lobes", *Acta Psychiatr. Neurol. Scand.*, 1939, Suppl. 20.

140. S. Ackerly, "Instinctive, emotional and mental changes following prefrontal lobe extirpation", *Am. J. Psychiatry*, 1935, 92:717–729.

141. R. M. Brickner, *The intellectual functions of the frontal lobes*, New York, Macmillan, 1936.

142. K. Goldstein, "The significance of the frontal lobes for mental performance", *J. Neurol. Psychopathol.*, 1936, 17:27–40.

143. I. C. Nichols & J. McV. Hunt, "A case of parietal bilateral frontal lobectomy: a psychopathological study", *Am. J. Psychiatry*, 1940, *96*:1063–1087.

144. W. C. Halstead, *Brain and intelligence. A quantitative study of the frontal lobes*, Chicago, University of Chicago Press, 1947.

145. D. O. Hebb, "Man's frontal lobes. A critical review", *Arch. Neurol. Psychiatry*, 1945, *54*:10–24.

146. M-M. Mesulam, "Frontal cortex and behavior", *Ann. Neurol.*, 1986, *19*:320–325.

147. F. Lhermitte, "Human autonomy and the frontal lobes. Part II: Patient behavior in complex and social situations: The 'environmental dependency syndrome'", *Ann. Neurol.*, 1986, *19*:335–343.

148. J. S. Janowsky, A. P. Shimamura & L. R. Squire, "Source memory impairment in patients with frontal lobe lesions", *Neuropsychologia*, 1989, *27*:1043–1056.

149. J. W. Brown, "Frontal lobe syndromes", in, J. A. M. Frederiks, (editor), *Handbook of clinical neurology*, Vol. 45, Amsterdam, Elsevier, 1985, pp. 23–41.

150. J. Bancaud, J. Talairach, S. Geier, A. Bonis, S. Trottier & M. Manrique, "Manifestations comportementales induites par la stimulation électrique du gyrus cingulaire antérieur chez l'homme", *Rev. Neurol.* (Paris), 1976, *132*:705–724.

151. S. Jonas, "The supplementary motor region and speech emission", *J. Commun. Dis.*, 1981, *14*:349–373.

152. A. B. Rubens, "Aphasia with infarction in the territory of the anterior cerebral artery", *Cortex*, 1975, *11*:239–250.

153. K. Poeck, "Temporal lobe syndromes", in, J. A. M. Frederiks, (editor), *Handbook of Clinical Neurology*, Vol. 45, Amsterdam, Elsevier, 1985, pp. 43–48.

154. P. Gloor, A. Olivier, L. F. Quesney, F. Andermann & S. Horowitz, "The role of the limbic system in experiential phenomena of temporal lobe epilepsy", *Ann. Neurol.*, 1982, *12*:129–144.

155. P. Gloor, "Experiential phenomena of temporal lobe epilepsy", *Brain*, 1990, 1673–1694.

156. J. Bancaud, F. Brunet-Bourgin, P. Chauvel & E. Halgren, "Anatomical origin of déja vu and vivid 'memories' in human temporal lobe epilepsy", *Brain*, *117*:71–90.

157. W. B. Scoville & B. Milner, "Loss of recent memory after bilateral hippocampal lesions", *J. Neurol. Neurosurg. Psychiatry*, 1957, *20*:11–21.

158. J. M. Nielsen, *Memory and amnesia*, Los Angeles, San Lucas Press, 1958.

159. H. Dimsdale, V. Logue & M. F. Piercy, "A case of persisting impairment of recent memory following right temporal lobectomy", *Neuropsychologia*, 1964, *1*:287–298.

160. M. L. Smith & B. Milner, "Right hippocampal impairment in the recall of spatial location: encoding deficit or rapid forgetting?", *Neuropsychologia*, 1989, *27*:71–81.

161. H. Hécaen & J. Ajuriaguerra, *Les gauchers. Préférence manuelle et dominance cérébrale*. Paris, Presses Universitaires Françaises, 1963.

162. R. J. Joynt, G. W. Honch, A. J. Rubin & R. G. Trudell, "Occipital lobe syndromes", in, J. A. M. Frederiks, (editor), *Handbook of clinical neurology*, Vol. 45, Amsterdam, Elsevier, 1985, pp. 49–62.

Appendix 1

The following list of annotated references to the history of cerebral localization deals mainly with cortical function. Although not intended to be exhaustive, it includes the more important contributions to this literature. With one or two exceptions articles on specific areas of cortex have been excluded.

Ackerknecht, E. H., "Contributions of Gall and the phrenologists to knowledge of brain function", in, F. N. L. Poynter (editor), *The history and philosophy of knowledge of the brain and its functions,* Oxford, Blackwell, 1958, pp. 149–153. A brief but useful summary of Gall's anatomy and physiology of the brain. 12 refs.

Adamkiewicz, A., "Zur Geschichte der Functionen der Grosshirnrinde und der Vorstellungen vom Substrat der 'Seele'", *Isis* (Amsterdam), 1896–1897, *1*:15–30. Brief historical introduction but mainly a report of the author's experiments and his ideas of functions of the cortex, mostly now disproved. 19 refs.

Ask-Upmark, E., "Swedenborg as a pioneer in cerebral localization", *J. Amer. med. Assoc.,* 1963, *183*:805–806. He notes omission by Gibson (1962) of Swedenborg. Makes chauvinistically oriented claims for S. as a pioneer though few if any of his statements were original.

Bailey, P. & G. von Bonin, *The isocortex in man,* Urbana, University of Illinois Press, 1951. Chapter 1 is "Historical introduction" (pp. 1–12). Meynert, Betz (with lengthy translations), Flechsig, cyto-architecture.

Bay, E., "Die Geschichte der Aphasielehre und die Grundlagen der Hirnlokalisation", *Dtsch. Z. Nervenheilk.,* 1961, *181*:634–646. Reliable, but nothing new except most recent material. Similar to Bay (1964).

Bay, E., "The history of aphasia and the principles of cerebral localization", in, G. Schaltenbrand & C. N. Woolsey (editors), *Cerebral localization and organization,* Madison & Milwaukee, University of Wisconsin Press, 1964, pp. 44–52. Aphasia the key problem in the localization of "higher psychic function" but this latter may be a chimera. The hazards of localizing psychic phenomena. 31 refs. and discussion pp. 53–65 [Meeting was in 1960].

von Bonin, G., *Essay on the cerebral cortex,* Springfield, Ill., C.C Thomas, 1950. There is a short but useful "Historical introduction" on pp. 5–16.

von Bonin, G., *Some papers on the cerebral cortex translated from the French and German,* Springfield, Ill., C. C Thomas, 1960. The classics: Flourens, Baillarger, Broca, Fritsch & Hitzig, Goltz, Flechsig, Brodmann, von Monakow, Sherrington, etc. Also, a good introduction, pp. vii–xix.

Bordier, A., "Revue critique des localisations cérébrales", *Rev. anthropol.,* 1877, *6*:265–288. Wide-ranging review of anatomy, human and comparative, physical anthropology, and physiology. 17 refs., mainly to French literature.

Brazier, M. A. B., "The historical development of neurophysiology", in, J Field (editor), *Handbook of physiology, Section I Neurophysiology,* Vol. 1, Washington, D.C., American Physiological Society, 1951, pp. 1–58. The best general survey of the history of neurophysiology available. Cortical localization is included. 320 refs. to primary, 50 to secondary, and 45 to biographical literature.

Brazier, M. A. B., "The history of the electrical activity of the brain as a method for localizing sensory function", *Med. Hist.*, 1963, *7*:199–211. The discovery of the brain's electrical activity, Richard Caton, Adolf Beck. Also brief but good survey of early history of cortical physiology. 47 refs.

Dodds, W. J., "On the localisation of the function of the brain: being an historical and critical analysis of the question", *J. Anat. & Physiol.*, 1878, *12*:340–363, 454–494, 636–660. An excellent and detailed review of the literature 1870–1878 grouped according to physiological, pathological and anatomical contributions. The best paper on the early history of cortical localization. 240 refs.

Donley, J. E., "On the early history of cerebral localization", *Amer. J. Sci.*, 1904, *128*(N.S.):711–721. From Antiquity to the 19th century. Competent survey with some unusual allusions and 37 refs.

Fiore, A., "La storia della dottrina della localizzazione cerebrale e l'emisfero dominante di Hudghlings [*sic*] Jackson", *Pag. Stor. Med.*, 1959, *3*(N.4):57–69. A slender effort, with no references and Jackson's name misspelt throughout.

Giannitrapani, D., "Developing concepts of lateralization of cerebral functions", *Cortex*, 1967, *3*:353–370. From Antiquity to end of 19th century and current theories. Detailed but not entirely reliable. 75 refs.

Gibson, W. C., "Pioneers in localization of function in the brain", *J. Amer. med. Assoc.*, 1962, *180*:944–951. From the Ancient Egyptians to the Yale School of Neurophysiology with diverse references to physiological and pathological data. No refs.

Gibson, W. C., "The early history of localization in the nervous system", in, P. J. Vinken & G. W. Bruyn, *Handbook of clinical neurology*, Vol. 2, *Localization in clinical neurology*, Amsterdam, North-Holland Publishing Co., 1969, pp. 4–14.

Halstead, W. C., *Brain and intelligence. A quantitative study of the frontal lobes*, Chicago, University of Chicago Press, 1947. History of neurological theories of intelligence: holistic (Goltz, Lashley, *et al.*), aggregation (Munk, von Monakow, Kleist, *et al.*), regional localization (Hitzig, Flechsig, Bianchi, *et al.*), 31 refs.

Hassler, R. "Die Entwicklung der Architektonik seit Brodmann und ihre Bedeutung für die moderne Hirnforschung", *D. med. Wschr.*, 1962, *87*:1180–1185. Useful follow-up of Brodmann's work, especially in Germany. 75 refs.

Head, H., *Aphasia and kindred disorders of speech*, Vol. 1, Cambridge, University Press, 1926, pp. 1–141. An excellent account of the history of the localization of language function, introduced by a brief survey of cerebral localization in general. 204 refs.

Hécaen, H. & J. Dubois (editors), *La naissance de la neuropsychologie du langage, 1825–1865. Textes et documents*, Paris, Flammarion, 1970. Mainly concerned with French contributions. The epoch-making papers of J. B. Bouillaud, P. Broca, and M. Dax on the cerebral localization of speech are reprinted.

Hollander, B., *In search of the soul and the mechanism of thought, emotion, and conduct, etc.*, London, K. Paul, Trench, Trübner, n.d. 2 vols. All of Vol. 1 (pp. 516) is a "history of philosophy & science" from ancient times to the 19th century which deals mainly with cerebral localization compiled by an ardent phrenologist. Exhaustive but uncritical and no references.

Hollander, B., *The mental functions of the brain. An investigation into their localization and their manifestation in health and disease*, London, G. Richards, 1901. "The revival of phrenology". A desperate attempt to equate phrenology with modern advances in cerebral localization. Historical material *passim*.

Horsley, V., "The function of the so-called motor area of the brain", *Brit. med. J.*, 1909, ii:125–132. Brief account of the first 10 years of physiological and anatomical cortical studies, but without reference to Sherrington. 51 refs.

Hunt, J., "On the localisation of the functions of the brain with special reference to the faculty of language", *Anthropological Rev.*, 1868, *6*:329–345; *ibid.*, 1869, *7*:100–116 and 201–214. Using data from physiology, pathology, psychology, and physiognomy the author, an anthropologist not medically qualified, presents a useful survey from Antiquity to Broca. It summarizes the position in 1868, just before the introduction of cortical stimulation in 1870. Ample footnotes. Our Figures 13, 32, 48 are reproduced. 40 refs.

Jasper, H. H., "Evolution of conceptions of cerebral localization since Hughlings Jackson", *World Neurology*, 1960, *1*:97–109. A valuable follow-up of Jackson's views with prominence given to Penfield's work. 33 refs.

Jaspers, K., in, *Allgemeine Psychopathologie*, 4th edition, Berlin & Heidelberg, Springer-Verlag, 1946, pp. 401–415.

Jefferson, G., "The prodromes of cortical localization", *J. Neurol. Neurosurg. Psychiat.*, 1953, *16*:59–72. A survey of studies up to mid-1880's of anatomy and histology of the brain and of stimulation and ablation experiments attempting to discover local signs of cortical function. 68 refs.

Jefferson, G., "Variations on a neurological theme—cortical localization", *Brit. med. J.*, 1956, *ii*:1405–1408. The contribution of Herbert Spencer to localization and his interest in phrenology. Literary and sociological effects of doctrines of localization: Charles Bray, George Eliot. 9 refs.

Kleist, K., "Die Lokalisation im Grosshirn und ihre Entwicklung", *Psychiat. Neurol. (Basel)*, 1959, *137*:289–309. Mainly developments in the 19th and 20th centuries in cortical structure and function. The most recent period (up to the 1950's) is detailed and useful. 69 refs.

Klingler, M., "Zur cerebralen Lokalisationslehre. Betrachtungen zur Geschichte einer Hypothese", *Schweiz. med. Wschr.*, 1967, *97*:725–731. A good survey from Hippocrates to Lashley & F. M. R. Walshe, but with nothing new. 26 refs.

Ladame, P., "Les localisations cérébrales d'après von Monakow", *Rev. Neurol.*, 1919, *35*:32–40. A review of von Monakow (1914).

Lorente de Nó, R., "Cerebral cortex: architecture, intracortical connections, motor projections", in, J. F. Fulton, *Physiology of the nervous system*, 3rd edition, New York, Oxford University Press, 1949, pp. 288–293. Brief but excellent "Historical note". 36 refs.

Luria, A. R., *Higher cortical functions in man*, London, Tavistock Publications, 1966, "I. The problem of localization of functions in the cerebral cortex. A. Psychomorphological concepts and their crisis—a historical survey", pp. 5–23. A good survey, well documented by an outstanding modern investigator of the cerebral cortex whose history, however, is influenced by his own contention of non-localization and by the Pavlovian school of physiology. See also, remainder of this Chapter.

Magoun, H. W., "Historical introduction", in, *The waking brain*, Springfield, Ill., C. C Thomas, 1958, pp. 3–14. Very brief but accurate lead-up to the reticular substance. 46 refs.

Magoun, H. W., "Early development of ideas relating the mind with the brain", in, G. E. W. Wolstenholme & C. M. O'Connor (editors), *The neurological basis of behavior*, London, J. A. Churchill, 1958, (Ciba Foundation Symposium), pp. 4–27. Excellent introduction to the history of cerebral localization.

Magoun, H. W., "Development of ideas relating the mind with the brain", in, C. Brooks & P. F. Cranefield (editors), *The historical development of physiological thought*, New York, Hafner, 1959, pp. 81–107. Cf. Magoun (1958). 14 refs.

Meyer, A., *Historical aspects of cerebral anatomy*, London, Oxford University Press, 1971. No one part of this excellent book deals with cerebral localization but there are many allusions to cortical anatomy. It can be used with the utmost confidence as an accurate, well documented source-book.

Mills, C. K., "A glance at the history of cerebral localization with some considerations regarding the subdivisions of the areas of representation of cutaneous and muscular sensibility and of concrete concepts" [Abstract only], *Proc. Philadelphia Co. Med. Soc.*, 1904, *25*:191–204. Useful for early views on cortical localization, but, like the author's other papers on the subject, historical perspective is lacking.

von Monakow, C., *Die Lokalisation im Grosshirn, und der Abbau der Funktion durch kortikale Herde*, Wiesbaden, J. F. Bergmann, 1914: pp. 75–135 is a review of literature detailed and copiously referenced; pp. 644–664, localization of speech function—Gall, Flourens, Broca, Pierre Marie and his students.

Neuburger, M., *Die historische Entwicklung der experimentellen Gehirn- und Rückenmarksphysiologie vor Flourens*, Stuttgart, F. Enke, 1897. Excellent and well-documented account of all aspects of cerebral localization before the early 19th century; *idem*, *The historical development of experimental brain and spinal cord physiology before Flourens*, translated and edited, with additional material by Edwin Clarke, Baltimore & London, Johns Hopkins University Press, 1981.

Olmsted, J. M. D., "Historical note on the *nœud vital* or respiratory center", *Bull. Hist. Med.*, 1944, *16*:343–350. The first example of punctate localization of brain function (Flourens, 1828). 28 refs.

Penfield, W. & E. Boldrey, "Somatic motor and sensory representation in the cerebral cortex of man as studied by electrical stimulation", *Brain*, 1937, *60*:389–443. Most of Dr Penfield's books and papers contain historical material. Here there is a historical introduction, pp. 390–396.

Penfield, W. & T. Rasmussen, *The cerebral cortex of man. A clinical study of localization of function*, New York, Macmillan, 1957. Historical introduction on pp. 1–4, 12–20.

Pick, A., "Das halbhundertjährige Jubiläum der Entdeckung der Rindencentren", *D. med. Wschr.*, 1920, *46*:18–19. Commemorating Fritsch & Hitzig's classic paper of 1870.

Polyak, S., *The vertebrate visual system*, Chicago, University of Chicago Press, 1967, Part 1. "History of investigations of the structure and function of the eye and the visual pathways and centers of the brain", pp. 9–203. Although only general accounts of the history of cerebral localization are included in this list, Dr Polyak's remarkable survey of a special part of the subject cannot be omitted. The text is exhaustive and accurate, the documentation is profuse and impeccable, and the illustrations excellent.

Rawson, N. R., "Early steps in cerebral localization" *Newcastle Med. J.*, 1926/27, *7*:95-112. Cortex not mentioned. Antiquity, Willis, Lorrey, Pourfour du Petit, Charles Bell. Accurate but no refs.

Révész, B., *Geschichte des Seelenbegriffes und der Seelenlokalisation*, Stuttgart, F. Enke, 1917. The history of the search for the soul is to a large extent the history of cerebral localization. Thorough survey to the end of the 19th century. Very few references.

Riese, W., "F.-J. Gall et le problème des localisations cérébrales", *L'Hygiène mentale*, 1936, *31*:105–136. Critical review of Gall's contribution and the general value of his doctrine. Refers mostly to Gall and Spurzheim (*Anatomie et physiologie du système nerveux*, Paris, Schoell, *et al.*, 1810–1814).

Riese, W., "Les discussions du problème des localisations cérébrales dans les sociétés savantes du XIXe siècle et leurs rapports avec des vues contemporaines", *ibid.*, 1936, *31*:137–158. The period immediately following Gall: Cuvier, Bouillaud, Broca, Flourens, etc.

Riese, W., "Changing concepts of cerebral localization", *Clio Medica*, 1967, *2*:189–230. Thorough, although somewhat diffuse, survey coloured by author's present concept of cortical functions. 27 refs.

Riese, W. & E. C. Hoff, "A history of the doctrine of cerebral localization. Sources, anticipations, and basic reasoning", *J. Hist. Med.*, 1950, *5*:50–71. Philosophical background: Descartes, Gassendi, Kant, Soemmerring, Lange, Bergson, dialectical materialism. An excellent survey in turgid style. 17 refs. "II. Methods and main results", *ibid.*, 1951, *6*:439–470. Anatomical, physiological, clinical localization history of aphasia; localization and the autonomic nervous system. 60 refs.

Sachs, H., "Die Entwicklung der Gehirnphysiologie im XIX. Jahrhundert", *Z. pädagogische Psychol. Pathol.*, 1901, *3*:255–280. Deals with cortical localization from Gall to Flechsig. French and German contributions only, mainly Flourens, Wernicke, Munk, Goltz. No references.

Scarff, J. E., "Primary cortical centres for movements of upper and lower limbs in man. Observations based on electrical stimulation", *Arch. Neurol. Psychiat.*, 1940, *44*:243–299. Excellent "Review of the literature" from 1870 to 1937 on pp. 245–280. Well-documented.

Schiller, J., "Histoire des localisations cérébrales", *Confrontations* [published by Laboratoire Choay, Paris] 1969. No. 4, pp. 39–56. Superficial, well-illustrated survey with no new material. Author follows Neuburger closely but French contributors are given undue prominence. No references and a profusion of misspellings of non-French proper names.

Sheer, D. E., "Brain and behavior: the background of interdisciplinary research", in, *Electrical stimulation of the brain*, Austin, University of Texas Press, 1961, pp. 3–21. This title is included merely to warn potential readers of the paper's wholly unreliable nature; even the portrait of Hughlings Jackson is incorrect!

Smith, G. Elliot, *The old and the new phrenology*, Edinburgh, Oliver & Boyd, 1924 (Henderson Trust lecture, No. 1). An evaluation of Gall's contributions to the anatomy and physiology of the brain in the light of modern (1924) studies of the cerebral cortex.

Soury, Jules, *Le système nerveux central, structure et fonctions. Histoire critique des théories et des doctrines*, Paris, G. Carré & C. Naud, 1899, 2 vols. This is the most detailed work on the history of neuro-anatomy and neurophysiology. Cerebral localization is dealt with in Vol. 1, *passim*, the latest period 1870–1899 being on pp. 607–631. Soury, however, was too close to give an accurate survey of the latter. References to the literature are scanty. See also, *idem*, in, C. Richet (editor), *Dictionnaire de physiologie*, Vol. 2, B–C, Paris, F. Alcan, 1897, pp. 611–670.

von Stauffenberg, G., "Der Wandel der Anschauungen über Gehirnlokalisation", *Münch. med. Wschr.*, 1913 *60*:2466–2469. Superficial review from Ancient Greeks to 19th century. Nothing new. No refs.

Stenvers, H. W., "On the function of the brain", *Folia Psychiat. Neurol. Neuroch. Neerland.*, 1955, *58*:8–25. Superficial survey from Antiquity to 20th century. 13 refs.

Stookey, B., "A note on the early history of cerebral localization", *Bull. N. Y. Acad. Med.*, 1954, *30*:559–578. Detailed consideration of the work of Gall, Bouillaud. Gratiolet, Aubertin, and Broca, especially the famous debates in Paris in the 1860's concerning the cortical localization of speech. The role of Aubertin in these is overstated. 22 refs.

Swazey, J. P., "Action propre and action commune: the localization of cerebral function", *J. Hist. Biol.*, 1970, *3*:213–234. Excellent review of conflict in 19th century between punctate localizers and those who upheld the field theory. 64 refs.

Tizard, B., "Theories of brain localization from Flourens to Lashley", *Med. Hist.,* 1959, *3*:132–145. Review of the localization and field theories. Author's preconceptions and inadequate background knowledge leads to poor history. More a review of the main literature and useful as such. 24 refs.

Trotter, W., "A landmark in modern neurology", *Lancet,* 1934, *ii*:1207–1210. First operation for removal of cerebral tumour, 25 November 1884. The influence on cerebral localization.

Vallois, H. V., "Le docteur Gall et le théorie des localisations cérébrales", *Rev. méd. Toulouse,* 1966, *2*:809–814. Gall's influence on the concept of cortical localization. No refs.

Walker, A. E., "The development of the concept of cerebral localization in the nineteenth century", *Bull. Hist Med.,* 1957, *31*:99–121. Excellent paper by an outstanding neuro-surgeon and neuro-scientist. 76 refs.

Walker, A. E., "Stimulation and ablation. Their role in the history of cerebral physiology", *J. neurophysiol.,* 1957, *20*:435–449. Excellent and reliable survey. 59 refs.

Walshe, F. M. R., "The brain-stem conceived as 'the highest level' of function in the nervous system with particular reference to the 'automatic apparatus' of Carpenter (1850) and the 'centrencephalic integrating system' of Penfield", *Brain,* 1957, *80*:510–539. (Also in, *Further critical studies in neurology and other essays and addresses,* Edinburgh & London, E. & S. Livingstone, 1965, pp. 61–95.) The search for Jackson's "highest level" in the brain. 29 refs.

Walshe, F. M. R., "Some reflections upon the opening phase of the physiology of the cerebral cortex, 1850–1900", F. N. L. Poynter (*op. cit.* reference above, Ackerknecht, 1958), pp. 223–234. Emphasizes the importance of the clinical approach, as exemplified by Hughlings Jackson. Walshe himself was basically a clinician. 14 refs.

Walshe, F. M. R., "An attempted correlation of the diverse hypotheses of functional localization in the cerebral cortex", *J. Neurol. Sci.,* 1964, *1*:111–128. (Also in, *Further clinical studies* (1965), pp. 115–142). Excellent review of current concepts by an outstanding contributor to them. Walshe always strongly opposed the punctate localizers, for example of 'discrete movement'. 58 refs.

Wilks, S., "Notes on the history of the physiology of the nervous system. Taken more especially from writers on phrenology", *Guy's Hosp.Rep.,* 1879, *24*(3rd Series):57–94. Brain and mind, double brain, aphasia and the seat of language, sense of weight and muscular resistance, sleep, cerebellum. No refs.

Williams, W. M., *A vindication of phrenology,* London, Chatto & Windus, 1894. Forlorn attempt to justify phrenology in the light of advances in scientific knowledge of brain function. Historical material *passim.*

Young, R. M., "The functions of the brain: Gall to Ferrier (1808–1886)", *Isis,* 1968, *59*:251–268. Relations among brain, mind, and behaviour in the investigation of Cartesian dualism as applied to the biological sciences.

Young, R. M., *Mind, brain and adaptation in the nineteenth century,* Oxford, Clarendon Press, 1970. Cerebral localization and its biological context from Gall to Ferrier. Given a mixed reception (see reviews in *T.L.S.,* 7 May 1970; *Science,* 10 September 1970; *Med. Hist.,* 1971, *15*:311).

Zangwill, O. L., "The cerebral localisation of psychological functions", *Advancement of Science,* 1963–1964. *20*(N.S.):335–344. An excellent survey by an outstanding contributor to modern concepts. 56 refs.

Appendix 2

Benton, A., "The 'minor' hemisphere", *J. Hist. Med.*, 1972, 27:5–14.

Benton, A., "The historical development of the concept of hemispheric cerebral dominance", in S. F. Spicker & H. T. Engelhardt (eds.), *Philosophical dimensions of the neuro-medical sciences*, Dordrecht, Reidel, 1976, pp. 35–57, 59–68.

Blakemore, C., *Mechanics of the mind. BBC Reith Lectures 1976*, Cambridge, Cambridge University Press, 1977. A remarkable survey of neuroscience up to the mid-1970s, with a galaxy of illustrations. Enthusiastically recommended.

Clarke, E. & L. S. Jacyna, *Nineteenth-century origins of neuroscientific concepts*, Berkeley, Los Angeles & London, University of California Press, 1987. See 6. "Brain functions", pp. 212-307. Review in History of Science, 1988, 26:427–437.

Cooter, R. J., *The cultural meaning of popular science. Phrenology and the organization of consent in nineteenth century Britain*, Cambridge, Cambridge University Press, 1985. An excellent survey of a diffuse and complex topic.

Cooter, R. J., "Phrenology and British alienists c. 1825–1845", *Med. Hist.*, 1976, 20:135–151.

Corsi, P. (ed.), *The enchanted loom. Chapters in the history of neuroscience*, New York & Oxford, Oxford University Press, 1991. A series of essays on ancient and modern aspects of neuroscience, with a vast array of excellent illustrations, some of which are in the present work. Many of them are in color.

Eccles, J. C. & W. C. Gibson, *Sherrington. His life and thought*, Heidelberg, Springer. An authoritative biography by two of his pupils.

Gregory, R. L., P. Heard, J. Harris, & D. Rose (eds.), *The artful eye*, Oxford, Oxford University Press, 1995. A fascinating discussion of science, art, and psychology, with novel links to art and science, and to mind and brain.

Hagner, M., "Die elektrische Erregbarkeit des Gehirns zur Konjunktur eines Experiments", in H.-J. Rheinberger & M. Hagner (eds.), *Experimentalsysteme in den biologischen Wissenschaften 1850–1950*, Berlin, Akademe Verlag, 1993.

Harrington, A., "A feeling for the 'whole': The holistic reaction in neurology from the *fin de siècle* to the interwar years", in M. Teich & R. Porter (eds.), *Fin de siècle and its legacy*, Cambridge, Cambridge University Press, 1989.

Harrington, A. "Beyond phrenology: localization theory in the modern era", in P. Corsi (ed.), *The enchanted loom. Chapters in the history of neuroscience*, New York & Oxford, Oxford University Press, 1991, pp. 207–239. 34 illustrations of cortex, many concerning recent research. Bibliography grouped with those of other authors, pp. 358–364.

Harrington, A., *Medicine, mind and the double brain*, Princeton, N.J., Princeton University Press, 1987. For review, see *Bull. Hist. Med.*, 1989, 62:308–309.

Harvey, E. R., *The inward wits. Psychological theory in the Middle Ages and the Renaissance*. London, Warburg Institute, 1975. Despite its prestigious origins, this review of the Cell Doctrine cannot be recommended.

Hughes, J. T., *Thomas Willis 1621–1675*, London & New York, Royal Society of medicine, 1991. Reviews have been less than enthusiastic.

Lesky, E. (ed.), *Franz Joseph Gall 1758–1828, Naturforscher und Anthropologe*, Stuttgart, Vienna, Huber, 1979. By an outstanding expert on Gall.

Mazzolini, R. G., "Schemes and models of the thinking machine", in P. Corsi (ed.), *The enchanted loom. Chapters in the history of neuroscience*, New York & Oxford, Oxford University Press, 1991, pp. 68–143. 89 illustrations, some on cortical function and structure. Bibliography, pp. 198–200.

Morsier, G. de, "Leonardo da Vinci et l'anatomie du cerveau humain", Physis, 1964, 6:335–346.

Oehler-Klein, S., *Die Schädellehre Franz Joseph Galls in Literatur und Kritik des 19. Jahrhunderts: zur Rezeptionsgeschichte einer medizinisch-biologisch begründeten Theorie der Physiognomik und Psychologie*, Stuttgart & New York, Fischer, 1990. (Soemmerring-Forschung, 8.)

Parssinen, T. M., "Popular science and society: the phrenology movement in early-Victorian Britain", *J. Soc. Hist.*, 1974, 7:1–20.

Pauly, P. J., "The political structure of the brain: cerebral localization in Bismarckian Germany", *Intern. J. Neuroscience*, 1983, 21:145–150. An excellent example of the influence of "external" historical factors.

Phelps, M. E., "The evolution of positron emission", in P. Corsi (ed.), *The enchanted loom. Chapters in the history of neuroscience*, New York & Oxford, Oxford University Press, 1991, pp. 347–357. 12 illustrations, all in color. Bibliography grouped with those of other authors, pp. 358–364.

Pogliano, C., "Between form and function: A new science of man", in P. Corsi (ed.), *The enchanted loom. Chapters in the history of neuroscience*, New York & Oxford, Oxford University Press, 1991, pp. 144–197. With 22 excellent illustrations, especially concerning phrenology. Bibliography, pp. 201–203.

Riese, W. *Selected papers on the history of aphasia*, Amsterdam, Swets & Zeitlinger, 1977. A useful sourcebook by a respected historian of neuroscience.

Roberts, K. B. and J. D. W. Tomlinson, *The fabric of the body*, Oxford, Clarendon Press, 1992. The only important contribution on this topic as it relates to the present work since 1972.

Smith, C.U.M., "A century of cortical architectonics", *J. Hist. Neurosci.*, 1992, 1:201–218. An excellent review of recent, radical views of cortical function.

Wolfson, H. A., "The internal senses in Latin, Arabic, and Hebrew philosophic texts", *Harvard Theological Review*, April, 1935, 28:69–133. The early history of the brain's internal psychological properties located in the ventricles, but confined to the meaning and classification of terms used to describe them. No illustrations. See "Preface to Second Edition", note 3.

York, G. K., & D. A. Steinberg, "Hughlings Jackson's theory of cerebral localization", *J. Hist. Neurosci.*, 1994, 3:153–168.

Young, R. M., *Mind, brain and adaptation in the nineteenth century. Cerebral localisation and its biological context from Gall to Ferrier*, New York & Oxford, Oxford University Press, 1990. A reprint of 1970 issue, with "New Preface".

Index

[Editor's Note: Both British- and American-English spellings occur in this work. American-English spellings have been used in the Index.]

Collaborators on *An Illustrated History of Brain Function*:
Heather Austin, Editorial Assistant
BookCrafters, Inc., Printer and Binder
Steve Renick/Anselm Design, Designer
Martha Nicholson Steele, Editor and Project Manager
Tiki Bob Publishing & Design, Typesetting

The text types are
Adobe Garamond and Frutiger
from Adobe Systems.

The edition is limited to 1000 copies.

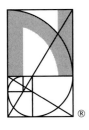